CASE FILES®
Critical Care

Eugene C. Toy, MD
Assistant Dean for Educational Programs
Director, Doctoring Courses
Professor and Vice Chair of Medical Education
Department of Obstetrics and Gynecology
McGovern Medical School at University of
   Texas Health Science Center (UTHealth)
   at Houston
Houston, Texas

Terrence H. Liu, MD, MPH
Physician/Surgeon
Sutter East Bay Medical Group
Berkeley, California

Manuel Suarez, MD, FACP, FACCP
Director of Cardiopulmonary Services
Administrative Director of Undergraduate
   Medical Education
Internal Medicine Residency Program Director
Assistant Clinical Professor of Internal
   Medicine
Assistant Clinical Professor of Pulmonary &
   Critical Care
Westchester General Hospital
Miami, Florida
Administrative Director of Medical Education
   Services of the Office of International Affairs
Associate Dean of the Clinical Medicine
   Certificate Program
Associate Professor of Medicine
Florida International University Herbert
   Wertheim College of Medicine
University Park, Florida
Adjunct Professor of Clinical Medicine
American University of Antigua College of
   Medicine
St. John's, Antigua, Antigua and Barbuda

New York   Chicago   San Francisco   Athens   London   Madrid
Mexico City   Milan   New Delhi   Singapore   Sydney   Toronto

Case Files®: Critical Care, Second Edition

1 2 3 4 5 6 7 8 9   LCR   22 21 20 19 18 17

ISBN 978-1-259-64185-5
MHID 1-259-64185-6

This book was set in Adobe Jenson Pro by Cenveo® Publisher Services.
The editors were Bob Boehringer and Cindy Yoo.
The production supervisor was Catherine Saggese.
Project management was provided by Raghavi Khullar, Cenveo Publisher Services.

Library of Congress Cataloging-in-Publication Data

Names: Toy, Eugene C., author. | Liu, Terrence H., author. | Suarez, Manuel,
    1957-author.
Title: Case files. Critical care / Eugene C. Toy, Terrence H. Liu, Manuel
    Suarez.
Other titles: Critical care
Description: Second edition. | New York : McGraw-Hill Education, [2017] |
    Includes bibliographical references and index.
Identifiers: LCCN 2017006769| ISBN 9781259641855 (pbk.) |
    ISBN 1259641856 (pbk.)
Subjects: | MESH: Critical Care—methods | Problems and Exercises | Case Reports
Classification: LCC RC86.7 | NLM WX 18.2 | DDC 616.02/8—dc23 LC record available at https://lccn.loc.gov/
    2017006769

To my dear friend and colleague Midge Haramis, who has assisted in
every one of my Case Files books. She recently retired from McGraw-Hill
after working there for nearly 47 years. She started as an editing assistant and
held other positions in the College Division, and then had roles in the
McGraw-Hill Professional Division as Administrative Assistant to the
Vice President, Assistant to the Director of Electronic Products,
Administrative Assistant and Editorial Assistant in the Computing and
Electronics Group, and Administrative Assistant to the Computing Marketing Manager,
and finally landed as Senior Editorial Assistant in the Medical Editorial Department,
where we met. Midge is caring, compassionate, the consummate professional,
and has a wonderful sense of humor. She is indeed the heart and soul
within the fibers of the pages of each of my case files books. Like a magician,
Midge coaxes the millions of rascally details of book publishing to fall
into place—allowing my works to breathe life and joy.

—ECT

I am grateful to all my teachers, colleagues, and patients who have taught me so much
over the years about the care of sick patients.

—THL

To the incredible staff, medical students, residents, and colleagues at
Westchester General Hospital. To the outstanding medical students of the
M.D. Certificate Program of the American University of Antigua in
collaboration with the Florida International University at WGH.
To Dr. Peter Bell, Dr. Eneida O. Roldan and Dean John A. Rock for creating and
allowing me to administer the program. To Mr. Alfredo "Fred" Sanchez,
for his ever present friendship, assistance and support. To my parents Manuel and
Teresa Suarez who gave me the world, and most especially,
to the two moons of my life, my daughters Alexia Teresa Suarez and
Melanie Nicole Suarez, who are my treasures.

—MS

CONTENTS

CONTRIBUTORS

Peter Bell, MD
Vice President of Global Medical Education
Manipal Education Americas
New York, New York
Executive Dean of Clinical Sciences
American University of Antigua College of Medicine
St. John's, Antigua, Antigua and Barbuda
Transfer of Critically Ill Patients

Catherine Bshouty
Medical Student
Class of 2017
American University of Antigua College of Medicine, in collaboration with the
    Florida International University Herbert Wertheim College of Medicine
St. John's, Antigua, Antigua and Barbuda/University Park, Florida
Acid-Base Disorders Part 1

Thomas R. Campi Jr., MD
Class of 2017
American University of Antigua College of Medicine, in collaboration with the
    Florida International University Herbert Wertheim College of Medicine
St. John's, Antigua, Antigua and Barbuda/University Park, Florida
Transfer of Critically Ill Patients

Neena Chandrasekaran, MD
Resident, Internal Medicine
University of Pittsburgh Medical Center Mercy
Pittsburgh, Pennsylvania
Respiratory Weaning

Arielle A. Dahlin, MD
Class of 2017
American University of Antigua College of Medicine, in collaboration with the
    Florida International University Herbert Wertheim College of Medicine
St. John's, Antigua, Antigua and Barbuda/University Park, Florida
Asthmatic Exacerbation
Cardiac Arrthymias

Victor Delgado, DNP, ARNP-BC
Clinical Assistant Professor
Florida International University
Nicole Wertheim College of Nursing and Health Sciences
University Park, Florida
Transfer of Critically Ill Patients

Shailvi Gupta, MD, MPH
Surgical Critical Care Fellow
R Adams Cowley Shock Trauma Center/University of Maryland Medical Center
Baltimore, Maryland
Pain Control and Sedation

Marcus K. Hernandez
Medical Student
Class of 2018
American University of Antigua College of Medicine, in collaboration with the
    Florida International University Herbert Wertheim College of Medicine
St. John's, Antigua, Antigua and Barbuda/University Park, Florida
Monitoring: Hemodynamic and Cardiovascular

Alan W. Jaziri, MD
Class of 2017
American University of Antigua College of Medicine, in collaboration with the
    Florida International University Herbert Wertheim College of Medicine
St. John's, Antigua, Antigua and Barbuda/University Park, Florida
Ventilator Management

Edward S. Johnson, MD
Senior Attending and Consultant in Infectious Diseases
Clara Maass Medical Center
Belleville, New Jersey
Senior Panel Physician/Consultant in Infectious Diseases
The Wound Care Center at Clara Maass Medical Center
FMR Dean of the Kingstown Medical College, St George's University School of Medicine
Saint Vincent and the Grenadines, Windward Islands
Immunosuppressed Patients
Meningitis/Encephalitis

Terrence H. Liu, MD, MPH
Physician/Surgeon
Sutter East Bay Medical Group
Berkeley, California
Acute Kidney Injury
Acute Liver Failure
Antimicrobial Use in ICU
DVT/Pulmonary Embolism
Fluid/Electrolyte Abnormalities
Imaging in Critical Care
Multiorgan Dysfunction
Nutritional Issues in ICU
Poisoning
Post-Resuscitation Management in the ICU
Postoperative Care in ICU
Sepsis

Diego Marin, DO
Chief Resident, Internal Medicine
Bayonne Medical Center
Bayonne, New Jersey
Status Epilepticus

Emily Miraflor, MD
Assistant Clinical Professor
University of California, San Francisco—East Bay
Alameda Health System
Oakland, California
University of California, San Francisco School of Medicine
San Francisco, California
Acute Gastrointestinal Bleeding
GI Bleeding
Scoring Systems and Patient Prognosis

Chase C. Parsons, MD
Class of 2017
American University of Antigua College of Medicine, in collaboration with the
    Florida International University Herbert Wertheim College of Medicine
St. John's, Antigua, Antigua and Barbuda/University Park, Florida
Airway Management/Respiratory Failure

Thea M. Recai
Medical Student
Class of 2018
American University of Antigua College of Medicine, in collaboration with the
    Florida International University Herbert Wertheim College of Medicine
St. John's, Antigua, Antigua and Barbuda/University Park, Florida
Immunosuppressed Patients
Meningitis/Encephalitis

Ronald Reis, MD, FACS
Chief of Staff, Chief of Thoracic Surgery
Westchester General Hospital
Miami, Florida
Clinical Instructor of Surgery
Florida International University Herbert Wertheim College of Medicine
University Park, Florida
Airway Management/Respiratory Failure

Mathew Resnick, CAPT, USAF, DO
Flight Surgeon
Tinker Air Force Base
Oklahoma City, Oklahoma
Altered Mental Status

Christopher R. Reyes, MS, EMT-B
Medical Student
Class of 2017
American University of Antigua College of Medicine, in collaboration with the
    Florida International University Herbert Wertheim College of Medicine
St. John's, Antigua, Antigua and Barbuda/University Park, Florida
Acid-Base Disorders Part 1
Acid-Base Disorders Part 2
Ethics/Do Not Resuscitate/Organ Donation

Eneida O. Roldan, MD, MPH, MBA
Chief Executive Officer
Florida International University Health Care Network
Associate Dean for International Affairs
Associate Professor Department of Pathology
Florida International University Herbert Wertheim College of Medicine
University Park, Florida
Ethics/Do Not Resuscitate/Organ Donation

Javid Sadjadi, MD
Associate Clinical Professor
University of California, San Francisco School of Medicine
Oakland, California
Blunt Trauma

Angela Fernandez Santiago, DO
Resident, Family Medicine
Saint Barnabas Medical Center
Livingston, New Jersey
Stroke

Aneesa Sataur, DO
Resident, Family Medicine
Westchester General Hospital
Miami, Florida
Florida International University Herbert Wertheim College of Medicine
University Park, Florida
Acute Cardiac Failure

Karim A. Sirsy, DO
Resident, Family Medicine
Westchester General Hospital
Miami, Florida
Non-invasive Methods of Ventilator Support

Randi Nicole Smith, MD, MPH
Assistant Professor
Emory University School of Medicine
Department of Surgery
Atlanta, Georgia
Hemorrhage and Coagulopathy
Trauma and Burns
Traumatic Brain Injury

Jose David Suarez, MD
Diplomate of the American Board of Family Medicine
Voluntary Assistant Clinical Professor
Florida International University Herbert Wertheim College of Medicine
University Park, Florida
Seneca District Hospital
Chester, California
Early Awareness of Critical Illness

Sammy A. Tayiem, MD
Class of 2017
American University of Antigua College of Medicine, in collaboration with the
  Florida International University Herbert Wertheim College of Medicine
St. John's, Antigua, Antigua and Barbuda/University Park, Florida
Early Awareness of Critical Illness

Allison L. Toy, RN
Registered Nurse
Baylor Scott & White Hillcrest Medical Center
Waco, Texas
Primary Manuscript Reviewer

Eugene C. Toy, MD
Assistant Dean for Educational Programs
Director, Doctoring Courses
Professor and Vice Chair of Medical Education
Department of Obstetrics and Gynecology
McGovern Medical School at University of Texas Health Science Center (UTHealth)
  at Houston
Houston, Texas
Hypertensive Emergencies in Obstetrics
Preeclampsia with Severe Features
Review Questions

Timothy D. Webb, DO
Family Medicine
Memorial Regional Hospital
Hollywood, Florida
Acute Coronary Syndrome

Jessica Weiss, DO
Class of 2017
Lake Erie College of Medicine
Bradenton, Florida
Vasoactive Drugs and Pharmacology

Hannah L. White
Medical Student
McGovern Medical School at University of Texas Health Science Center (UTHealth)
  at Houston
Houston, Texas
Endocrinopathies in ICU
ICU Patients with Obstetrical Issues

ACKNOWLEDGMENTS

The curriculum that evolved into the ideas for this series was inspired by Philbert Yau and Chuck Rosipal, two talented and forthright students, who have since graduated from medical school. It has been a tremendous joy to work with my excellent coauthors, especially Dr. Manny Suarez, who exemplifies the qualities of the ideal physician—caring, empathetic, and avid teacher—and who is intellectually a giant. It was on the island of St. Vincent and the Grenadines, while reviewing the curriculum of the fledgling Trinity School of Medicine, that Manny and I conceived the idea of this book, a critical care book for students. I also enjoy collaborating with Dr. Terry Liu, my long-time friend and colleague whose expertise and commitment to medical education is legendary. This second edition has three new cases and includes updates on nearly every case. I appreciate McGraw-Hill's believing in the concept of teaching through clinical cases, and I would like to especially acknowledge Cindy Yoo for her editing expertise and Catherine Saggese and Raghavi Khullar, Cenveo Publisher Services for the excellent production. It has been amazing to work together with my daughter Allison, who is an extremely talented registered nurse at the Baylor Scott and White Hillcrest Medical Center in Waco, Texas. She is an astute manuscript reviewer and diligently read and helped me to edit each case. Already in her early career, she has a good clinical acumen. I appreciate the excellent support from the Office of Educational Programs at McGovern Medical School, especially Dr. Sean Blackwell, Chair of the Department of Ob/Gyn, and Dr. Patricia Butler, the Vice Dean for Educational Programs. Most of all, I appreciate my ever-loving wife Terri, and our four wonderful children: Andy and his wife Anna, Michael, Allison, and Christina for their patience and understanding.

Eugene C. Toy

Mastering the cognitive knowledge within a field such as critical care is a formidable task. It is even more difficult to draw on that knowledge, procure and filter through the clinical and laboratory data, develop a differential diagnosis, and, finally, to make a rational treatment plan. In critical care, a detailed understanding of hemodynamics, cardiovascular and pulmonary medicine, and pharmacology are important. Sometimes, it is prudent to initiate therapy for significant derangements rather than finding out the precise underlying disorder. For instance, in a patient with respiratory failure, therapy to increase oxygenation and ventilation is initiated while simultaneously determining the etiology. It is done through a more precise understanding of the pathophysiology that allows for rational and directed therapy. The critical care setting does not allow for much error. A skilled critical care physician must be able to quickly assess the patient's situation and produce an efficient diagnostic and therapeutic plan.

These skills the student learns best at the bedside, guided and instructed by experienced teachers, and inspired toward self-directed, diligent reading. Clearly, there is no replacement for education at the bedside, especially because in "real life," delay in correct management leads to suboptimal outcome. Unfortunately, clinical situations usually do not encompass the breadth of the specialty. Perhaps the best alternative is a carefully crafted patient case designed to stimulate the clinical approach and the decision-making process. In an attempt to achieve that goal, we have constructed a collection of clinical vignettes to teach diagnostic and therapeutic approaches relevant to critical care medicine.

Most importantly, the explanations for the cases emphasize the mechanisms and underlying principles, rather than merely providing rote questions and answers. This book is organized for versatility; it allows the student "in a rush" to go quickly through the scenarios and check the corresponding answers, and it allows the student who wants thought-provoking explanations to obtain them. The answers are arranged from simple to complex: the bare answers, an analysis of the case, an approach to the pertinent topic, a comprehension test at the end, clinical pearls for emphasis, and a list of references for further reading. The clinical vignettes are placed in a systematic order to better allow students to gain an understanding of the pathophysiology and mechanisms of disease. A listing of cases is included in Section III to aid the student who desires to test his/her knowledge of a certain area, or to review a topic, including basic definitions. Finally, we intentionally did not use a multiple-choice question format in the opening case scenarios because clues (or distractions) are not available in the real world.

LISTING BY CASE NUMBER

LISTING BY DISORDER (ALPHABETICAL)

How to Approach Clinical Problems

Part 1. Approaching the Patient

The transition from the textbook or journal article to the clinical situation is one of the most challenging tasks in medicine. Retention of information is difficult; organization of the facts and recall of a myriad of data in precise application to the patient is crucial. The purpose of this text is to facilitate in this process. The first step is gathering information, also known as establishing the database. This includes taking the history (asking questions), performing the physical examination, and obtaining selective laboratory and/or imaging tests. Of these, the historical examination is the most important and useful. Sensitivity and respect should always be exercised during the interview of patients.

CLINICAL PEARL

▶ The history is the single most important tool in obtaining a diagnosis. All physical findings, laboratory, and imaging studies are first obtained, and then interpreted, in the light of the pertinent history.

HISTORY

1. **Basic information:**

   a. **Age, gender, and ethnicity:** These should be recorded because some conditions are more common at certain ages; for instance, pain on defecation and rectal bleeding in a 20-year-old may indicate inflammatory bowel disease, whereas the same symptoms in a 60-year-old would more likely suggest colon cancer.

2. **Chief complaint:** What is it that brought the patient into the hospital or office? Is it a scheduled appointment, or an unexpected symptom? The patient's own words should be used if possible, such as, "I feel like a ton of bricks are on my chest." The chief complaint, or real reason for seeking medical attention, may not be the first subject the patient talks about (in fact, it may be the last thing), particularly if the subject is embarrassing, such as a sexually transmitted disease, or highly emotional, such as depression. It is often useful to clarify exactly what the patient's concern is; for example, they may fear their headaches represent an underlying brain tumor.

3. **History of present illness:** This is the most crucial part of the entire database. The questions one asks are guided by the differential diagnosis based on the chief complaint. The duration and character of the primary complaint, associated symptoms, and exacerbating/relieving factors should be recorded. Sometimes, the history will be convoluted and lengthy, with multiple diagnostic or therapeutic interventions at different locations. For patients with chronic illnesses, obtaining prior medical records is invaluable. For example,

when extensive evaluation of a complicated medical problem has been done elsewhere, it is usually better to first obtain those results than to repeat a "million-dollar workup." When reviewing prior records, it is often useful to review the primary data (eg, biopsy reports, echocardiograms, serologic evaluations) rather than to rely upon a diagnostic label applied by someone else, which then gets replicated in medical records and by repetition acquires the aura of truth, even when it may not be fully supported by data. Some patients will be poor historians because of dementia, confusion, or language barriers; recognition of these situations and querying of family members is useful. When little or no history is available to guide a focused investigation, more extensive objective studies are often necessary to exclude potentially serious diagnoses.

4. **Past history:**

   a. **Any illnesses** such as hypertension, hepatitis, diabetes mellitus, cancer, heart disease, pulmonary disease, and thyroid disease should be elicited. If an existing or prior diagnosis is not obvious, it is useful to ask exactly how the condition was diagnosed; that is, what investigations were performed. Duration, severity, and therapies should be included.

   b. **Any hospitalizations and emergency room visits** should be listed with the reason(s) for admission, intervention, and the location of the hospital.

   c. **Transfusions** with any blood products should be listed, including any adverse reactions.

   d. **Surgeries:** The year and type of surgery should be recorded and any complications documented. The type of incision and any untoward effects of the anesthesia or the surgery should be noted.

5. **Allergies:** Reactions to medications should be recorded, including severity and temporal relationship to the medication. An adverse effect (such as nausea) should be differentiated from a true allergic reaction.

6. **Medications:** Current and previous medications should be listed, including dosage, route, frequency, and duration of use. Prescription, over-the-counter, and herbal medications are all relevant. Patients often forget their complete medication list; thus, asking each patient to bring in all their medications— both prescribed and nonprescribed—allows for a complete inventory.

7. **Family history:** Many conditions are inherited or are predisposed in family members. The age and health of siblings, parents, grandparents, and others can provide diagnostic clues. For instance, an individual with first-degree family members with early onset coronary heart disease is at risk for cardiovascular disease.

8. **Social history:** This is one of the most important parts of the history. It includes the patient's functional status at home, social and economic circumstances, and goals and aspirations for the future. These are often critical in determining the best way to manage a patient's medical problem. Living arrangements, economic situations, and religious affiliations may provide

important clues for puzzling diagnostic cases or suggest the acceptability of various diagnostic or therapeutic options. Marital status and habits such as alcohol, tobacco, or illicit drug use may be relevant as risk factors for the disease.

9. **Review of systems:** A few questions about each major body system ensure that problems will not be overlooked. The clinician should avoid the mechanical "rapid-fire" questioning technique that discourages patients from answering truthfully because of fear of "annoying the doctor."

PHYSICAL EXAMINATION

The physical examination begins as one is taking the history, by observing the patient and beginning to consider a differential diagnosis. When performing the physical examination, one focuses on body systems suggested by the differential diagnosis and performs tests or maneuvers with specific questions in mind; for example, does the patient with jaundice have ascites? When the physical examination is performed with potential diagnoses and expected physical findings in mind ("one sees what one looks for"), the utility of the examination in adding to diagnostic yield is greatly increased, as opposed to an unfocused "head-to-toe" physical.

1. **General appearance:** A great deal of information is gathered by observation, as one notes the patient's body habitus, state of grooming, nutritional status, level of anxiety (or perhaps inappropriate indifference), degree of pain or comfort, mental status, speech patterns, and use of language. This forms your impression of "who this patient is."

2. **Vital signs:** Temperature, blood pressure, heart rate, and respiratory rate. Height and weight are often placed here. Blood pressure can sometimes be different in the two arms; initially, it should be measured in both arms. In patients with suspected hypovolemia, pulse and blood pressure should be taken in lying and standing positions to look for orthostatic hypotension. It is quite useful to take the vital signs oneself, rather than relying upon numbers gathered by ancillary personnel using automated equipment, because important decisions regarding patient care are often made using the vital signs as an important determining factor.

3. **Head and neck examination:** Facial or periorbital edema and pupillary responses should be noted. Funduscopic examination provides a way to visualize the effects of diseases such as diabetes on the microvasculature; papilledema can signify increased intracranial pressure. Estimation of jugular venous pressure is very useful to estimate volume status. The thyroid should be palpated for a goiter or nodule, and carotid arteries auscultated for bruits. Cervical (common) and supraclavicular (pathologic) nodes should be palpated.

4. **Breast examination:** Inspect for symmetry, skin or nipple retraction with the patient's hands on her hips (to accentuate the pectoral muscles), and also with arms raised. With the patient sitting and supine, the breasts should then be palpated

systematically to assess for masses. The nipple should be assessed for discharge and the axillary and supraclavicular regions should be examined for adenopathy.

5. **Cardiac examination:** The point of maximal impulse (PMI) should be ascertained for size and location, and the heart auscultated at the apex as well as at the base. Heart sounds, murmurs, and clicks should be characterized. Murmurs should be classified according to intensity, duration, timing in the cardiac cycle, and changes with various maneuvers. Systolic murmurs are very common and often physiologic; diastolic murmurs are uncommon and usually pathologic.

6. **Pulmonary examination:** The lung fields should be examined systematically and thoroughly. Wheezes, rales, rhonchi, and bronchial breath sounds should be recorded. Percussion of the lung fields may be helpful; hyperresonance may indicate tension pneumothorax, while dullness may point to a consolidated pneumonia or a pleural effusion.

7. **Abdominal examination:** The abdomen should be inspected for scars, distension, and discoloration (eg, the Grey-Turner sign of flank discoloration indicates intra-abdominal or retroperitoneal hemorrhage). Auscultation of the bowel can identify normal versus high-pitched, and hyperactive versus hypoactive sounds. The abdomen should be percussed, including assessing for liver and spleen size, and for the presence of shifting dullness (indicating ascites). Careful palpation should begin initially away from the area of pain, involving one hand on top of the other, to assess for masses, tenderness, and peritoneal signs. Tenderness should be recorded on a scale (eg, 1 to 4 where 4 is the most severe pain). Guarding, whether it is voluntary or involuntary, should be noted.

8. **Back and spine examination:** The back should be assessed for symmetry, tenderness, and masses. The flank regions are particularly important to assess for pain on percussion, which might indicate renal disease.

9. **Genitalia:**
    a. **Females:** The pelvic examination should include an inspection of the external genitalia, and with the speculum, evaluation of the vagina and cervix. A pap smear and/or cervical cultures may be obtained. A bimanual examination to assess the size, shape, and tenderness of the uterus and adnexa is important.
    b. **Males:** An inspection of the penis and testes is performed. Evaluation for masses, tenderness, and lesions is important. Palpation for hernias in the inguinal region with the patient coughing to increase intra-abdominal pressure is useful.

10. **Rectal examination:** A digital rectal examination is generally performed for individuals with possible colorectal disease or gastrointestinal bleeding. Masses should be assessed, and stool for occult blood should be tested. In men, the prostate gland can be assessed for enlargement and for nodules.

11. **Extremities:** An examination for joint effusions, tenderness, edema, and cyanosis may be helpful. Clubbing of the nails might indicate pulmonary diseases such as lung cancer or chronic cyanotic heart disease.

12. **Neurological examination:** Patients who present with neurological complaints usually require a thorough assessment, including examination of the mental status, cranial nerves, motor strength, sensation, and reflexes.

13. **Skin:** The skin should be carefully examined for evidence of pigmented lesions (melanoma), cyanosis, or rashes that may indicate systemic disease (malar rash of systemic lupus erythematosus).

LABORATORY AND IMAGING ASSESSMENT

1. **Laboratory:**

    a. Complete blood count (CBC) to assess for anemia and thrombocytopenia.

    b. Chemistry panel is most commonly used to evaluate renal and liver function.

    c. For cardiac conditions, the electrocardiogram (ECG), rhythm strip, and/or cardiac enzymes are critically important.

    d. For pulmonary disorders, the oxygen saturation level and/or arterial blood gas findings provide excellent information.

    e. Lipid panel is particularly relevant in cardiovascular diseases.

    f. Urinalysis is often referred to as a "liquid renal biopsy" because the presence of cells, casts, protein, or bacteria provides clues about underlying glomerular or tubular diseases.

    g. Gram stain and culture of urine, sputum, and cerebrospinal fluid, as well as blood cultures, are frequently useful to isolate the cause of infection.

2. **Imaging procedures:**

    a. Chest radiography is extremely useful in assessing cardiac size and contour, chamber enlargement, pulmonary vasculature and infiltrates, and the presence of pleural effusions.

    b. Ultrasonographic examination is useful for identifying fluid–solid interfaces and for characterizing masses as cystic, solid, or complex. It is also very helpful in evaluating the biliary tree, kidney size, and evidence of ureteral obstruction, and it can be combined with Doppler flow to identify deep venous thrombosis. Ultrasonography is noninvasive and has no radiation risk, but it cannot be used to penetrate through bone or air and is less useful in obese patients.

CLINICAL PEARL

> ▶ Ultrasonography is helpful in evaluating the biliary tree, looking for ureteral obstruction, and evaluating vascular structures, but it has limited utility in obese patients.

    c. Computed tomography (CT) is helpful in possible intracranial bleeding, abdominal and/or pelvic masses, and pulmonary processes, and it may help delineate the lymph nodes and retroperitoneal disorders. CT exposes the patient to radiation and requires the patient to be immobilized during the procedure. Generally, CT requires administration of a radiocontrast dye, which can be nephrotoxic.

d. Magnetic resonance imaging (MRI) identifies soft-tissue planes very well and provides the best imaging of the brain parenchyma. When used with gadolinium contrast (which is not nephrotoxic), MR angiography (MRA) is useful for delineating vascular structures. MRI does not use radiation, but the powerful magnetic field prohibits its use in patients with ferromagnetic metal in their bodies (eg, many prosthetic devices).

e. Cardiac procedures:

  i. **Echocardiography:** Uses ultrasonography to delineate the cardiac size, function, ejection fraction, and presence of valvular dysfunction.

  ii. **Angiography:** Radiopaque dye is injected into various vessels, and radiographs or fluoroscopic images are used to determine vascular occlusion, cardiac function, or valvular integrity.

  iii. **Stress treadmill tests:** Individuals at risk for coronary heart disease are asked to run on a treadmill. This increases oxygen demands on the heart. Meanwhile, the patient's blood pressure, heart rate, presence of chest pain, and EKG are monitored. Nuclear medicine imaging of the heart can be added to increase the sensitivity and specificity of the test. Individuals who cannot run on the treadmill (such as those with severe arthritis), may be given medications such as adenosine or dobutamine, which cause a mild hypotension to "stress" the heart.

Part 2. Approach to Clinical Problem Solving

There are typically four distinct steps to the systematic solving of clinical problems:

1. Making the diagnosis
2. Assessing the severity of the disease (stage)
3. Rendering a treatment based on the stage of the disease
4. Following the patient's response to the treatment

MAKING THE DIAGNOSIS

Introduction

There are two ways to make a diagnosis. Experienced clinicians often make a diagnosis very quickly using **pattern recognition**, that is, the features of the patient's illness match a scenario the physician has seen before. If it does not fit a readily recognized pattern, then one has to undertake several steps in diagnostic reasoning:

1. The first step is to **gather information with a differential diagnosis in mind.** The clinician should start considering diagnostic possibilities after recording the chief complaint and present illness. This differential diagnosis is continually refined

as information is gathered. Historical questions and physical examination tests and findings are all pursued tailored to the potential diagnoses one is considering. This is the principle that "you find what you are looking for." When one is trying to perform a thorough head-to-toe examination, for instance, without looking for anything in particular, one is much more likely to miss findings.

2. The next step is to try to move from subjective complaints or nonspecific symptoms to focus on objective abnormalities in an effort to **conceptualize the patient's objective problem with the greatest specificity one can achieve.** For example, a patient may come to the physician complaining of pedal edema, a relatively common and nonspecific finding. Laboratory testing may reveal that the patient has renal failure, a more specific cause of the many causes of edema. Examination of the urine may then reveal red blood cell casts, indicating glomerulonephritis, which is even more specific as the cause of the renal failure. The patient's problem, then, described with the greatest degree of specificity, is glomerulonephritis. The clinician's task at this point is to consider the differential diagnosis of glomerulonephritis rather than that of pedal edema.

3. The last step of the diagnostic process is to **look for discriminating features** of the patient's illness. This means the features of the illness, which by their presence or their absence must narrow the differential diagnosis. This is often difficult for junior learners because it requires a well-developed knowledge base of the typical features of disease, so the diagnostician can judge how much weight to assign to the various clinical clues present. For example, in the diagnosis of a patient with a fever and productive cough, the finding by chest x-ray of bilateral apical infiltrates with cavitation is highly discriminatory. There are few illnesses besides tuberculosis that are likely to produce that radiographic pattern. A negatively predictive example is a patient with exudative pharyngitis who also has rhinorrhea and cough. The presence of these features makes the diagnosis of streptococcal infection unlikely as the cause of the pharyngitis. Once the differential diagnosis has been constructed, the clinician uses the presence of discriminating features, knowledge of patient risk factors, and the epidemiology of diseases to decide which potential diagnoses are most likely.

CLINICAL PEARL

There are three steps in diagnostic reasoning:

1. Gathering information with a differential diagnosis in mind.

2. Identifying the objective abnormalities with the greatest specificity.

3. Looking for discriminating features to narrow the differential diagnosis.

Once the most specific problem has been identified and a differential diagnosis of that problem is considered using discriminating features to order the possibilities, the next step is to consider using diagnostic testing, such as laboratory, radiologic, or pathologic data, to confirm the diagnosis. Quantitative reasoning in the use and interpretation of tests were discussed in the previous section. Clinically, the timing and effort with which one pursues a definitive diagnosis using objective data depends on several factors: the potential gravity of the diagnosis in question, the clinical state of the patient, the potential risks of diagnostic testing, and the potential benefits or harms of empiric treatment. For example, if a young man is admitted to the hospital with bilateral pulmonary nodules on chest x-ray, there are many possibilities including metastatic malignancy, and aggressive pursuit of a diagnosis is necessary, perhaps including a thoracotomy with an open-lung biopsy. The same radiographic findings in an elderly bed-bound woman with advanced Alzheimer dementia who would not be a good candidate for chemotherapy might be best left alone without any diagnostic testing. Decisions like this are difficult, require solid medical knowledge as well as a thorough understanding of one's patient and the patient's background and inclinations, and constitute the art of medicine.

Assessing the Severity of the Disease

After ascertaining the diagnosis, the next step is to characterize the severity of the disease process; in other words, it is describing "how bad" a disease is. There is usually prognostic or treatment significance based on the stage. With malignancy, this is done formally by cancer staging. Most cancers are categorized from stage I (localized) to stage IV (widely metastatic). Some diseases, such as congestive heart failure, may be designated as mild, moderate, or severe based on the patient's functional status, that is, their ability to exercise before becoming dyspneic. With some infections, such as syphilis, the staging depends on the duration and extent of the infection and follows along the natural history of the infection (ie, primary syphilis, secondary, latent period, and tertiary/neurosyphilis).

Treating Based on Stage

Many illnesses are stratified according to severity because prognosis and treatment often vary based on the severity. If neither the prognosis nor the treatment was affected by the stage of the disease process, there would not be a reason to subcategorize as to mild or severe. As an example, a man with mild chronic obstructive pulmonary disease (COPD) may be treated with inhaled bronchodilators as needed and advice for smoking cessation. However, an individual with severe COPD may need around-the-clock oxygen supplementation, scheduled bronchodilators, and possibly oral corticosteroid therapy.

The Treatment Should Be Tailored to the Extent or "Stage" of the Disease

In making decisions regarding treatment, it is also essential that the clinician identify the therapeutic objectives. When patients seek medical attention, it is generally because they are bothered by a symptom and want it to go away. When physicians institute therapy, they often have several other goals besides symptom relief, such as prevention of short- or long-term complications or a reduction in mortality. For example, patients with congestive heart failure are bothered by the symptoms of edema and dyspnea. Salt restriction, loop diuretics, and bedrest are effective at reducing these symptoms. However, heart failure is a progressive disease with a high mortality, so other treatments such as angiotensin-converting enzyme (ACE) inhibitors and some β-blockers are also used to reduce mortality in this condition. It is essential that the clinician know what the therapeutic objective is so that one can monitor and guide therapy.

> ### CLINICAL PEARL
>
> ▶ The clinician needs to identify the objectives of therapy: symptom relief, prevention of complications, or reduction in mortality.

Following the Response to Treatment

The final step in the approach to disease is to follow the patient's response to the therapy. The "measure" of response should be recorded and monitored. Some responses are clinical, such as the patient's abdominal pain, or temperature, or pulmonary examination. Obviously, the student must work on being more skilled in eliciting the data in an unbiased and standardized manner. Other responses may be followed by imaging tests, such as CT scan of a retroperitoneal node size in a patient receiving chemotherapy, or a tumor marker such as the prostate-specific antigen (PSA) level in a man receiving chemotherapy for prostatic cancer. For syphilis, it may be the nonspecific treponemal antibody test rapid plasma reagent (RPR) titer over time. The student must be prepared to know what to do if the measured marker does not respond according to what is expected. Is the next step to retreat, or to repeat the metastatic workup, or to follow up with another more specific test?

Part 3. Approach to Reading

The clinical problem-oriented approach to reading is different from the classic "systematic" research of a disease. Patients rarely present with a clear diagnosis; hence, the student must become skilled in applying the textbook information to the clinical setting. Furthermore, one retains more information when one reads with a purpose. In other words, the student should read with the goal of answering specific questions. There are several fundamental questions that facilitate **clinical thinking**. These questions are:

1. What is the most likely diagnosis?
2. What should be your next step?
3. What is the most likely mechanism for this process?
4. What are the risk factors for this condition?
5. What are the complications associated with the disease process?
6. What is the best therapy?
7. How would you confirm the diagnosis?

> ## CLINICAL PEARL
>
> ▶ Reading with the purpose of answering the seven fundamental clinical questions improves retention of information and facilitates the application of "book knowledge" to "clinical knowledge."

WHAT IS THE MOST LIKELY DIAGNOSIS?

The method of establishing the diagnosis was discussed in the previous section. One way of attacking this problem is to develop standard "approaches" to common clinical problems. It is helpful to understand the most common causes of various presentations, such as "the most common causes of pancreatitis are gallstones and alcohol." (See the *Clinical Pearls* at end of each case.)

The clinical scenario would entail something such as:

A 28-year-old man presents to the emergency room with abdominal pain, nausea and vomiting, and an elevated amylase level. What is the most likely diagnosis?

With no other information to go on, the student would note that this man has a clinical diagnosis of pancreatitis. Using the "most common cause" information, the student would make an educated guess that the patient has either alcohol abuse or gallstones. "The ultrasonogram of the gallbladder shows no stones."

> ## CLINICAL PEARL
>
> ▶ The two most common causes of pancreatitis are gallstones and alcohol abuse.

Now, the student would use the phrase "patients without gallstones who have pancreatitis most likely abuse alcohol." Aside from these two causes, there are many other etiologies of pancreatitis.

WHAT SHOULD BE YOUR NEXT STEP?

This question is difficult because the next step may be more diagnostic information, staging, or therapy. It may be more challenging than "the most likely diagnosis" because there may be insufficient information to make a diagnosis and the next step may be to pursue more diagnostic information. Another possibility is that there is enough information for a probable diagnosis and the next step is to stage the disease. Finally, the most appropriate action may be to treat. Hence, from clinical data, a judgment needs to be rendered regarding how far along one is on the road of:

Make a diagnosis → stage the disease → treat based on stage → follow response

Frequently, the student is "taught" to regurgitate the same information that someone has written about a particular disease but is not skilled at giving the next step.

This talent is learned optimally at the bedside, in a supportive environment, with freedom to make educated guesses, and with constructive feedback. A sample scenario may describe a student's thought process as follows.

1. **Make the diagnosis:** "Based on the information I have, I believe that Mr. Smith has stable angina *because* he has retrosternal chest pain when he walks three blocks, but it is relieved within minutes by rest and with sublingual nitroglycerin."

2. **Stage the disease:** "I don't believe that this is severe disease because he does not have pain lasting for more than 5 minutes, angina at rest, or congestive heart failure."

3. **Treat based on stage:** "Therefore, my next step is to treat with aspirin, β-blockers, and sublingual nitroglycerin as needed, as well as lifestyle changes."

4. **Follow response:** "I want to follow the treatment by assessing his pain (I will ask him about the degree of exercise he is able to perform without chest pain), perform a cardiac stress test, and reassess him after the test is done."

In a similar patient, when the clinical presentation is unclear or more severe, perhaps the best "next step" may be diagnostic in nature such as thallium stress test or even coronary angiography. The **next step** depends upon the **clinical state of the patient** (if unstable, the next step is therapeutic), the **potential severity** of the disease (the next step may be staging), or the **uncertainty of the diagnosis** (the next step is diagnostic).

CLINICAL PEARL

▶ Usually, the vague question, "What is your next step?" is the most difficult question because the answer may be diagnostic, staging, or therapeutic.

WHAT IS THE LIKELY MECHANISM FOR THIS PROCESS?

This question goes further than making the diagnosis by also requiring the student to understand the underlying mechanism for the process. For example, a clinical scenario may describe an "18-year-old woman who presents with several months of severe epistaxis, heavy menses, petechiae, and a normal CBC except for a platelet count of 15,000/mm^3." Answers that a student may consider to explain this condition include immune-mediated platelet destruction, drug-induced thrombocytopenia, bone marrow suppression, and platelet sequestration as a result of hypersplenism.

The student is advised to learn the mechanisms for each disease process and not merely memorize a constellation of symptoms. In other words, rather than solely committing to memory the classic presentation of idiopathic thrombocytopenic purpura (ITP) (isolated thrombocytopenia without lymphadenopathy or offending drugs), the student should understand that ITP is an autoimmune process whereby the body produces IgG antibodies against the platelets. The platelets-antibody complexes are then taken from the circulation in the spleen. Because the disease process is specific for platelets, the other two cell lines (erythrocytes and leukocytes) are normal. Also, because the thrombocytopenia is caused by excessive platelet peripheral destruction, the bone marrow will show increased megakaryocytes (platelet precursors). Hence, treatment for ITP includes oral corticosteroid agents to decrease the immune process of antiplatelet IgG production and if refractory, then splenectomy.

WHAT ARE THE RISK FACTORS FOR THIS PROCESS?

Understanding the risk factors helps the practitioner to establish a diagnosis and to determine how to interpret tests. For example, understanding the risk factor analysis may help manage a 45-year-old obese man with sudden onset of dyspnea and pleuritic chest pain following an orthopedic surgery for a femur fracture. This patient has numerous risk factors for deep venous thrombosis and pulmonary embolism. The physician may want to pursue angiography even if the ventilation/perfusion scan result is low probability. Thus, the number of risk factors helps categorize the likelihood of a disease process.

CLINICAL PEARL

▶ When the pretest probability of a test is highly likely based on risk factors, even with a negative initial test, more definitive testing may be indicated.

WHAT ARE THE COMPLICATIONS OF THIS PROCESS?

A clinician must understand the complications of a disease so that one may monitor the patient. Sometimes the student has to make the diagnosis from clinical clues and then apply his/her knowledge of the sequelae of the pathological process. For example, the student should know that chronic hypertension may affect various end organs, such as the brain (encephalopathy or stroke), the eyes (vascular changes), the kidneys, and the heart. Understanding the types of consequences also helps the clinician to be aware of the dangers to a patient. The clinician is acutely aware of the need to monitor for end-organ involvement and undertakes the appropriate intervention when involvement is present.

WHAT IS THE BEST THERAPY?

To answer this question, the clinician needs to reach the correct diagnosis, assess the severity of the condition, and weigh the situation to reach the appropriate intervention. For the student, knowing exact dosages is not as important as understanding the best medication, the route of delivery, mechanism of action, and possible complications. It is important for the student to be able to verbalize the diagnosis and the rationale for the therapy. A common error is for the student to "jump to a treatment," like a random guess, and therefore receive "right or wrong" feedback. In fact, the student's guess may be correct, but for the wrong reason; conversely, the answer may be a very reasonable one, with only one small error in thinking. Instead, the student should verbalize the steps so that feedback may be given at every reasoning point.

For example, consider the question, "What is the best therapy for a 25-year-old man who complains of a cough, fever, and a 2-month history of 10 lb weight loss?" The incorrect manner of response is for the student to blurt out "trimethoprim/sulfa." Rather, the student should reason it out in a way similar to this: "The most common cause of a cough and fever and weight loss in a young man is either HIV infection with *Pneumocystis jiroveci* pneumonia or malignancy such as lymphoma. Therefore, the best treatment for this man is either antimicrobial therapy such as with trimethoprim/sulfa, or chemotherapy after confirmation of the diagnosis."

CLINICAL PEARL

▶ Therapy should be logical and based on the severity of disease. Antibiotic therapy should be tailored for specific organisms.

HOW WOULD YOU CONFIRM THE DIAGNOSIS?

In the previous scenario, there is a wide differential diagnosis involving the man with a weight loss, fever, and cough, but two common disorders are *Pneumocystis carinii* pneumonia (PCP) or malignancy. Chest radiograph or CT imaging of the chest with possible Gallium scanning may be helpful. Knowing the limitations of diagnostic tests and the manifestations of a disease aid in this area.

Summary

1. There is no replacement for a careful history and physical examination.

2. There are four steps to the clinical approach to the patient: making the diagnosis, assessing severity, treating based on severity, and following response.

3. Assessment of pretest probability and knowledge of test characteristics are essential in the application of test results to the clinical situation.

4. There are seven questions that help bridge the gap between the textbook and the clinical arena.

REFERENCES

Bordages G. Elaborated knowledge: a key to successful diagnostic thinking. *Acad Med.* 1994;69(11): 883-885.

Gross R. *Making Medical Decisions.* Philadelphia, PA: American College of Physicians; 1999.

Hall JB, Schmidt GA, Wood LDH. An approach to critical care. In: *Principles of Critical Care.* 4th ed. New York, NY: McGraw-Hill; 2015:3-10.

Marino PL, Sutin KM. *The ICU Book.* 3rd ed. Philadelphia, PA: Lippincott Williams & Wilkins; 2007.

Mark DB. Decision-making in clinical medicine. In: Fauci AS, Braunwald E, Kasper KL, et al, eds. *Harrison's Principles of Internal Medicine.* 19th ed. New York, NY: McGraw-Hill; 2015:16-23.

Cases

A 39-year-old African-American woman with sickle cell disease (SSD) is admitted for fever, chills, and difficulty breathing. The patient has become more lethargic and confused upon admission to the intensive care unit (ICU). On physical examination, the patient's vital signs are: temperature 100.0°F, heart rate (HR) 110 beats/min, respiratory rate (RR) 28 breaths/min, blood pressure (BP) 90/50 mm Hg, and oxygen saturation (O$_2$ Sat) 89% on ambient air. Pulmonary examination reveals rhonchi and dullness to percussion in the right base. Cardiac examination reveals regular tachycardia. Laboratory studies are shown in the following table.

Laboratory Studies	Measured Values
WBC	10.3 ×10^3 per μL (4.5-11.0 × 10^3 per μL)
HgB	10.2 10^3 per μL (13.5-17.5 g/dL)
Sodium	143 mEq/L (135-145 mEq/L)
Potassium	4.1 mEq/L (3.5-5.0 mEq/L)
Chloride	102 mEq/L (95-105 mEq/L)
BUN	39 mg/dL (7-18 mg/dL)
Creatinine	2.9 mg/dL (0.6-1.2 mg/dL)
pH	7.28 (7.35-7.45)
Paco$_2$	28 (35-45 mm Hg)

► What is the most likely diagnosis?
► How would one gauge the severity of the patient's condition?
► What are the next steps in treatment?

ANSWERS TO CASE 1:
Early Awareness of Critical Illness

Summary: A 39-year-old woman with pneumonia and sickle cell disease (SSD) with a quick sepsis-related organ failure (qSOFA) score of 3 is admitted for signs of sepsis with multiorgan involvement.

- **Most likely diagnosis:** Sepsis secondary to pneumonia in a patient with underlying SSD.

- **Assessment of severity:** The sequential (sepsis-related) organ failure assessment (SOFA) score and the quick SOFA (qSOFA) score (Table 1–1) are useful objective tools used to assess the severity of potentially and critically ill patients, especially those with sepsis. In contrast to other evaluation systems, such as the simplified acute physiology score (SAPS II) and acute physiology and chronic health evaluation (APACHE II), the SOFA score was designed to focus more on organ dysfunction and morbidity and less on mortality prediction, although it can also be used to predict the risk of mortality in critically ill patients. Both SOFA and qSOFA are based on deviations of easily obtained and frequently monitored vital signs. The SOFA score is used to track a patient's status throughout their hospital course in an ICU. A score of 2 or higher is associated with in-hospital mortality of 10%. The qSOFA is a simplified version of the full SOFA score that includes only three *clinical criteria* from the full SOFA score, which not only has more criteria but also relies on laboratory studies. Another important distinction is the use of the Glasgow coma scale (requiring a score ≤13) in the SOFA score, while any altered mental status meets the qSOFA criteria. Due to the qSOFA's quickness and ease of use, the qSOFA score will aid in earlier recognition and management of patients with sepsis or patients at the risk of developing sepsis.

A qSOFA score of 2 or more suggests a diagnosis of sepsis; therefore, if the qSOFA score is 2 or more, clinicians should further investigate for organ dysfunction using the full SOFA score. **In this case, the qSOFA score of 3 indicates this patient needs acute care and ICU admission.**

Table 1–1 · COMPARING qSOFA VS SIRS CRITERIA	
qSOFA Criteria (Two or More of the Following)	SIRS Criteria (Two or More of the Following)
• Respiratory rate >22 breaths/min • Systolic blood pressure ≤100 mg Hg • Altered mental status	• Temperature: >38.0°C (100.4°F) or <36.0°C (96.8°F) • Heart rate: >90 beats/min • Respiratory rate: >20 breaths/min or P_{CO_2} <32 mm Hg • WBC: >12,000/μL or <4000/μL or >10% band forms

- **Next steps in treatment:** Administer oxygen to raise O_2 saturation >90% and give a fluid bolus of 20 to 30 mL/kg of normal saline. Transfer the patient to the ICU and start IV fluids and the correct antibiotic (within 1-6 hours). **Antibiotic choice should be influenced by the patient's SSD and probable autosplenectomy.**

ANALYSIS

Objectives

1. To recognize the early signs of critical illnesses.

2. To be familiar with the treatment strategies to correct abnormal vital signs and to initiate early goal-directed therapy.

3. To understand the role of the rapid response team (RRT) in managing deteriorating clinical status in hospitalized patients.

Considerations

The clinical presentation and the qSOFA score of 2 points or greater identifies the patient's organ dysfunction. The patient has an obvious focus of infection in the lung and underwent rapid deterioration soon after admission. Although systemic inflammatory response syndrome (SIRS) score was formerly widely used, it is being replaced by qSOFA because SIRS score has been shown to exclude 12.5% of otherwise similar patients with infection, organ failure, and significant mortality, while also failing to define a transition point in early intervention and prevention of death. Consequently, the qSOFA score has largely replaced the SIRS score since the latter has been found to be too sensitive (many patients may meet criteria but are not septic) and not specific enough. Overall, a qSOFA evaluation score has been found to work better than SIRS in better predicting those patients requiring rapid response and ICU care. A rapid response team with an efficient protocol should respond to high qSOFA score patients with clinical instability by rapidly giving required basic support, including IV fluids and monitoring of the patient. A delay in assessment, recognition, or therapy could lead to adverse consequences, including cardiac arrest and death. The SOFA score is a mortality prediction score based on the degree of dysfunction in six separate organ systems and is calculated on admission and again every 24 hours until discharge using the worst parameters measured during the prior 24 hours. The scores can be used in a number of ways: as individual scores for each organ to determine progression of organ dysfunction, as the sum of scores on one single ICU day, or as the sum of the worst scores during the ICU stay. It is believed to provide a better stratification of the mortality risk in ICU patients, given that the data used to calculate the score are not restricted to admission values. The SOFA score can be used on all patients admitted to an ICU. It is not clear if the score can be reliably used in patients who were transferred from another ICU. In summary, the SOFA score can be used to determine the level of organ dysfunction and the mortality risk in ICU patients.

APPROACH TO:

Early Recognition of Critical Illness

Early awareness of a critical illness is crucial in order to reduce both morbidity and mortality. The mortality rate among all hospitalized patients is about 5% and increases to 15% in patients admitted to an ICU. In cases of sepsis and acute lung injury, the death rate can approach 50%. Critical care is extremely costly, and ICU costs represent about 15% of all hospital expenses. The recently developed rapid response teams or medical emergency teams, consist of a group of clinicians and nurses who bring critical care expertise to the bedside. Their early intervention with IV fluids and antibiotics for patients who show early signs of sepsis with hemodynamic deterioration (such as tachycardia, low blood pressure, low urine output, fever, and changes in mental status) has markedly lowered both morbidity and mortality (Table 1–2).

Scoring systems utilizing routine observations and vital signs taken by the nursing and ancillary staff are used to evaluate the possible deterioration of patients. This deterioration is frequently preceded by a decline in physiological parameters. Furthermore, a failure of the clinical staff to recognize this failure in respiratory or cerebral function will put patients at risk of cardiac arrest. Suboptimal care prior to admission to an ICU leads to increased mortality. Because of resource limitations, the number of patients that can be monitored and treated in an ICU is limited. The selection of patients who might benefit most from critical care is crucial. The early identification of patients at risk of deterioration based on measurements of physiological parameters will reduce the number of pre-ICU resuscitations required.

Rapid response teams (RRTs). Earlier detection of a patient's clinical deterioration provides a great opportunity to prove Ben Franklin's adage that "an ounce of prevention is worth a pound of cure." Rapid response teams aim at intervening as soon as possible before the patient's condition deteriorates and helping ensure optimal outcomes. They use protocols that recognize deteriorating hemodynamics as quickly as possible. The result has been early referrals to the ICU or, in many cases, an avoided ICU admission when the patient has a good early response and reaches clinical stability quickly while still being closely monitored. Since most patients in

Table 1–2 • SIGNS OF SIGNIFICANT HEMODYNAMIC INSTABILITY	
Instability Indicated by One or More of the Following	Inadequate Perfusion Indicated by One or More of the Following
Hypotension	Lactic acidosis, >2 mmol
Tachycardia unresponsive to treatment	New abnormal capillary refill (>3 s)
Orthostatic vital sign changes	Reduced urine output
Multiple IV fluid boluses required to maintain adequate blood pressure or perfusion	New altered mental status
IV inotropic or vasopressor medication to maintain adequate blood pressure or perfusion	Cool, mottled extremities, body

this situation require respiratory care and evaluation, respiratory therapists (RTs) are considered key team members. In addition, a critical care nurse, a physician, a physician's assistant, and/or a pharmacist are all important members of the team. Their expertise has drastically reduced the incidences of both cardiac arrests and subsequent deaths. RRTs have also decreased the number of days in an ICU, overall hospital days, and the number of in-patient deaths. This has resulted in an increase in the number of patients who are discharged in a functional state.

Basic early interventions include measures to prevent aspiration, such as elevating the head of the bed to 30° to 45°. This should be instituted whenever there is a change in mental status or increased risk of aspiration, provided the current blood pressure allows this. The patient should be transferred to the ICU for further treatment and provided continuous monitoring and goal-directed therapy based on the surviving sepsis guidelines. Cardiac arrest has been associated with the failure to correct physiological derangement in oxygenation, hypotension, and mental status. These features may be apparent up to 8 hours prior to eventual cardiac arrest.

VITAL SIGNS

Respiratory rate. The respiratory rate (RR) varies with age, but the normal reference range for an adult is 12 to 20 breaths/min. The respiratory rate is an indicator of potential respiratory dysfunction. An **elevated RR >22 breaths/min is a poor prognostic factor** in patients with pneumonia, congestive heart failure (CHF), and other illnesses such as chronic obstructive pulmonary disease (COPD).

Blood pressure. Blood pressure (BP) is measured by two readings: a high systolic (ventricular contraction) pressure and the lower diastolic (ventricular filling) pressure. A BP (mm Hg) of 120 systolic over 80 diastolic is considered normal. The difference between the systolic and diastolic pressure is called the pulse pressure (PP). A low or narrow PP suggests significant intravascular volume loss. If the pulse pressure is extremely low, <25 mm Hg, the cause may be a decreased low stroke volume as in CHF or shock. A narrow pulse pressure value is also caused by aortic stenosis and cardiac tamponade. **There is no absolute natural or "normal" value for BP; rather, there is a range of values.** When excessively elevated, these values are associated with an increased risk of stroke and heart disease. Blood pressure is usually taken at the arms but may also be taken at the lower level of the legs, which is called segmental BP and evaluates blockage or arterial occlusion in a limb. **Be aware of falsely elevated or low blood pressures due to inappropriate blood pressure cuff sizes.** Too small of a cuff will result in high false readings, while too large of a cuff will result in low false readings.

Pulse. The pulse is the result of the physical expansion of the artery. The pulse rate is usually measured at the wrist or at the ankle and is recorded as beats per minute. The pulse is commonly taken at the radial artery. If the pulse cannot be taken at the wrist, it may be taken at the elbow (brachial artery), at the neck against the carotid artery (avoid carotid massage), behind the knee (popliteal artery), or in the foot (dorsalis pedis or posterior tibial arteries). It can also be measured by listening directly to the heartbeat using a stethoscope. Rates <60 or >100 are defined as bradycardia and tachycardia, respectively. When there is a rapid, regular pulse, sinus tachycardia and supraventricular tachycardia should be considered. An irregularly irregular pulse is very suggestive of atrial fibrillation.

Temperature. An elevated temperature is an important indicator of illness, especially when preceded by **chills.** Systemic infection or inflammation is indicated by the presence of a fever (temperature >38.5°C or sustained temperature >38°C) or a significant elevation of the temperature above the individual's normal temperature. Fever will increase the heart rate by 10 beats/min with every Fahrenheit (F) degree above normal. **Temperature depression (hypothermia),** <95°F, should also be evaluated since it is an ominous sign for severe disease and is more threatening than hyperthermia. Body temperature is maintained through a balance of heat produced by and lost from the body. Antipyretics should not be withheld. The patient should be made comfortable, and fluid repletion should be used to counter fever-induced fluid losses. The absence of fever does not indicate the absence of infection. High, spiking fevers in the 104°F to 105°F range may represent a drug allergy or blood transfusion reaction. Fever and other vital signs are keys to the diagnosis of SIRS, albeit many patients fit this criterion without actually being septic.

The fifth vital sign. The phrase "fifth vital sign" usually refers to **pain** or **oxygen saturation measurement.** Pupil size, equality in pupil size, and reactivity to light can also be used as vital signs. A **pulse oximetry saturation of 90% to 92% represents a Pao$_2$ near 60 mm Hg** and should be the minimal goal of O$_2$ supplementation. The 90% O$_2$ sat point represents the elbow of the hemoglobin dissociation curve, whereas below this number there is rapid hemoglobin desaturation. Above this number there is little gain in O$_2$-carrying capacity of hemoglobin.

SEPSIS

Sepsis is defined as life-threatening organ dysfunction caused by a dysregulated host response to infection. Severe sepsis is now considered to be redundant, and the term will no longer be used. **Septic shock,** a subset of sepsis, is defined as **a non-response to initial fluid resuscitation and the need for vasopressors in which profound circulatory, cellular, and metabolic abnormalities contribute to a greater risk of mortality.**

PROTOCOL-BASED CARE

Protocols are decision-making tools in which differential interventions are applied based on explicit directions and regular patient assessments. Protocols serve to standardize care practices and aid in the implementation of evidence-based therapies. Protocols have been associated with improvements in the quality of critical care. These include protocols for sedation, weaning from mechanical ventilation, lung protective ventilation in acute lung injury, early adequate resuscitation in severe sepsis, and moderate glucose control in post-cardiac surgery patients.

Protocol-based care offers a unique opportunity to improve the care of patients who do not have access to an intensivist. Nurses, pharmacists, and respiratory therapists can implement protocols successfully. Protocols are not superior to major decisions made by a qualified intensivist or physician. In settings with optimal physician staffing, protocols have not consistently resulted in improved outcomes; however, few ICUs are staffed with the trained intensivists and multidisciplinary clinicians necessary to provide such optimal care. **Because of the shortage of trained intensivists, the evidence suggests that outcomes are improved when routine care decisions are standardized and taken out of the hands of individuals.**

There is a myriad of diagnostic tests that can be obtained quickly to aid in the diagnosis and treatment of patients. Electrocardiography, arterial and venous blood gases, serum and urine electrolyte levels, O_2 saturation, cardiac enzyme analyses, echocardiography, CT scans, and ultrasound are all examples of such tests. The proper evaluation of the patient's physical condition and vital signs will enable a quick and correct application of the proper treatment. **The differential diagnosis of a patient's problems should immediately identify the most catastrophic but reversible and treatable events.**

The current gold standard for the organization of critical care services is the incorporation of an intensivist in the multidisciplinary care team. The intensivist is responsible for overseeing the multidisciplinary collaborative team that is endorsed as a key to successful evidence-based practice for the management of critically ill patients.

CLINICAL CASE CORRELATION

- See also Case 2 (Transfer of Critically Ill Patients), Case 3 (Scoring Systems and Patient Prognosis), and Case 4 (Monitoring).

COMPREHENSION QUESTIONS

1.1 A 34-year-old man was admitted earlier in the day with kidney stones and possible pyelonephritis that presented with hematuria, fever, pain, and chills. IV fluids and broad-spectrum antibiotics were administered 7 hours ago. Vital signs are: temperature (101.6°F), blood pressure 110/65 mm Hg, respiratory rate 32 breaths/min, heart rate 150 beats/min, and O_2 saturation 95% on ambient air. Heart rate upon admission was 92 beats/min. The skin is very warm and dry. The rest of the physical examination is unremarkable.

Activation of a rapid response team would be expected to decrease which of the following adverse outcomes in this patient?

A. Chance of cardiopulmonary arrest

B. ICU utilization

C. Intubation

D. Length of hospital stay

1.2 A patient presents to the ER with dyspnea and fever. Vital signs include: blood pressure 98/60 mm Hg, respiratory rate 24 breaths/min, temperature of 101.5°F, and a new onset of altered mental status. According to the qSOFA score, which of these findings is most predictive of an adverse outcome?

A. Dyspnea and respiratory rate >22 breaths/min

B. Systolic blood pressure <100 mm Hg

C. Temperature >101.4°F

D. New onset of altered mental status

ANSWERS

1.1 **A.** Activation of a rapid response team would be expected to decrease the risk of cardiopulmonary arrest in this patient. Unrecognized or delayed recognition of a deteriorating clinical status may lead to a very poor prognosis and survival rate. The signs and symptoms of deterioration are typically present with a median time of 6 hours prior to arrest. A number of indicators have been identified with an increased risk of clinical deterioration (Tables 1–1 and 1–2). The patient's persistent tachycardia suggests possible instability that necessitates further evaluation. Studies of rapid response teams have shown reduced rates of cardiopulmonary arrest and reduced mortality; however, they have not been consistently shown to reduce rates of intubation, ICU utilization, or length of hospital stay.

1.2 **A.** Recent studies have found that a significant number of patients on the medical wards may meet SIRS criteria, yet they do not need acute care. Application of qSOFA score to such patients would be more effective in evaluating these patients' clinical status, providing better early management and subsequent outcomes. Studies have shown that abnormal vital signs are strong predictors for both ICU admissions and in-hospital mortality. Both the number and the types of abnormal vital signs are predictive for adverse outcomes. **In one study, the highest in-hospital mortality rate was associated with dyspnea, followed by altered level of consciousness.**

CLINICAL PEARLS

▶ Early recognition of changes in vital signs and mental status is critical to the early detection of patient's deterioration and the prevention of cardiac arrest and death.

▶ SIRS score has been shown to be overly sensitive and replaced by the qSOFA bedside evaluation tool.

▶ The qSOFA is a simplified version of the full SOFA score that includes only three *clinical criteria* and does not require laboratory studies.

▶ The qSOFA criteria include two or more of respiratory rate >22/min, sBP ≤ 100 mm Hg, and/or altered mental status.

▶ A SOFA score >2 indicates an overall mortality risk of ~ 10%, while those advancing to septic shock have a mortality risk of 40%.

▶ Protocol-driven rapid response teams have significantly decreased the mortality and morbidity of patients.

REFERENCES

Kaukonen KM, Bailey M, Pilcher D, Cooper DJ, Bellomo R. Systemic inflammatory response syndrome criteria in defining severe sepsis. *N Engl J Med*. 2015;372:1629-1638.

Singer M, Deutschman CS, Seymour C, et al. The Third International Consensus Definitions for Sepsis and Septic Shock (Sepsis-3). *JAMA*. 2016;315(8):801-810.

Vincent JL. qSOFA (Quick SOFA Score) for Sepsis Identification MDCalc. 2016. http://www.mdcalc.com/qsofa-quick-sofa-score-for-sepsis-identification/. Accessed May 13, 2016.

Winters BD, Weaver SJ, Pfoh ER, et al. Rapid-response systems as a patient safety strategy: a systematic review. *Ann Intern Med*. 2013;Mar 5;158(5 Pt 2):417-425.

A 72-year-old woman is admitted to the ICU for progressive chest pain that began 2 hours ago. She has not had recent surgery or stroke and takes amlodipine for hypertension. On physical examination, blood pressure is 154/88 mm Hg, and pulse rate is 88 beats/min. Cardiac and pulmonary examinations are normal. Initial electrocardiogram shows a 2-mm ST-segment elevation in leads V1 through V5. Chest radiograph shows no cardiomegaly and no evidence of pulmonary edema. The patient is given aspirin, clopidogrel, unfractionated heparin and, as the nearest hospital with primary percutaneous coronary intervention (PCI) capabilities is more than 120 minutes away, she is also given a bolus dose of tenecteplase.

► What are the key conditions that must be stabilized when transferring a critically ill patient in both an inter- and intra-hospital setting?
► What other arrangements should be conducted prior to inter-hospital (between facilities) transfer?
► What monitoring is needed for inter-hospital transfers?

ANSWERS TO CASE 2:

Transfer of Critically Ill Patients

Summary: This 72-year-old woman presents with an ST-elevation myocardial infarction (STEMI) of acute onset and needs transfer for a percutaneous coronary intervention (PCI) and possible percutaneous transluminal coronary angioplasty (PTCA) with possible stenting, which are not available at the present facility.

- **What are the next steps in transportation process?** Stabilize the patient's vital signs, begin indicated emergency therapy, and arrange transfer to a new facility with the same treatments and personnel available in the ICU. Personnel qualified and experienced in transferring critically ill patients should be incorporated into the transfer.

- **Other arrangements prior to arrival at the new facility:** (1) Acceptance should be prearranged prior to arrival at the accepting facility. (2) Activation of key personnel is important to avoid an interruption in patient care. (3) An agreement regarding optimal transfer methods should be reached. The fastest and safest route of transfer is the best choice. (4) The transport method chosen should have all the equipment needed to conduct a safe transfer.

- **Inter-hospital transfer (IHT) of the critically ill:** (1) Transport the patient safely with the appropriate documented reason for leaving the ICU. (2) The same monitoring that the patient received in the ICU must continue during the patient's transport and stay outside the ICU.

ANALYSIS

Objectives

1. Describe how to assess the benefits and risks of transferring the critically ill patient.

2. Discuss the modalities of inter-hospital transfer and their advantages and disadvantages.

3. Describe the key requirements for transfer of the critically ill patient.

4. List the adverse effects of intra- and inter-hospital transfer of ICU patients.

Considerations

Patients with STEMI should be transferred to the nearest hospital with primary PCI capabilities for emergency PCI or rescue PCI. Before transfer, it must be demonstrated that there is a clear benefit in the treatment available at the receiving facility compared to the current facility. After ensuring stabilization and the absence of life-threatening conditions or arrhythmias, the patient can be transferred with appropriate monitoring and personnel. If providing a clinical escort, it is the responsibility of the transferring hospital to ensure that the appropriate clinical support is available for the patient during the transfer. Communication and coordination are keys to a successful transfer. PCI in patients with STEMI should ideally be performed within 90 minutes of presentation to a facility with PCI capability or within 120 minutes if the patient requires transfer from a non-PCI-capable hospital. **PCI is most effective if completed within 12 hours of chest pain onset; the earlier the intervention, the better the outcome. PCI may still be reasonable in selected patients beyond this window.**

APPROACH TO:
Transferring the Critically Ill Patient

Critical care transport has become a common occurrence. The centralization of therapeutic specialties and an expanding number of diagnostic and therapeutic options outside of the ICU are major reasons why transport is necessary. Bringing improved diagnostic testing and medical-surgical services to the patient reduces the adverse effects that accompany transportation outside the ICU. Infection rates are also lower in patients who are transported less often in the ICU setting. Most instances of critical care transport occur within the hospital itself and are referred to as intra-hospital (in-house transport). Nevertheless, **critical care transport is a high-risk undertaking, regardless of the setting.** Adequate planning, proper equipment, and appropriate staffing can minimize the transportation risks. Inter-hospital transport (IHT) of the critically ill patient presents more problems than intra-hospital (in-house) transport because of the distance, different hospital settings, and at times, inability to coordinate prior planning. Guidelines for personnel needs, such as physicians, nurses, and paramedics, have come from these experiences. **Alternative advantages and disadvantages of the mode of transport (by air or ground) are also necessarily weighed.** Specific treatments such as pre-transfer tracheal intubation and other advanced life support measures may be required.

Significant physiological disturbances occur frequently in patients during IHT, including variations in heart rate, blood pressure, and O_2 saturation. Physiological variability is also common in critically ill patients in stationary circumstances, occurring in 60% of such patients compared with 66% in transported patients. An appropriately trained transport team can safely manage these physiologic changes, but even then, serious adverse events occur. Cardiac arrest rates of 1.6% have been noted during IHT. Reduction in the Pao_2/Fio_2 ratio occurred in patients when transported while using a transport ventilator, and severe changes (ie, >20% reduction from baseline) were common. These changes persisted for >24 hours in 20% of the transported patients. Out-of-unit transport was an independent risk factor for ventilator-associated pneumonias (VAP). IHT is also one of the factors associated with unplanned extubation in the mechanically ventilated patient. Compared to matched controls of patients not requiring transport, IHT individuals had a higher mortality rate (28.6% vs 11.4%) and a longer length of stay in the ICU.

Table 2–1 • PREDICTIVE ADVERSE EVENTS DURING INTRA-HOSPITAL TRANSPORT BY RISK FACTORS	
1. Pre-transport secondary insults in head-injury patients	2. F_{IO_2} levels >50% are predictive of respiratory deterioration on transport
3. High injury severity score, age >43 years	4. The number of intravenous pumps and infusions
5. High therapeutic interventions severity score (TISS) but not acute physiology and chronic health evaluation scoring system (APACHE II) score	6. The time spent outside the unit has been shown to correlate with the number of technical mishaps

Serious adverse events, however, occurred in 6% of all transports. See Table 2–1. Rechecking the patient and equipment and assurance of skilled assistance prior to transfer are important preventative measures.

Transport from the operating room to the ICU: Hemodynamic variability is more common in patients being transferred from the operating room to the ICU than those transported for diagnostic procedures outside the ICU. This is probably related to the patient's emergence from anesthesia. Accurate and complete information is important in these transfers. Ideally, both the medical team (surgeon and anesthesiologist) and nursing team should communicate important information to the ICU team. A directed form to ensure that proper information is transmitted can be useful. Likewise, a clear understanding of which physician will be responsible for what aspect of the patient's care is vital.

Management of transport: Ventilators used in transport are known to reduce variability in blood gas parameters when compared with manual bagging. Manual bagging with a tidal volume monitor was shown to be superior to mechanical ventilation (MV). No significant variations in blood gas parameters were noted in transport patients who received MV when under supervision by a respiratory therapist. Changes in blood gas parameters correlate with hemodynamic disturbances like arrhythmias and hypotension. Capnometry ($Etco_2$) monitoring clearly reduces $Paco_2$ variability in adults. In children, less than one-third of patients undergoing manual ventilation without $Etco_2$ monitoring had ventilator parameters within the intended range.

Inter-hospital transfer: The benefits to the patient of the higher care at another facility should be weighed against the considerable risks of the transport process.

Adverse effects: The inter-hospital transport of critically ill patients is associated with an increased morbidity and mortality during and after the journey. Even with specialist mobile intensive care teams, the mortality before and during transport is substantial (2.5%). A reduced Pao_2/Fio_2 ratio (hypoxemia), arterial hypotension, and tachycardia occur, respectively. **Transported patients have a higher ICU mortality and longer ICU stays than do controls.** Studies have found a 4% increase in mortality in the transferred group despite adjustments for diagnosis.

Prediction of adverse events: The prediction of patient deterioration during inter-hospital transport has proven difficult. The variables that predict deterioration in adults include **old age, high F_{IO_2}** requirements, **multiple injuries, and inadequate stabilization.**

Planning of the transport: Poor plans lead to an increased incidence of adverse events and mortality. In an audit of transfers to a neurosurgical center, 43% of patients were found to have inadequate injury assessment and 24% of individuals received inadequate resuscitation. Deficiencies in assessment and resuscitation before transfer were identified in all patients who died. Guidelines have been developed to address this issue in many jurisdictions, but inadequate assessment and resuscitation remain a problem. Some found that the application of national guidelines led to only modest improvements in patient care, with an incidence of hypoxia and hypotension that remains unacceptably high.

Selection of personnel: A **minimum of two people** in addition to the vehicle operators should accompany a critically ill patient during transport. The team leader can be a nurse or a physician, depending on clinical and local circumstances. It is imperative that the team leader has adequate training in transport medicine and advanced cardiac life support (ACLS). Adequately trained nurses and physicians are acceptable in transporting critically ill children. Appropriately staffed and equipped specialist retrieval teams are superior to impromptu teams in transferring critically ill adults and children; these have recorded up to an 80% reduction in critical incidents during pediatric inter-hospital transport.

Mode of transport: The choice among the three options of ground, helicopter, and fixed wing transport is affected by three main factors: distance, patient status, and weather conditions. A retrospective review of adult transfers demonstrated no difference in mortality or morbidity between patients transferred by air versus ground transportation. A prospective cohort study revealed that air transport is faster than ground transport, and for transfers of <225 km (140 miles), helicopter transport is faster than fixed wing. Severely injured patients undergoing inter-hospital transport had a reduced mortality when carried by air compared to ground transport.

Equipment and monitoring: Comprehensive lists of equipment and medications needed for the transport of critically ill patients should be identical to that of an ICU environment. The transport ventilators used in intra-hospital transfers create less ventilatory fluctuation than hand ventilation (Ambu bagging). However, when compared to standard ICU ventilators, transport ventilators were inferior in delivering set tidal volume (V_t) and had a tendency to trap gas. Extra care in ventilatory monitoring is warranted when changing from an ICU to a transport ventilator. Arterial blood gas (ABG) analysis during inter-hospital transfer allows for early identification and treatment of changes in gas exchange and metabolic parameters.

When pre-hospital care is delayed for more than 60 minutes, severely injured patients are at higher risk for complications, increased length of hospital stay, and death. There is a reduction in mortality for severely injured trauma patients when they are transferred directly to a Level I trauma center. In summary, the careful, organized, and coordinated transfer to critically ill patients is important.

CLINICAL CASE CORRELATION

- See also Case 1 (Early Awareness of Critical Illness), Case 3 (Scoring Systems and Patient Prognosis), and Case 4 (Monitoring).

COMPREHENSION QUESTIONS

2.1 A 21-year-old man was admitted to the surgical ICU 17 days ago for multiple gunshot wounds and needs surgical intervention, which is scheduled for tomorrow. He is mechanically ventilated and has a central line catheter placed in the right femoral vein. *Acinetobacter baumannii* has been isolated from blood cultures. His ICU room has another patient with pneumonia. Which of the following is most likely to reduce spread of this patient's *Acinetobacter* infection upon transfer to the operating room?

A. Clean the patient's room with bleach.

B. Ensure strict staff adherence to hand hygiene practices and contact precautions.

C. Give prophylactic antimicrobial agents active against *Acinetobacter* species to the patient's roommate in the ICU.

D. Replace the patient's central line catheter and endotracheal tube.

2.2 A 22-year-old man has been "saved" from an automobile fire after he was knocked unconscious and is currently resting in the ICU of a rural hospital with 35% of body surface burns. The patient is breathing spontaneously and maintaining 98% O_2 saturation on 4 L/min oxygen delivered by nasal cannula. IV fluid hydration with lactated Ringer's (LR) has been started with a delivery amount of 9.8 L as the first 24-hour total fluid requirement, and 4.9 L to be delivered within the first 8 hours (1/2 of total), according to the Parkland formula. His sputum is noted to be black (carbonaceous). The current facility does not have mechanical ventilation (MV) capacity or a burn center with a barometric pressure chamber. The patient's blood carbon monoxide level is 30%. His family requests transfer to a tertiary care facility with a burn unit. The next most appropriate step in the management of this patient is:

A. Check his carboxyhemoglobin level.

B. Give 100% F_{IO_2} and transfer to the nearest facility with burn center care facililities.

C. Monitor the patient closely for respiratory distress.

D. Take the patient to the operating room for immediate debridement and grafting.

E. Transfer the patient to a burn center via ambulance or helicopter.

ANSWERS

2.1 **B.** Hand hygiene is the single most important measure to prevent infections, including those from multidrug-resistant organisms. Hand hygiene, performed before and after patient contact, consists of handwashing with soap and water for at least 15 to 30 seconds. Alcohol-based hand disinfectants are also acceptable alternatives to soap and water. In addition to hand hygiene, standard precautions include the use of barrier protection (eg, wearing gloves and personal protective equipment for the mouth, nose, and eyes), appropriate handling of patient care equipment and instruments/devices, and proper handling, transporting, and processing of used/contaminated linen. Removal of any contaminated catheters and drains from a source patient has not been demonstrated to reduce the risk for spread of pathogens to other patients.

2.2 **E.** Stabilization in the operating room (OR) or ICU is key to a safe transport to a hospital that can treat burn victims and carbon monoxide poisoning where MV and hyperbaric oxygen are available. Despite his 100% oxygen saturation, the presence of carbonaceous sputum is an ominous sign and should be considered an indication that the patient may require intubation and MV. The good neurological status suggests that the carboxyhemoglobin and carbon monoxide levels have decreased with 2 hours on high-flow O_2. Decompensation may require intubation for upper airway obstruction secondary to edema. Once intubated and stable, the patient should be transferred via the fastest route available to a hospital with a burn center, accompanied by skilled personnel and all the necessary equipment for a safe transfer. The Parkland formula is used to calculate total IV hydration. The total amount of fluid in 24 hours is calculated as *(4 mL × Kg × BSA%)*, and the first 8-hour delivery is calculated as *(4 mL × Kg × BSA%)/2.* Lactated Ringer's (LR) is the preferred solution of choice to avoid a hyperchloremic metabolic acidotic state.

CLINICAL PEARLS

► Patients with thrombolytic therapy failure following an ST—elevation myocardial infarction (STEMI) should be immediately transferred for rescue percutaneous coronary intervention (PCI).

► PCI is most effective if completed within 12 hours of the onset of chest pain. The earlier the intervention, the better the outcome. PCI may still be reasonable in selected patients beyond this time window.

► Physiological derangements during transport are seen slightly more frequently than in stationary ICU patients.

► Transport risk can be reduced by appropriate planning, including arranging for trained transport personnel and achieving pre-transport stabilization.

► The pre-hospital interventions associated with improved outcome are:

   ► Helicopter transport of severely injured patients

   ► The presence of a physician on the pre-hospital transport team

   ► A short injury-to-hospital time of less than 60 minutes

   ► Transfer directly to a Level I trauma center

► Correct transfer of the most severely injured, critically ill patients has shown long-term benefit, evaluated at 1 year post transfer.

► Hand hygiene is the single most important measure to prevent the spread of hospital acquired infections, especially when transporting patients.

REFERENCES

Burke JP. Infection control—a problem for patient safety. *N Engl J Med.* 2003;348(7):651-656.

Deutschman CC, Neligan PJ. *Evidence Based Practice of Critical Care, Expert Consult.* Philadelphia, PA: Saunders Publishers; 2011.

Koppenberg J, Taeger K. Inter-hospital transport: transport of critically ill patients. *Curr Opin Anaesthesiology.* 2002;15:211-215.

A 78-year-old man is admitted to the intensive care unit (ICU) for an exacerbation of congestive heart failure (CHF). During the first 2 days of his ICU stay, his clinical condition further deteriorates and he subsequently requires intubation and mechanical ventilation. At a patient care conference with family members, his family members inquire regarding his prognosis and your assessment of his chances for recovery with meaningful survival.

▶ What can be used to predict recovery or death in this patient?
▶ What are the types of prognostic systems to determine severity of conditions in the ICU?

ANSWERS TO CASE 3:

Scoring Systems and Patient Prognosis

Summary: A 78-year-old man is admitted to the ICU for CHF exacerbation. By day two in the ICU, the patient has shown signs of continued deterioration and is placed on mechanical ventilation. The family is hoping you can help them understand his potential for meaningful recovery.

- **Severity and prognostic scoring models to predict outcome:** A variety of models are available for disease severity stratification and outcomes prognostication. These models are necessary for quality control and management in the ICU. Although these systems are helpful for outcome prediction in various ICU cohorts, the models generally are not intended to be used for outcome prediction in individual patients.

- **Prognostic systems available for severity determination in the ICU:** There are four broad categories of prognostic scoring systems that are used in the ICU setting: general risk-prognostic scores, disease-specific scores, organ dysfunction scores, and trauma severity scores. Examples of *general risk-prognostic scores* include the acute physiology and chronic health evaluation (APACHE), the mortality probability model (MPM), and the simplified acute physiology score (SAPS). The APACHE, MPM, and SAPS can be used to predict either ICU length of stay or mortality, but they are most often used to compare quality outcomes in the ICU. *Disease- and organ-specific prognostic scores* attempt to predict outcome based on the level of function or dysfunction in a specific organ system. Examples include the Glasgow coma score (GCS) for neurological function, the Child-Pugh classification for liver disease, and the RIFLE (Risk, Injury, Failure, Loss of kidney function, and End-stage kidney disease) classification for acute kidney injury. *Organ dysfunction scores* grade the severity of dysfunction when more than one organ system is affected by a disease process. The sepsis-related organ failure score (SOFA), multiple-organ dysfunction score (MODS), and the logistic organ dysfunction system (LODS) are commonly used multiorgan dysfunction scores. Lastly, predictors of outcome after a *traumatic injury* include the injury severity score (ISS) and the revised trauma score (RTS).

ANALYSIS

Objectives

1. Learn the various scoring systems that are applicable to patient population in the ICU.

2. Learn the applicability and limitations of prognostic systems in clinical practice.

Considerations

When we care for a critically ill patient, we are frequently approached by the patient's family members to predict how likely the patient is to recover. It is important in these situations to clearly communicate to those involved that **there are no tools to accurately predict an individual's clinical course or outcome.** In this case, there are several models that estimate the probability of in-hospital mortality and 1-year mortality for heart failure patients, and these models may provide some insight into what events could transpire during the patient's ICU and hospital stay (Table 3–1). These predictive models take into account a variety of clinical and laboratory values like age, comorbidities, vital signs, left ventricular function, serum sodium, and serum blood urea nitrogen (BUN). These variables can be entered into a risk-prediction model to calculate the probability of in-hospital and long-term survival. When discussing risk prediction with family members, it is important to remind them that the results produced by predictive models are based on prior observations of similar patients and that these projections based on historical observations of large population or patients may not reliably predict a single individual's outcome.

Table 3–1 • HEART FAILURE PROGNOSTIC MODELS				
Study	Patient Population	Variables	Outcomes	Reference
AHA-GWTG-HF (2010)	Hospitalized patients	Age, SBP, HR, serum sodium, BUN, COPD, patient race	In-hospital mortality stratification based on number of points	*Circ Cardiovasc Qual Outcomes.* 2010;3:25-32.
OPTIMIZE-HF (2008)	Hospitalized patients	Age, HR, SBP, sodium, creatinine, LV function, and HF as the reason for admission	In-hospital mortality prediction based on nomogram	*J Am Coll Cardiol.* 2008;52:347-356.
EFFECT (2003)	Hospitalized patients	Age, SBP, respiratory rate, BUN, serum sodium, comorbidities (CVA, COPD, cirrhosis, dementia, or cancer)	30-d and 1-y mortality calculation based on points	*JAMA.* 2003;290: 2581-2587.
Seattle Heart Failure Model (2006)	Outpatients and hospitalized patients	Age, gender, AHA classification, weight, LVEF, SBP, medications, diuretic doses, laboratory data, and ventricular assist devices use	1-, 2-, and 3-y survival	*Circulation.* 2006;113: 1414-1433.

Abbreviations: SBP: systolic blood pressure; HR: heart rate; HF: heart failure; COPD: chronic obstructive pulmonary disease; CVA: cerebral vascular accident; LV: left ventricular; LVEF: left ventricular ejection fraction; BUN: blood urea nitrogen.

APPROACH TO:
Scoring Systems and Patient Prognosis

DEFINITIONS

GENERAL RISK-PROGNOSTICATION SYSTEMS: These systems were developed based on the assumption that acute disease severity can be measured by the patients' characteristics and degree of abnormality of various physiologic variables. The general risk-prognostication systems include the APACHE II model introduced in 1985, one of the most commonly applied prognostic systems of this type in the ICU. These systems are designed to help determine outcomes in populations and are useful for quality assurance and outcome assessment in cohorts of patients. *These scoring systems can provide a good estimate of the number of patients who are predicted to die in a population of similar patients; however, these systems cannot be used to predict exactly which of the patients will die.*

DISEASE- AND ORGAN-SPECIFIC PROGNOSTIC SCORES: These are scoring systems used to quantify single-organ failure or disease-specific outcomes. Examples of these include the GCS, Child-Pugh classification, model for end-stage liver disease (MELD), RIFLE, and the variety of heart failure predictive models discussed earlier. Unlike the general risk-prognostic scores, these scoring systems are reasonably accurate for organ-specific risk prognostication and are commonly applied in clinical decision making.

ORGAN DYSFUNCTION SCORING SYSTEMS: There are several scoring systems that are used to quantify and serially follow the progression of patients with multiple organ dysfunction syndromes. These include SOFA, MODS, and LODS. These systems are not only useful at the bedside for clinical decision making, but they are also useful for quality assurance and outcome assessment in cohorts of patients.

TRAUMA SCORES: The two most commonly used trauma scoring systems are the RTS and ISS. The RTS is based on three physiological parameters (GCS, systolic blood pressure, and respiratory rate). The ISS is an anatomy-based scoring system based on accumulated injuries and the severity of injuries in six distinct body regions (head, face, chest, abdomen, extremity, and external). The RTS is a useful system for the serial assessment of trauma patients, particularly during the initial assessment phase. The ISS is more useful for quality assurance and outcome assessment in cohorts of patients, and this scoring system is not used for clinical decision making.

CLINICAL APPROACH

Quantitative assessment of disease severity and prognostication of outcomes in the ICU have become increasingly important. From the standpoint of individual patient care, the ability to accurately assess the severity of illness and accurately determine the level of function of specific organs is very helpful in clinical decision making and in determining the level of medical resources that the individual patient may require. Scoring systems that have become integral part of day-to-day care for critically ill patients include the GCS, MODS, MELD, and SOFA. The major reasons why these scoring systems have gained popularity in direct patient care are that these scores can easily be calculated by care providers and the calculations are reproducible between observers. The drawback of using any scoring system for outcome prognostication is that while all scoring systems are useful to trend improvement or deterioration, the scores are in no way predictive of individual outcomes. As all scoring systems are mathematical models, the usefulness of each model is influenced by its *discrimination* and *calibration*.

The **discrimination** of a predictive model measures the ability to distinguish patients who would have one outcome versus another (eg, which patients with heart failure can be expected to survive). **Discrimination is most commonly expressed by a receiver operating curve (ROC). The ROC plots the sensitivity of a test (y-axis) against one specificity (x-axis). The area under the ROC (reported as aROC or area under the curve [AUC]) represents the combined performance of the model (Figure 3–1).** A perfect model has an aROC of 1, whereas an aROC of 0.5 suggests that the model is no better than chance alone. Most predictive models that are useful have an aROC >0.7. An aROC >0.8 is considered good, and an aROC of >0.9 is considered excellent. With further discrimination, the curve will have a more vertical initial rise followed by a more horizontal extension.

The **calibration** of a scoring system is a measurement of its accuracy at different levels of risk. The calibration of a system can be examined using **goodness-of-fit** statistics, which looks at the difference between the observed frequency and the expected frequency for a wide range of patients. The Hosmer-Lemeshow test is a statistical goodness-of-fit test for logistical regression models used to test whether the expected outcomes match the observed outcomes in various population subgroups. A *P* value can be calculated, and if it is large, the model is well calibrated or fits the data well (Figure 3–2).

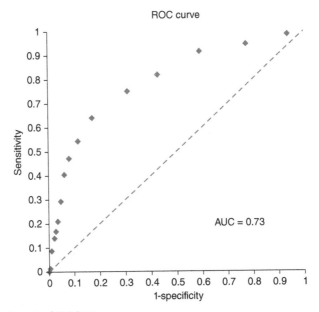

Figure 3–1. Example of ROC Curve.

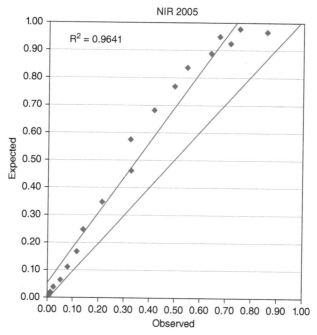

Figure 3–2. An Example of Goodness-of-fit Curve. The diagonal line that bisects the graph is the curve expected when the observed outcomes are equal to the expected outcomes. Deviation away from this line indicates a mismatch between the expected and the observed outcomes. In this example, the observed outcomes are closer to the expected outcome in the low-risk cohorts in comparison to the cohorts in the higher risk groups.

APPLICATIONS OF SCORING SYSTEMS

As predictors of individual outcomes in the ICU, organ-specific prognostic scores are frequently used to follow patient progress and guide clinical decisions. These scores are generally easily calculated and have good inter-observer reproducibility. For the purpose of outcome prediction, most scoring systems that are available will provide estimates of outcome in a specific population of patients; however, most systems are not designed to predict outcomes for individual patients. Mortality prediction using serial severity scores have been evaluated by a number of groups. These results have demonstrated that with the assessment of serial scores such as APACHE II and APACHE III, the specificity of the predictive models can be improved. The values of most scoring systems are used to evaluate the performance of the ICU care system for quality assurance purposes. When scoring systems are used for ICU performance evaluation, it is important that the model chosen for outcome prediction is appropriate. For example, an ICU with a lower actual mortality in comparison to the expected mortality does not necessarily indicate that the care is better. Multiple factors can influence ICU mortality, including case-mix, admission and discharge policies, and resource availability such as staffing (Table 3–2).

	Year Introduced	Origin of System	Age of Population	aROC of Original Report	Parameters	Applications
APACHE II	1985	United States	> 16	0.86	17 variables selected by panel of experts: age, physiologic status, acute conditions, and chronic disease processes	Research, benchmarking for quality improvement
APACHE III	1991	United States	> 16	0.90	26 variables selected based on multiple logistic regression: age, chronic conditions and acute conditions	Research, benchmarking for quality improvement; sequential application to monitor clinical progress
APACHE IV	2006	United States	> 16	0.88	Improved over APACHE III in that it can be used to provide for ICU length of stay prediction, which can provide benchmarks for comparison of ICU efficiency and resources	Research, benchmarking for quality improvement; sequential application to monitor clinical progress
SAPS II	1993	Europe and North America	> 18	0.86	17 variables developed from multiple logistic regression based on data collected during the first 24 hours of ICU admission	Research, benchmarking for quality improvement; sequential application to monitor clinical progress
SAPS III	2005	Multinational	> 16	0.85	Modified from SAPS II. 20 variables are divided into three subscores relating to the patient: characteristics prior to ICU admission, circumstances for ICU admission, and derangements that occurred during the first hour after admission	Research, benchmarking for quality improvement; sequential application to monitor clinical progress
MPM II 0	1993	North America and Europe	> 18	0.82	A score at admission; 5 admission variables	Research; bench marking for quality improvement
MPM II 24	1993	North America and Europe	> 18	0.84	A second score at 24 hours after admission; includes 8 additional variables	Research; bench marking for quality improvement

Table 3-2 • GENERAL-RISK PROGNOSTIC SYSTEMS FOR MORTALITY PREDICTION

Abbreviations: APACHE: acute physiology and chronic health evaluation; SAPS: simplified acute physiology score; MPM: mortality prediction model; ROC: receiver operating curve.

> ## CLINICAL CASE CORRELATION
>
> - See also Case 1 (Early Awareness of Critical Illness), Case 2 (Transfer of Critically Ill Patient), and Case 4 (Invasive and Hemodynamic Monitoring).

COMPREHENSION QUESTIONS

3.1 Which of the following scoring systems has been found directly correlating with change in patient's condition and is most useful for bedside decision-making?

A. Injury severity score (ISS)

B. Revised trauma score (RTS)

C. Multiple organ dysfunction score (MODS)

D. APACHE II

E. APACHE III

3.2 Which of the following is NOT a general risk-prognostication scoring system?

A. APACHE II

B. SAPS II

C. MPM II

D. APACHE III

E. GCS

3.3 Which of these scoring systems is most useful for the maintenance of quality control in a general medical-surgical ICU?

A. MODS

B. ISS

C. MELD score

D. RIFLE

E. APACHE III

ANSWERS

3.1 **B.** The revised trauma score (RTS) is a physiology-based scoring system. This is based on the patient's GCS, systolic blood pressure, and respiratory rate. A drop in RTS of ≥ 2 during the early post-injury observational period generally indicates a worsening condition and would require re-assessment of the patient. The ISS is an anatomy-based trauma scoring system that is most useful when assessing population outcome and quality management of trauma services. The MODS is a scoring system to document the severity of organ dysfunction. It is used to direct care when there is a pattern of change that is unexpected. It is, however, not as useful as the RTS in direct decision-making in the ICU. The APACHE II and APACHE III scores are general prognostication scores that are mainly applied for quality management. Some groups have shown that serial measurements of APACHE II and III scores can be used for individual outcome prognostication.

3.2 **E.** The GCS is not a general risk-prognostication scoring system, whereas all other scoring systems listed are general-risk prognostication scores.

3.3 **E.** In a combined medical-surgical ICU population, the APACHE III scoring system would be the most useful for outcome prognostication and quality control. The MODS score is an organ dysfunction scoring system that may not capture all the patient outcomes in a mixed ICU population. Similarly, ISS is for trauma severity grading. The MELD and RIFLE are organ-specific scoring systems for liver and kidney injury quantification, and these scoring systems would not capture all the important variables that might influence outcome.

CLINICAL PEARLS

▶ Most general risk-prognostic scoring systems are designed for population-risk prognostication and lack specificity for individual-risk prognostication.

▶ Some of the disease-specific scoring systems are useful for bedside decision making; these include GCS, RIFLE, and MELD scores.

▶ Some predictors of outcome after a *traumatic injury* include the ISS and RTS.

REFERENCES

Capuzzo M, Moreno RP, Le Gall JR. Outcome prediction in critical care: the simplified acute physiology score models. *Curr Opin Crit Care*. 2008;14:485-490.

Gartman EJ, Casserly BP, Martin D, Ward NS. Using serial severity scores to predict death in ICU patients: a validation study and review of the literature. *Curr Opin Crit Care*. 2009;15:578-582.

Russell JA. Assessment of severity of illness. In: Schmidt GA, Kress JP, Hall JB, eds. *Principles of Critical Care*. 4th ed. New York, NY: McGraw-Hill; 2015:83-96.

Strand K, Flaatten H. Severity scoring in the ICU: a review. *Acta Anesthesiol Scan*. 2008;52:467-478.

Vincent JL, Bruzzi de Carvalho F. Severity of illness. *Semin Resp Crit Care Med*. 2010;31:31-38.

Vincent JL, Moreno R. Clinical review: scoring systems in the critically ill. *Crit Care*. 2010;14:207-215.

A 20-year-old woman is admitted to the ICU for a blood pressure of 88/52 mm Hg, which has persisted despite fluid challenge. She has a positive blood culture secondary to a UTI. Her condition deteriorates and she develops increasing respiratory distress with adult respiratory distress syndrome (ARDS) that requires intubation for mechanical ventilation (MV). The resident on staff inserts a right heart catheter to measure the pulmonary vascular pressure to assist with fluid management. The following hemodynamic readings were obtained:

Hemodynamic Studies	
Central Venous Pressure	2 mm Hg (0-5 mm Hg)
Pulmonary Artery Pressure	20/5 mm Hg (20-25/5-10 mm Hg)
Pulmonary Capillary Occlusion "wedge" Pressure	7 mm Hg (6-12 mm Hg)
Cardiac Output	3.0 L/min (4-8 L/min)

► What is the most likely diagnosis?
► What are the best next steps in the treatment of this patient?

ANSWERS TO CASE 4:

Hemodynamic Monitoring of the Unstable Patient

Summary: This 20-year-old woman has acute hemodynamic instability, secondary to septic shock with severe dehydration and low pulmonary capillary wedge pressure (PCWP). The patient's cardiac output is also decreased, which is likely caused by hypovolemia and endotoxins from gram negative bacteria acting as a cardiosuppressant.

- **Most likely diagnosis:** Dehydration/septic shock, urinary tract related sepsis.

- **Best treatment steps:** The best initial treatment for acute septic shock is to administer fluids and start the patient on appropriate antibiotics within 6 hours of hospital admission. Vasopressors may be indicated to correct hypoperfusion, and dobutamine may also be indicated to improve cardiac output.

ANALYSIS

Objectives

1. To understand the goals of hemodynamic monitoring.

2. To appreciate various forms of acute hemodynamic monitoring.

3. To be able to interpret data from hemodynamic monitoring.

Considerations

Septic shock is present when there is systemic hypotension and evidence of end-organ hypoperfusion that is not responsive to fluid therapy. In septic shock, the patient should be started on norepinephrine if the fluid challenge has failed; if needed, dobutamine may be administered to correct the decreased cardiac output. Both dobutamine and milrinone are used to increase cardiac output; however, **in the setting of kidney dysfunction, dobutamine would be the appropriate choice** because milrinone is metabolized by the kidneys. The provider should also continue with aggressive hydration and follow hemodynamic parameters. A low central venous pressure (CVP) usually indicates decreased preload to the heart and decreased intraventricular volume. A right heart catheterization can be used to guide therapy of volume status and cardiac output.

APPROACH TO:

Hemodynamic Monitoring and Goals

The goal of hemodynamic monitoring (HM) is to evaluate the vital signs needed to **maintain adequate tissue perfusion.** HM can be accomplished by noninvasive (preferred) or invasive means. Continuous monitoring allows for early recognition

✷ MAP + Urine out = indic. of organ perfusion.

of poor tissue perfusion based on low blood flow. Invasive pulmonary artery catheter (PAC) use provides data on systemic, pulmonary arterial and venous pressures, and measurements of cardiac output (CO). Since the flow of blood into organs cannot be measured directly, blood pressure (more specifically, mean arterial pressure [MAP > 65 mm Hg]) and urine output are used as indirect indicators of adequate tissue perfusion. In the ICU, **hypotension has been identified as the most common cause of hemodynamic instability.** Assuming that the CVP and the PCWP are adequate estimates of the systemic and pulmonary volumes, respectively, one can create a working relationship between CVP and PCWP, with further consideration of the CO or stroke volume (SV). This can be plotted on a Starling curve, allowing for the optimum range of the end-diastolic volume and CO for each patient. Misleading readings can occur with abnormal pressure/volume relationship (compliance) of the right ventricle (RV) or left ventricle (LV), increased intrathoracic pressure (positive end expiratory pressure [PEEP], auto PEEP, intra-abdominal pressure), and valvular heart disease (mitral stenosis). CVP is often used as the sole guide to monitor hemodynamic function. Techniques such as echocardiography, transesophageal echocardiography, doppler, and volume-based monitoring can be used. No single monitoring technique has been demonstrated to improve a patient's outcome. Time is crucial for an early diagnosis of a hemodynamic catastrophe and application of effective therapy. **Assuring accuracy of the data is the key to correct interpretation. Trends of data are more reliable than single data points ("the direction of the trend is your friend" – A Manny Suarez saying, or "Suarezism").**

Monitoring

Critically ill patients require continuous monitoring to diagnose and manage their complex medical conditions. This is most commonly achieved by using direct pressure monitoring systems. Pulmonary artery pressure (PaP) measurements are much less commonly used today since their use has not shown a decrease in mortality. Monitoring central venous pressure (CVP) and BP are common approaches to evaluating hemodynamic functioning. Most facilities use noninvasive monitoring of hemodynamic functions of BP and other basic vital signs.

Continuous Vital Signs

Modern electronic devices regularly monitor a minimum of five vital signs (heart rate, respiration rate, temperature, oxygen saturation, and blood pressure). The data are entered into a five-point index that is constantly on display. Nursing staff can review these vital signs and the patient status index to enable early response and identify a patient who is experiencing distress. This should lead to fewer unplanned admissions to ICUs and minimize cardiac arrests occurring in out-of-intensive care units, thereby significantly improving cost and survival rate.

Monitoring of Cardiac Function

The assessment of ventricular function is based on both blood volume and BP. The left ventricular ejection fraction (EF), dp/dt_{max}, has been widely accepted as an index of the left ventricle's contractile performance. Measurement of left ventricular dp/dt_{max} is a satisfactory index of ventricular contractility.

ECG Monitoring

All ICU patients must have continuous ECG monitoring. The diagnosis of arrhythmias and the commencement of rapid treatment is a goal of hemodynamic monitoring. The wave form display is arranged to monitor Leads I, II, or V1-V2, whichever provides the **tallest QRS complex and best p-wave morphology.** Alarms must be set and placed in the "on position" at all times. High- and low-alarm settings are assessed and documented in a graphic record. Upper and lower alarm limits are selected for each patient. The rhythm strip allows only for rhythm interpretation; for the evaluation of morphology, a 12-lead ECG is needed.

Intra-arterial Blood Pressure Monitoring

Intra-arterial BP monitoring is used to obtain direct and continuous BP measurements in ICU patients who have hypertension or hypotension. Arterial blood gas (ABG) measurements and blood sampling can also be obtained repeatedly via arterial lines. To check collateral circulation to the hand, one can use the Allen test to evaluate the radial and ulnar arteries' circulation status or use an ultrasonic Doppler to evaluate any of the arteries. When obtaining an ABG, it is important to note that if no collateral circulation exists and the cannulated artery becomes occluded, ischemia and infarction of the area distal to that artery could occur. In the Allen test, the radial and ulnar arteries are compressed simultaneously. The Allen test confirms the presence of collateral circulation. If this collateral circulation is not confirmed, arterial blood gases (ABGs) using that site should be avoided. Site preparation for arterial lines and their subsequent care are the same as for CVP catheters. **Complications of arterial lines include local obstruction with distal ischemia, external hemorrhage, massive ecchymosis with compartmental syndrome, dissection, air embolism, blood loss, pain, arteriospasm, and infection.** Blood pressure readings are more commonly obtained by automatic self-inflating cuff devices. Under most circumstances, these produce comparable blood pressure results when compared to arterial lines. BP cuffs should be avoided on arms with arteriovenous shunts for hemodialysis to avoid occlusion.

To Catheterize or Not to Catheterize?

Previously, PAC was the gold standard for evaluating the circulatory function of patients in the ICU. Recent studies show that PAC has no impact on mortality and is not recommended for routine use of hemodynamic monitoring. Although its benefits are not seen in the ICU, PAC-based hemodynamic management is successful in improving patient outcome in instances of planned major surgery. However, it should be noted that **PAC-based monitoring has its limitations; the most significant being the misinterpretation of the data being produced, even by well-trained intensivists and cardiologists.** PAC monitoring provides measurements of PaP and right atrial pressure. Flow variables such as CO and mixed venous O_2 (Svo_2) are also measured. Calculations of systemic and pulmonary vascular resistance (SVR, PVR), right ventricular stroke work, and left ventricular stroke work (LVSW) are obtained. There was no significant difference regarding outcome or postoperative complications whether managed with a CVP or a PAC (Table 4–1).

Table 4-1 · HEMODYNAMIC CHANGES WITH VARIOUS DISORDERS

	Right Atrial (mm Hg)	Right Ventricle Systolic (mm Hg)	Right Ventricle Diastolic (mm Hg)	Pulmonary Artery Systolic (mm Hg)	Pulmonary Artery Diastolic (mm Hg)	Pulmonary Capillary Wedge (mm Hg)	Cardiac Index (L/min)/m²	Systemic Vascular Resistance (dyne · sec/cm⁵)
Normal values	<6	<25	0-12	<25	0-12	<6-12	2.5	(800-1600)
Myocardial infarction without pulmonary edema	—	—	—	—	—	13 (5-18)	2.7 (2.2-4.3)	—
Pulmonary edema	No Δ/Increased	No Δ/Increased	No Δ/Increased	Increased	Increased	Increased	No Δ/Decreased	Increased
Cardiogenic shock — Left ventricular failure	No Δ/Increased	No Δ/Increased	No Δ/Increased	No Δ/Increased	Increased	Increased	Decreased	No Δ/Increased
Cardiogenic shock — Right ventricular failure	Increased	Decreased/No Δ/Increased	Increased	Decreased/No Δ/Increased*	Decreased/No Δ/Increased*	Decreased/No Δ/Increased*	Decreased	Increased
Cardiac tamponade	Increased	No Δ/Increased	Increased	No Δ/Increased	No Δ/Increased	No Δ/Increased	Decreased	Increased
Acute mitral regurgitation	No Δ/Increased	Increased	No Δ/Increased	Increased	Increased	Increased	No Δ/Decreased	No Δ/Increased
Ventricular septal rupture	Increased	No Δ/Increased	Increased	No Δ/Increased	No Δ/Increased	No Δ/Increased	Increased Pulm BF† / Decreased System BF†	No Δ/Increased
Hypovolemic shock	Decreased	No Δ/Decreased	No Δ/Decreased	Decreased	Decreased	Decreased	Decreased	Increased
Septic shock	Decreased	No Δ/Decreased	No Δ/Decreased	Decreased	Decreased	Decreased	Increased	Decreased

*Different subsets of diseases have different values.
†Pulm BF, pulmonary blood flow; System BF, systemic blood flow.

Svo_2 = Global. Oxygenation.

Central Venous Catheter

PAC has not improved survival or organ function and has been associated with more complications than CVP-guided therapy. Some newer CVP catheters provide a continuous recording of O_2 saturation, which helps monitor **venous O_2 sat (goal >70%)**. CVP catheters should be placed with guidance from ultrasound. Peripherally inserted central catheter (PICC) lines are also an option and can serve as a central line with fewer complications than a CVP catheter.

The CVP and PCWP parallel each other closely in patients with EF >50%. In EF <40%, the correlation between the CVP and PCWP decreases due to changes in myocardial compliance. Patients with PAC placement receive more fluid in the first 24 hours and have an increased incidence of renal failure and thrombocytopenia than those with CVP use. Also, a line infection is an important risk that must be considered. Complications arose in approximately 20% of the instances in which a catheter was left in place for more than six days.

Mixed Venous Oxygen Saturation

Continuous monitoring of venous oxygen saturation (Svo_2) by reflectometry immediately detects trends and abrupt changes in the oxygen supply-to-demand ratio. Svo_2 has been promoted as an indicator of changes in CO. **Normal values for Svo_2 range from 70% to 75%.** A linear correlation has been demonstrated between the CO and Svo_2. Svo_2 reflects the overall oxygen reserve of the whole body. A normal Svo_2 value does not rule out an impaired oxygen supply to individual organs. The pulmonary artery carries blood from all vascular beds in the body; thus, Svo_2 represents the amount of oxygen in the systemic circulation that is left after passage of the blood through all tissues. Svo_2 thus serves as a measure of global oxygenation. The determinants of Svo_2 are Sao_2, systemic VO_2, CO, and Hb.

$$Svo_2 = Sao_2 - [(VO_2)/(Hb \times 1.36 \times CO)]$$

An increase in VO_2, Hb, or CO and/or a decrease in arterial oxygenation will result in a decrease of Svo_2. Interpretation of Svo_2 values might be difficult in conditions where oxygen delivery to oxygen consumption (DO_2/VO_2) relationships are altered. Arterial-venous microcirculatory shunting in sepsis may increase Svo_2 tissue oxygenation while regional tissue dysoxia is present.

Monitoring of the Right Ventricle

The right ventricle is responsible for accepting venous blood and pumping it through the pulmonary circulation. Circulatory homeostasis depends on an adequate function and synchronization of both ventricles. Changes in the dimensions of one ventricle influence the geometry of the other. Monitoring CVP has demonstrated its value in judging right ventricular function. The use of right ventricular end-diastolic volume (RVEDV) and right ventricular ejection fraction (RVEF) are unaffected by arbitrary variations.

Measurement of Extravascular Lung Water and Intrathoracic Blood Volume

Depressed left ventricular performance increases hydrostatic pressure in the pulmonary circulation, influencing fluid flux across a damaged pulmonary microvascular membrane.

Extravascular lung water (EVLW) can be measured at the bedside using a double-dye technique with indocyanine green. Intrathoracic blood volume appears to be a more reliable indicator of preload than cardiac filling pressure.

Echocardiography

Assessing global and regional LVF is the domain of echocardiography, via transthoracic echocardiography (TTE) or transesophageal echocardiography (TEE). Two-dimensional echocardiography provides significant information, including left ventricular cavity size, fractional shortening, and abnormalities in regional wall motion. Two-dimensional colored echocardiography enables a quantification of shunts, CO, and provides a noninvasive assessment of concomitant valvular disease. The **presence and extent of ischemic heart disease is determined by monitoring segmental wall motion.** These abnormalities are indirect markers of myocardial perfusion that can persist for prolonged periods in the absence of infarction. TEE provides more accurate information on ventricular size than standard TTE. Left ventricular end-diastolic volume (LVEDV) is a better predictor of myocardial performance than PCWP. **If immediately available, TEE is the first diagnostic method which should be used when aortic dissection, endocarditis, or pulmonary embolism with hemodynamic instability are suspected.** Hypovolemia, left ventricular failure, global systolic function, and the size of both the ventricles can be rapidly identified using TTE/TEE. Valvular abnormalities and functionally important heart disease can also be readily determined using these methods.

Monitoring of Organ Perfusion and Microcirculation

Monitoring of tissue oxygenation and organ function in the clinical setting is based on measuring variables of global hemodynamics like pulse oximetry, capillary refill, and urine output, or by the use of indirect biochemical markers. These parameters are insensitive indicators of dysoxia and are considered poor surrogates for measuring O_2 at the tissue levels. The net balance between cellular O_2 supply and O_2 demand determines the status of tissue oxygenation. Regional tissue dysoxia can persist despite the presence of adequate systemic blood flow, pressure, and arterial oxygen content.

Oxygen Delivery and Oxygen Consumption

Total body perfusion and oxygenation relies on an adequate arterial oxygen saturation (Sao_2), appropriate hemoglobin (Hb) concentration, and cardiac output. The total amount of oxygen delivered to the peripheral tissue per minute (DO_2) can be calculated as $DO_2 = CO \times Cao_2$, with arterial oxygen content, $Cao_2 = (Hb \times 1.39 \times Sao_2)$. In steady state the uptake of oxygen from the arterial blood (VO_2) represents the sum of all oxidative metabolic reactions in the body. VO_2 can be measured by analysis of the expired gas or calculated from CO and arterial and mixed venous blood samples. The VO_2/DO_2 is the oxygen extraction ratio. VO_2/DO_2 dependency occurs when the increase in oxygen extraction can no longer fully compensate for the fall in DO_2. The relationship between DO_2 and VO_2 can therefore be used to assess the adequacy of tissue oxygenation. The determination of DO_2 and VO_2 requires right heart catheterization to measure CO.

Blood Lactate Level

Arterial blood lactate levels in critically ill patients have proven very useful. Lactate is formed from pyruvate by the cytosolic enzyme lactate dehydrogenase. A lactate concentration >2 mmol/L is generally considered a biochemical indicator of inadequate oxygenation. Circulatory failure with impaired tissue perfusion is the most common cause of lactic acidosis. Mechanisms other than impaired tissue oxygenation may cause an increase in blood lactate, including an activation of glycolysis, a reduction in pyruvate dehydrogenase activity, or liver failure. The complex process of tissue lactate production and its utilization mandates an understanding of the usefulness and limitations of blood lactate levels. Elevated lactate levels should prompt the clinician to initiate procedures for assessment of the circulatory status.

Respiratory Monitoring

A breathing wave pattern is generated by the standard three ECG leads used in the ICU for ECG rhythm monitoring. A change in breathing rate disturbs the electrical triangle formed by the leads, measuring respiratory rate and apneas. **This method is not accurate and is predisposed to deliver incorrect data.** Noninvasive monitoring of pulmonary function is most important in the mechanically ventilated patient. The respiratory system requires the generation of pressure for the inflation needed to overcome resistive and elastic properties of the lung. Resistance is located mainly in the central airways. Several techniques are available to measure respiratory mechanics, but the most practical method is the rapid airway occlusion technique. This technique estimates the elastic recoil pressure of the alveoli by measuring the inspiratory plateau airway pressure (Pplat). Functional lung monitoring has questionable prognostic value and is of limited use in daily clinical practice. Bedside monitoring of static compliance and Pplat should be used routinely to detect the presence of alveolar overdistention and at least to qualitatively assess the risk for volume-induced lung injury (VILI). An important factor in respiratory mechanics is intrinsic positive end-expiratory pressure (PEEPi). This is commonly measured using end-expiratory airway occlusion. PEEPi causes decreased cardiac output, alveolar overdistention, increased work of breathing, and patient-ventilator asynchrony. If neglected, PEEPi leads to an underestimation of compliance.

O_2 Saturation

The determination of O_2 saturation (O_2 sat) via pulse oximeters is a valuable adjunct to clinical oxygen monitoring. When properly applied, it reliably indicates the patient's heart rate and arterial oxygen saturation. ECG synchronization reduces motion artifacts when the ECG R wave is detected. The **diagnosis of hypoxemia requires an arterial blood gas analysis and is commonly defined as a P_{AO_2} of <60 mm Hg or O_2 sat <90%.** Pulse oximetry is commonly used for assessing hypoxemia ("A poor man's blood gas" -Suarezism). However, this modality measures the saturation of hemoglobin and not Pao_2, reflecting oxygen dissolved in the blood, which includes both bound and unbound O_2. Thus, a patient with severe anemia may have a normal Pao_2 but a low O_2 content. Low pulse oximetry values <90% coincide with significant hypoxemia, but normal oxygen saturation does not exclude hypoxemia, especially in patients receiving a high FiO_2. Normal Pao_2

levels are 80 to 100 mm Hg in a healthy patient. Pulse oximetry values may remain normal until Pao_2 decreases to <60 mm Hg. For this reason, the alveolar-arterial oxygen gradient should be evaluated in patients receiving a high Fio_2. **A widening alveolar-arterial oxygen gradient (A-a) is a sign of an increasing hypoxemia. Pulse oximetry may be unreliable in cases of severe anemia, carbon monoxide poisoning, methemoglobinemia, or peripheral vasoconstriction.**

End-Tidal CO₂ Monitoring

End-tidal CO_2 monitoring is now standard in intraoperative care. Although pulse oximetry monitoring (oxygenation) is useful, bedside monitoring of carbon dioxide is likewise important. Capnometry or end-tidal volume CO_2 ($Etco_2$) monitoring is used to evaluate the $Paco_2$ level during surgery and in intubated patients in the ICU. In children, manual ventilation with $Etco_2$ monitoring resulted in increased $Paco_2$ readings falling within the intended range.

Urinary Bladder Pressure

Measurement of intra-abdominal pressure (IAP) is accomplished via the use of Foley bladder balloons in critically ill patients. Monitoring IAP to avoid and detect abdominal compartment syndrome is increasingly recommended, especially for inpatients who have undergone abdominal surgery. IAP is usually estimated, indirectly, by measuring intrabladder pressure (IBP).

Electroencephalographic Monitoring

Continuous EEG monitoring (CEEG) is a powerful tool for evaluating cerebral function in obtunded and comatose patients. Ongoing analysis of CEEG data is a major task because of the amount of data generated and the near real-time interpretation of a patient's EEG. Methods such as the computerized detection of seizures have increasingly allowed focused reviews of EEG epochs of interest. These allow personnel and inexperienced staff to recognize significant EEG changes in a timely fashion.

Esophageal Pressure Measurement

The chest wall includes the abdomen. The use of a pressure monitor in the esophagus can help to approximate pleural pressure. Abdominal pathology affects respiratory mechanics. Esophageal pressure and airway pressure affects respiratory mechanics and particularly compliance. Supine measurements are less reliable.

Near-Infrared Spectroscopy

Near-infrared spectroscopy (NIRS) is a noninvasive way to measure oxygenated and deoxygenated Hb as well as the redox state of cytochrome 3 as an average value of arterial, venous, and capillary blood. It has been used primarily in studies of cerebral or muscle oxygenation after different types of hypoxic injuries.

CLINICAL CASE CORRELATION

- See also Case 5 (Vasoactive Drugs) and Case 16 (Acute Cardiac Failure).

COMPREHENSION QUESTIONS

4.1 A 61-year-old man with heart failure is admitted to the ICU for chest pain, increasing dyspnea and fatigue. Jugular venous distention was noted at the angle of the jaw while sitting, and cardiac examination reveals an S3. Chest radiograph shows cardiomegaly and vascular congestion. A catheter was placed in his pulmonary artery and provided the following hemodynamic readings: central venous pressure (CVP) 15 mm Hg (0-5 mm Hg), pulmonary artery pressure (PAP) 40/15 mm Hg (20-25/5-10 mm Hg), pulmonary capillary occlusion "wedge" pressure (PCWP) 18 mm Hg (6-12 mm Hg), and cardiac output (CO) 3.0 L/min (4-8 L/min). The CVP pressure is 18 mm Hg. What is the most likely cause?

A. Congestive heart failure, Stage 1

B. Noncompressible arterial disease

C. Peripheral venous disease

D. Cardiogenic shock

E. COPD

4.2 A 75-year-old man with long-standing history of coronary artery disease is admitted to the ICU with hypotension and a 24-hour episode of intermittent chest pain. Physical examination reveals a new S3 gallop and bilateral pitting edema. The lower extremities are also cool on palpation and have weak pulses. Which of the following modalities will most likely *worsen* this patient's condition?

A. Positive inotropes

B. Aortic balloon pump

C. Continuous positive airway pressure (CPAP)

D. Afterload reducing agents

E. IV fluid modulation

ANSWERS

4.1 **D.** This 61-year-old man has an acute decompensation of his congestive heart failure (CHF). There is a new S3 gallop. The CVP of 18 mm Hg indicates a volume overload, with an elevated central venous and PCWP. Stage 1 CHF indicates no limitations of physical activity, whereas decompensated CHF limits physical activity. Patient with decompensated CHF should be started on dobutamine for probable cardiogenic shock and on IV fluids.

4.2   **C.** Right heart catheterization can be helpful to guide volume as well as medical therapy if volume status or cardiac output is uncertain. However, CPAP have not been shown to improve outcomes in most ICU patients and can perhaps exacerbate the cardiac condition. This patient has clinical evidence of volume overload, as indicated by the pitting edema and new onset of an S3 gallop. Additionally, he has evidence of low cardiac output (hypotension and cool extremities). Together, these clinical presentations insinuate heart failure. Initiating inotropic therapy, afterload reducing agents, IV fluid modulation, and an aortic balloon pump have been shown to decrease mortality of patients with heart failure.

CLINICAL PEARLS

▶ There is no specific monitoring technique that is known to improve patient outcome.

▶ Pulmonary artery catheter (PAC) use has not been associated with improvement in patient outcomes and is now rarely used except in selected cases.

▶ A MAP of 65 mm Hg is a target associated with signs of adequate urine output and mental status.

▶ CVP and PCWP are comparable in patients with EF >50% and indicate end-diastolic volume.

▶ Maintaining plateau alveolar pressures at <30 cm H_2O reduces alveolar strain and barotrauma.

▶ PEEP is clinically titrated by measuring its effects on gas exchange and hemodynamics.

▶ The mechanical characteristics of the respiratory system are compliance, resistance, and intrinsic PEEP; all can be measured using standard ventilators and bedside maneuvers.

▶ Monitoring esophageal pressure can help assess the extent of alveolar strain from PEEP.

▶ Cardiogenic shock usually requires treatment with intravenous vasoactive medications and, in severe cases, device-based hemodynamic support.

REFERENCES

Nativi-Nicolau J, Selzman CH, Fang JC, Stehlik J. Pharmacologic therapies for acute cardiogenic shock. *Curr Opin Cardiol.* 2014 May;29(3):250-257.

Schorr CA, Zanotti S, Dellinger RP. Severe sepsis and septic shock: management and performance improvement. *Virulence.* 2014 Jan;5(1):190-199. doi:10.4161/viru.27409.

Summerhill EM, Baram M. Principles of pulmonary artery catheterization in the critically ill. *Lung.* 2005;183:209-219. [PMID: 16078042]

A 67-year-old woman is admitted to the intensive care unit (ICU) from a nursing home for a 24-hour onset of new altered mental status that has been progressively worsening. On arrival to the ICU, she was disoriented, febrile with a temperature of 101°F, had a heart rate of 115 beats/min, and was hypotensive with a blood pressure of 80/40 mm Hg. A chest radiograph showed a right lower lobe infiltrate. Central venous access was obtained, and she was started on broad-spectrum antibiotics. A 20 mL/kg normal saline fluid challenge was administered over 30 minutes. Blood pressure is now 85/45 mm Hg, and heart rate is 110 beats/min. Her urine output has been 10 mL/h since arrival. Laboratory studies are as follows:

	Results	Normal Range
Blood		
Hemoglobin	11g/dL	13.5-17.5 g/dL
Leukocyte Count	33,000/µL Differential: 85% Neutrophils 10% Bands 5% Lymphocytes	4,500-11,000 µL (4.5-11 x 10⁹/L)
Urine		
Dipstick	(+)nitrites (+)leukocyte esterase	Negative nitrites and leukocyte esterase

▶ What is the next step in addressing the blood pressure?
▶ What other measures should be undertaken in this patient?

ANSWERS TO CASE 5:

Vasopressor Drugs and Pharmacology

Summary: This 67-year-old woman has decreased blood pressure (BP) as well as signs of decreased intravascular volume and cardiac output. After failing adequate fluid challenge, she now needs vasopressor support to correct her hypotension for what is considered septic shock.

- **Next step in addressing blood pressure:** The first step should incorporate efforts to increase the BP with isotonic IV fluids, mainly normal saline or Ringer's lactate. A starting bolus of 20 mL/kg followed by maintenance fluids is standard. If the hemodynamic parameters fail to respond to hydration, as in this case, the next best step is to begin proper vasopressor therapy to elevate BP. Vasopressor therapy is indicated to maintain a mean arterial pressure (MAP) of ≥65 mm Hg or central venous pressure measurement of 8 to 12 mm Hg in patients with sepsis who have failed to respond to an initial crystalloid fluid challenge. The BP should be supported to ensure that the blood flow to target organs is sufficient with this combination. Ideal MAP is ≥65 mm Hg.

  The MAP is calculated with the following equation:

  $$MAP = ([2 \times \text{diastolic blood pressure}] + \text{systolic blood pressure}) \div 3$$

- **Other measures:** Fluid and blood volume should be maintained appropriately with adherence to goal-directed therapy. Usually, a minimum pH of 7.20 is needed for vasopressors to be effective. Vasopressors are classically delivered via a central line, although recent data has shown delivery via peripheral access can be safe as well.

ANALYSIS

Objectives

1. To describe the indications for the use of IV fluids and vasopressors.

2. To understand the pharmacological mechanisms of action of the vasopressors available.

Considerations

This 67-year-old woman is admitted to the ICU with pneumonia and urosepsis. The patient's fluid-unresponsive hypotension and need for norepinephrine (NE) confirms septic shock. Improving survival requires rapidly addressing the abnormal hemodynamic parameters and early correction of the underlying cause of the sepsis, including administration of correct antibiotics in a timely fashion (within 1 hour for hospital inpatients and up to 6 hours for outpatients).

APPROACH TO:

Fluid and Vasopressor Use

IV FLUIDS

IV fluids are usually the **first-line therapy for hypotension.** Fluid therapy is effective in increasing intravascular volume (IVC), which in turn increases the BP and MAP. An ideal fluid would maintain IVC without expanding the interstitial space (eg, blood). There are two types of IV fluids used: crystalloid and colloid. Crystalloid solutions are composed of water with added electrolytes. Colloid solutions are typically based on crystalloid fluid with added substances that cannot freely cross semi-permeable membranes (eg, albumin). The crystalloid solutions include lactated Ringer's solution and 0.9% sodium chloride; the primary colloid solution is albumin.

Crystalloids

Crystalloid solutions are universally used for initial volume resuscitation and may be isotonic, hypotonic, hypertonic or balanced solutions. The determination of which crystalloid to use still remains controversial; however, most studies favor the use of normal saline (0.9%) as the fluid of choice. In sepsis, capillary permeability is increased, and significant tissue accumulation of resuscitation fluid occurs, resulting in adverse effects. Aggressive resuscitation with crystalloids induces a dramatic increase in extracellular fluid (ECF), alterations in acid–base balance, electrolyte composition, colloid balance, and coagulation. Combinations of crystalloids and colloids have proven effective because significantly greater tissue perfusion occurs when compared with crystalloid alone. During sepsis, up to 80% of the crystalloid solutions given cause edema that varies linearly with the volume of crystalloid that is administered.

The volume distribution of 1 L of 0.9% NaCl would put 250 mL in the IVC and 750 mL in the extracellular fluid volume (EFV), a 1:3 ratio. **Isotonic saline, when administered in large volumes, is associated with hyperchloremic non-anion gap acidosis.** The tendency for crystalloids to extravasate out of the vascular space may lead to relative hypoperfusion. There is **emerging evidence that intravenous fluids may have an indigenous pro-inflammatory property.** In contrast, findings on injured soldiers in Iraq who were resuscitated from a hypotensive state with low volume hypertonic 3% saline demonstrated an elevation in BP without an increase in inflammatory markers. Thus, hypertonic low-volume repletion may emerge as the resuscitation of choice.

Lactated Ringer's Solution

Buffered crystalloid solutions such as lactated Ringer's can also be used in septic shock. A 2012 meta-analysis examining the use of lactated Ringer's solution perioperatively over normal saline showed a lower incidence of hyperchloremia and metabolic acidosis.

Hypertonic Saline

The osmolality of normal plasma is 280 to 295 mOsm/L. Any solution with an osmolality exceeding 310 mOsm/L is considered to be a hypertonic fluid. Hypertonic saline (HS) and sodium bicarbonate are examples of hypertonic fluids. The most commonly used concentrations of HS are 1.8%, 3%, 7.5%, and 23.4%. The higher the concentration of Na^+ in HS, the larger the amount that stays in the IVC. HS dramatically increases the osmotic pressure in the compartment where it is injected. Water flows along the osmotic gradient into the compartment, expanding the compartment's fluid volume for several hours. There are two well-defined uses of hypertonic fluid. The first is to expand the IVC in patients in hypovolemic shock as a means of low-volume and high-impact resuscitation (eg, war victims with closed trauma). The second use is a corollary of the first, namely intracellular volume depletion. This second advantage is widely appreciated in neurosurgery and neurocritical care, where the reduction of cerebral volume and intracranial pressure (ICP) is especially important. HS may also increase myocardial contractility. The metabolic consequences of HS are hypernatremia, hyperosmolality, and hyperchloremic non-gap acidosis.

Some studies and case reports suggest that patients have better hemodynamic profiles when given HS than when given isotonic crystalloid. No study of the prehospital administration of HS has shown an overall statistically significant benefit. Survival benefit has been noted for patients requiring surgery and receiving prehospital administration of HS plus dextran (HSD) versus an equal volume of isotonic crystalloid. Wade and colleagues reported an improved survival in patients who had suffered penetrating trauma if they were given HS. The major controversy in trauma is not the utility of HS but the timing of its use. There are no large prospective studies on the use of HS in sepsis. Hypothetically, HS should improve overall systemic perfusion and presumably oxygen delivery, and in addition it may modulate the inflammatory response.

Colloids

High molecular-weight solutions (colloids) are used widely as plasma substitutes. Colloid solutions remain in the intravascular space because of their large molecular size and low membrane permeability. Colloids may also plug leaky capillaries and increase colloid oncotic pressure (COP), thus expanding the intravascular volume (IVC). Using colloids, one can achieve a volume expansion equal to or greater than the volume administered, which reduces tissue edema. There is a strong argument that colloid solutions are not only expensive but also leak into the extracellular space and affect blood coagulation. Blood products are discussed in another section.

Albumin

Albumin is a volume expander that comes in vials of 250 and 500 mL; it is also available as a 25% solution in 50- and 100-mL vials. Albumin products contain 130 to 160 mEq of sodium per liter of solution. The 5% solution is iso-oncotic with respect to human plasma; the 25% solution is four to five times more oncotically active. Albumin solutions do not appear to alter blood coagulation. The administration of albumin is associated with a rapid but unpredictable expansion of the plasma volume. Concerns that albumin therapy may increase mortality appear to be unfounded. Albumin is safe to use, but it is costly. There is no evidence that the administration of albumin improves patient recovery from sepsis or reduces mortality when compared to crystalloids. However, in contrast to the relative hypoperfusion potentially caused by crystalloids, the administration of 5% albumin will increase plasma volume by 52% of the volume infused. Albumin increases the cardiac index significantly more than saline and has a significant effect on hemoglobin dilution. As a result, some sepsis patients may have a better BP response. Current recommendations are to use colloid solutions only in patients with septic shock who require substantial amounts of crystalloid fluid.

VASOPRESSOR AGENTS

Vasopressor therapy is used when hypotension, such as that caused by sepsis, is unresponsive to fluid therapy. Vasopressors are less effective in the setting of hypovolemia. See Table 5–1 for a summary of the most commonly used vasopressor medications. There are two situations in which intravenous hydrocortisone in stress doses is indicated. First, it is indicated when hypotension remains unresponsive to adequate fluid resuscitation and vasopressor therapy; second, it is indicated if there is concern for possible underlying adrenal insufficiency. The recommended vasopressors for initial treatment are centrally administered norepinephrine or dopamine. Vasopressors should be administered into large veins, preferably via a central line in order to avoid potential extravasation. Recent research supports the safety of peripheral use in the first 48 to 72 hours of intervention when good peripheral IV access exists.

Vasopressors are used to assist in the maintenance of MAP, whereas inotropes are used to increase cardiac output, cardiac index, stroke volume, and Svo_2. The exact MAP target in patients is uncertain because each patient autoregulates within his/her own individualized limits. Autoregulation in various vascular beds can be lost below a certain MAP. This could lead to conditions in which tissue perfusion becomes linearly dependent on blood pressure. **The titration of norepinephrine (NE) to a MAP of ≥65 mm Hg is known to preserve tissue perfusion.** A patient with preexisting hypertension may well require a higher MAP to maintain adequate tissue perfusion. The ideal "pressor" would restore blood pressure while maintaining cardiac output and preferentially perfuse the brain, heart, splanchnic organs, and kidneys. All vasopressors are associated with adverse effects.

Dobutamine

Dobutamine is a synthetic catecholamine with primarily β_1 agonist activity, leading to increased cardiac contractility. The increase in heart rate caused by dobutamine is offset by its vasodilation effect with little net effect on BP. Dobutamine is primarily used in patients with refractory CHF, hypotension, or septic patients with hypoperfusion in whom vasodilators cannot be used because of their effect on BP. The onset of dobutamine action is 1 to 10 minutes after its administration, with its peak effect being reached in 10 to 20 minutes. The usual drip rate for adults is at 2.5 to 20 μg/kg/min with a recommended maximum of 40 μg/kg/min. It is important to titrate the dosage to achieve the desired target of increased cardiac output.

Table 5–1 • COMMON VASOACTIVE DRUGS AND THEIR ACTIONS				
Drug Name	Receptor	Action	Uses	Comments
Dobutamine	β_1 agonist	Inotrope Vasodilator (mild)	Cardiogenic shock, Right-sided heart failure	Minimal effects on heart rate
Dopamine	$\alpha_1 \beta_1 \beta_2$ DA agonist	Vasoconstrictor Inotrope Chronotrope	Hypotension (second line)	May cause tachyarrhythmia
Norepinephrine	$\alpha_1 \alpha_2$ and β_1 agonist	Vasoconstrictor Inotrope	Septic shock	First-line therapy
Epinephrine	$\alpha_1 \alpha_2 \beta_1 \beta_2$ agonist	Vasoconstrictor Inotrope Chronotrope	Anaphylaxis, cardiac arrest	Increases myocardial O_2 demand, calorigenic effects
Phenylephrine	pure α agonist	Vasoconstrictor	Hypotension in anesthesia	May cause reflex bradycardia
Vasopressin	V1 agonist	Vasoconstrictor	Refractory hypotension	Can be used in cardiac arrest

Abbreviation: DA: dopaminergic

Dobutamine has less effect on heart rate than dopamine. Dobutamine also appears particularly effective in splanchnic resuscitation, increasing pH (gastric mucosal pH), and improving mucosal perfusion when compared to dopamine. As part of an early goal-directed resuscitation protocol that combined close medical and nursing attention with aggressive fluid and blood administration, dobutamine was associated with a significant absolute reduction in the risk for mortality.

Dopamine

Dopamine has predominantly β-adrenergic effects in low-to-moderate dose ranges (up to 10 μg/kg/min). It is converted to norepinephrine in the myocardium and activates adrenergic receptors. In higher doses, it sensitizes α-adrenergic receptors to cause vasoconstriction. **Dopamine is a mixed inotrope and vasoconstrictor.** At all dose ranges, dopamine is a potent chronotrope, an agent increasing heart rate. **Dopamine causes more tachycardia and is more arrhythmogenic than NE.** Evidence suggests that dopamine does not have a net substantial effect on the kidneys. It may interfere with thyroid and pituitary function and may have an immunosuppressive effect. The use of "renal-dose" dopamine has been proven false. **Dopamine-resistant septic shock (DRSS),** a well-described condition, is defined as MAP <70 mm Hg despite administration of dopamine at 20 μg/kg/min. **In some research the incidence of DRSS was 60%, and those patients had a mortality rate of 78%, compared with 16% in the dopamine-sensitive group.**

Norepinephrine

Norepinephrine (NE) has pharmacologic effects on both α_1- and β_1-adrenergic receptors. NE is used to maintain BP in hypotensive states and is a more potent vasoconstrictor than its relative, phenylephrine. The usual maintenance dose is

2 to 4 µg/min. Doses as high as 0.5 to 1.5 µg/kg/min for 1 to 10 days have been used in patients with septic shock. **NE is currently considered the agent of choice** for the patient requiring vasopressor therapy, although this is controversial. Both vasoconstriction and increased MAP are evident when NE is used in the normal dosage range. NE does not increase heart rate. The main beneficial effect of NE is an increase in organ perfusion by increasing vascular tone. Studies that have compared NE to dopamine have favored NE in terms of overall improvement in oxygen delivery, organ perfusion, and oxygen consumption. Although NE was favored, oxygen delivery and oxygen consumption was increased in both the dopamine and NE patient study groups. Norepinephrine is less metabolically active than epinephrine and reduces serum lactate levels. Norepinephrine significantly improves renal perfusion and splanchnic blood flow in sepsis, particularly when combined with dobutamine.

Epinephrine

Epinephrine has potent β_1-, β_2-, and α_1-adrenergic activity; however, the increase in MAP in sepsis is mainly due to an increase in cardiac output (stroke volume). There are three major drawbacks to using epinephrine: (1) epinephrine increases myocardial oxygen demand; (2) it increases serum glucose and lactate, which is largely a calorigenic effect (increased release and anaerobic breakdown of glucose); (3) epinephrine appears to have adverse effects on splanchnic blood flow, redirecting blood to peripheral tissues as part of the sympathetic autonomic response. There is little data that distinguishes epinephrine from norepinephrine in the ability to achieve hemodynamic goals, and epinephrine is a superior inotrope. The impact of epinephrine on splanchnic perfusion needs to be considered. Concern about the effect of increased serum lactate and hyperglycemia has limited the use of epinephrine. Hypokalemia and arrhythmia are the result of the β_2 agonist action of epinephrine, which drives potassium into the cell.

Phenylephrine

Phenylephrine is an almost pure α_1-adrenergic agonist with moderate potency. Although widely used in anesthesia to treat iatrogenic hypotension, it is often an ineffective agent in treating sepsis. Phenylephrine is especially useful in counteracting the hypotensive effect of epidural and subarachnoid anesthetics. Phenylephrine is the adrenergic agent least likely to cause tachycardia. It is a less effective vasoconstrictor than norepinephrine or epinephrine. With its pure α activity, phenylephrine lacks inotropic or chronotropic activity, causing an elevation in blood pressure without increasing the heart rate or contractility. Reflex bradycardia may result from the elevation of blood pressure, and this effect may be useful in hypotensive patients that present with a tachyarrhythmia. Compared with NE, phenylephrine is more effective in reducing splanchnic blood flow, oxygen delivery, and lactate uptake. Phenylephrine may be a good therapeutic option when tachyarrhythmias limit therapy with other vasopressors. Phenylephrine and neosynephrine are selective α_1-adrenergic receptor agonists used primarily as decongestants and in ophthalmology to dilate the pupil, but they can also increase BP. Myocardial infarction can occur from the frequent- or over-use of these compounds in nasal sprays.

The response of blood pressure and the side effect profiles of these compounds render them inadequate for use in the ICU.

Vasopressin

Arginine-vasopressin is an endogenous hormone that is released in response to decreases in intravascular volume and increased plasma osmolality. Vasopressin constricts vascular smooth muscle directly through V1 receptors. It also increases the responsiveness of the vasculature to catecholamines. Vasopressin is an antidiuretic hormone analog secreted from the posterior pituitary. **It is no longer the first drug administered to adults in asystole (cardiac arrest).** Vasopressin or its analogue, terlipressin, may be used in patients with refractory shock in which adequate fluid and pressor resuscitation has failed to increase BP. Vasopressin has emerged as an additive vasoconstrictor in septic patients who have become resistant to catecholamines. There appears to be a quantitative deficiency of this hormone in sepsis, and administration of vasopressin in addition to NE increases splanchnic blood flow and urinary output. It also allows for a lower dosage of NE to be used. Vasopressin does not increase myocardial oxygen demand significantly, and its receptors are unaffected by acidosis.

Midodrine

Midodrine is a peripheral selective α_1-adrenergic agonist indicated for the treatment of chronic orthostatic hypotension. Its pressor effect is due to both arterial and venous vasoconstriction. Small studies have also shown that midodrine can be used to prevent excessive drops in blood pressure in people requiring dialysis. Midodrine may reduce the duration of IV vasopressors during the recovery phase from septic shock and may be associated with a reduction in length of stay in the ICU. Midodrine has been used in complications of cirrhosis. It is also used with octreotide for hepatorenal syndrome; the proposed mechanism is constriction of splanchnic vessels and dilation of renal vasculature.

Levosimendan

Levosimendan acts by increasing the sensitivity of the heart to calcium, thereby increasing cardiac contractility without forcing a rise in intracellular calcium. The combined inotropic and vasodilatory actions result in an increased power of contraction with decreased preload and decreased afterload. A recent meta-analysis comparing levosimendan and standard inotropic therapy with dobutamine for patients in septic shock found a significant reduction in mortality in patients given levosimendan.

Other Vasopressors

A variety of other vasopressors are available, including phosphodiesterase inhibitors, such as milrinone and enoximone. These appear to be alternatives to dobutamine as a treatment for cardiomyopathy of critical illness while restoring splanchnic blood flow, but they are not currently recommended therapy for acutely hypotensive patients. Trials of several types of pressor medications in the treatment of acute heart failure failed to show an incremental benefit over placebo; these drugs included inotropic agents and other vasoactive agents such as tolvaptan, tezosentan, levosimendan, rolofylline, and nesiritide.

CLINICAL CASE CORRELATION

- See also Case 4 (Hemodynamic Monitoring), Case 16 (Acute Cardiac Failure), Case 28 (Blunt Trauma), and Case 41 (Hemorrhage, Coagulopathy).

COMPREHENSION QUESTIONS

5.1 A 47-year-old man is admitted to the hospital following a penetrating stab wound to the abdomen. Surgical repair is successful, and he remains stable in the ICU. On postoperative day four, he develops fever, tachypnea, and tachycardia. His vital signs are temperature of 103.7°F, respirations 24/min, pulse 115 beats/min, and BP 86/60 mm Hg. Physical examination shows a well-healing abdominal wound and crackles at the base of the right lung. His urine output is 110 mL over the last 12 hours. Arterial blood gas (ABG) studies show an anion gap metabolic acidosis, and lactic acid level is found to be elevated. He is started on IV antibiotics. Which of the following is the next step in managing this patient's condition?

A. Give IV hypertonic saline

B. Give IV normal saline

C. Administer epinephrine IV

D. Administer sodium bicarbonate

E. Continue to monitor the patient on antibiotics alone

5.2 You are called to the ICU to evaluate a 67-year-old man who has been undergoing chemotherapy treatment for multiple myeloma. During the night, his blood pressure dropped from 110/76 to 84/48 mm Hg. His temperature was 102°F, respirations were 26/min and pulse was 122 beats/min. IV fluids were given, and his blood pressure was raised to 90/50 mm Hg in the past 6 hours. Which vasopressor agent is most appropriate to administer at this time?

A. Norepinephrine

B. Epinephrine

C. Phenylephrine

D. Dopamine

E. Vasopressin

ANSWERS

5.1 **B.** This patient has developed postoperative pneumonia and is at risk of septic shock. The patient's hypotension has resulted in hypoxia and increased anaerobic respiration, causing lactic acidosis. In addition to antibiotics, this patient's vital signs indicate the need for IV fluids to maintain intravascular pressure. Normal saline would be the correct answer here, as hypertonic saline would increase intravascular pressure using fluid from the extravascular space. Vasopressors may be considered if the patient's BP fails to improve on IV fluids.

5.2 **A.** This patient failed to respond adequately to fluid resuscitation efforts and requires vasopressor therapy to maintain adequate perfusion. The goal of vasopressor therapy is to maintain a MAP of 65 or greater with adequate urine output and mentation. The first-line drug given to patients with hyperdynamic septic shock who fail initial fluid therapy is norepinephrine. Phenylephrine can be given if NE is not initially successful. Dopamine is associated more with arrhythmia and tachycardia and is used more in hypodynamic shock. Vasopressin may be used in refractory hypotension. Additionally, the cause of the patient's sepsis should be addressed.

CLINICAL PEARLS

► It is essential that patients be fluid-resuscitated before commencing vasopressor therapy.

► Crystalloid solutions are universally used for initial volume resuscitation in sepsis and septic shock to compensate for fluid debt.

► Isotonic saline, when administered in large volumes, is associated with hyperchloremic acidosis; this may affect splanchnic blood flow and may be nephrotoxic.

► Colloid solutions achieve hemodynamic goals faster than crystalloids with lower volumes and without chloride overload, but they are much more expensive.

► The goal of vasopressor support is to maintain BP in the autoregulation range of organs.

► Dobutamine is a potent inotrope used as an adjunct to fluids in early sepsis.

► Norepinephrine is a potent vasoconstrictor that maintains CO and restores blood flow to dependent organs; it is currently the first-line vasopressor treatment.

► Epinephrine is a potent vasoconstrictor and inotrope. It causes an early lactic acidosis secondary to aerobic glycolysis and may reduce splanchnic blood flow.

► Phenylephrine may be a good therapeutic option when tachyarrhythmia limits therapy with other vasopressors.

REFERENCES

Dellinger RP, Levy MM, Rhodes A, et al. Surviving sepsis campaign: international guidelines for management of severe sepsis and septic shock: 2012. *Crit Care Med*. 2013 Feb;41(2):580-637.

Loscalzo J. *Harrison's Pulmonary and Critical Care Medicine*. New York, NY: McGraw-Hill; 2013.

Roberts I, Alderson P, Bunn F, et al. Colloids versus crystalloids for fluid resuscitation in critically ill patients. *Cochrane Database Syst Rev*. 2004;CD000567.

Zangrillo A, Putzu A, Monaco F, et al. Levosimendan reduces mortality in patients with severe sepsis and septic shock: a meta-analysis of randomized trials. *J Crit Care*. 2015 Oct;30(5):908-913. doi: 10.1016/j.jcrc.2015.05.017. Epub 2015 May 29.

A 44-year-old man with subarachnoid hemorrhage and GCS of nine is admitted to the ICU after initial assessment in the emergency department. In the emergency department, he is intubated and placed on a ventilator. A CT of the brain reveals subarachnoid hemorrhage and intracerebral hemorrhage. Several hours after his arrival to the ICU, the patient is noted to have increased ventilatory pressures and decreased breath sounds on the left. His O_2 saturation remains at 100%.

▶ What are the possible causes for the patient's change in condition?
▶ What imaging modalities can you use to further assess the patient's problem?

ANSWERS TO CASE 6:

Imaging in Critical Care

Summary: An intubated and mechanically ventilated 44-year-old man with a subarachnoid hemorrhage develops increased airway pressures and decreased left-sided breath sounds.

- **Possible causes for the patient's condition:** Right mainstem intubation, left-sided mucous plug, and left pneumothorax.

- **Imaging studies:** Portable chest radiograph to determine whether the patient has developed a pneumothorax, loss of lung volume on the left, or if the endotracheal tube has advanced into the right mainstem bronchus. Bedside ultrasound can also be used to determine the presence (or absence) of visceral/parietal pleural sliding. The presence of this tissue interface would confirm a fully expanded left lung and exclude the diagnosis of left pneumothorax.

ANALYSIS

Objectives

1. Learn the values and indications of portable chest radiographs in the ICU.

2. Learn the indications and applications of bedside ultrasound in the ICU (diagnostic and procedure-guidance).

3. Learn to apply echocardiography and CT scans for the management of patients in the ICU.

Considerations

This patient is receiving positive pressure ventilation and has been recently transported from the emergency department to the CT scanner and then to the intensive care unit. Additionally, patients with traumatic brain injuries often undergo invasive procedures, such as placement of central venous catheters for central venous pressure monitoring. Such events place patients at risk for both malpositioning of the endotracheal tube into the right mainstem bronchus and the development of pneumothorax. Both of these conditions can present clinically with decreased left-sided breath sounds. In addition, the development of a mucous plug in the left mainstem bronchus can also present with a decrease in right-sided breath sounds and increased airway pressures.

> # APPROACH TO:
> ## Imaging in ICU Patients

DEFINITIONS

Portable Chest Radiography: It is a modality for performing chest radiographs at the patient's bedside. Patients are often supine or semi-supine for these studies. Portable radiographs are performed using antero-posterior technique, where x-ray beams penetrate from the anterior position. This orientation decreases the quality of the image and impairs detection of small pneumothoraces and hemothoraces due to the supine position. Portable x-rays are helpful for confirmation of endotracheal tube positions and infiltrates or effusions that may signify pathology.

Ultrasound: Tissue interfaces reflect sound waves. These "acoustic signals" can be translated into two-dimensional images that represent the anatomy beneath the ultrasound probe. The images are displayed with those structures closest to the probe at the top of the image, whereas those farthest away from the probe appear at the bottom of the image. Subcutaneous air and dense structures (eg, bones, gallstones, foreign bodies) can create artifacts that distort the ultrasound images. Body habitus and lack of skin-to-probe interface secondary to surgical dressings or wounds can also limit visibility and quality of images. Ultrasonography in the ICU is useful for diagnostic purposes (detection of pneumothorax, intraperitoneal fluid, bladder volume) or for the guidance of bedside procedures (central venous catheter placement, arterial line placement, peripheral venous catheter placement, drainage of intraperitoneal or intrapleural fluid collections).

Echocardiography: Ultrasound that is used specifically to evaluate cardiac anatomy and function. Modern day echocardiography adds computerized functions, such as color-flow doppler and waveform analysis to quantify flow patterns across (and within) anatomic regions of the heart. The addition of flow analysis and volume measurement software enhances the diagnostic range of echocardiograms. As with other forms of ultrasound, subcutaneous air, wounds and body habitus all can affect the quality of images obtainable in individual patients. Echocardiography is especially useful for the bedside assessment of cardiac performance and intravascular volume statuses, especially in patients with clinical shock.

CLINICAL APPROACH

Portable Chest Radiography in the ICU

Portable chest radiographs allow for assessment of ICU patients with acute or progressive respiratory changes. One of the major advantages of these bedside procedures is that transport during instability is avoided. Despite a reduction in image quality, bedside chest radiographs are helpful in determining many different conditions that warrant prompt intervention (Table 6–1).

Table 6–1 • IMAGING STUDIES FOR VARIOUS CLINICAL SITUATIONS		
Symptoms	Diagnosis	Imaging Study
Fever Leukocytosis Hemodynamic Instability	Sepsis	Portable chest radiograph (infiltrate suggests pneumonia) Ultrasound (especially for suspected biliary tract pathology) Computed tomography (full anatomic assessment possible)
Fever Leukocytosis Hemodynamic Instability	Systemic Inflammatory Response Syndrome	Computed tomography (if no new findings after source control, likely SIRS)
Altered Mental Status	Stroke	Non-contrast computed tomography of brain
Acute Respiratory Deterioration	Pneumothorax Hemothorax Pneumonia Pulmonary Embolism	Portable chest radiograph (pneumonia, pneumo/hemothorax) Computed tomography of the chest (CT angiogram if suspicion for PE)

Portable chest radiographs are less helpful in determining if the respiratory decompensation is due to pulmonary embolism (PE). Patients with seemingly "normal" radiographs can have venous embolic disease as the source of their ventilation/perfusion mismatch. If the findings on portable chest films do not elucidate a cause, and the patient is at risk for PE, CT angiography can be helpful to rule in or out embolic disease.

Historically, the practice of daily "routine" chest films was common in the ICU. In a recent meta-analysis, this practice was compared to the practice of only performing chest radiographs when clinically indicated (ie, "on demand"). There was no difference in mortality, ICU length of stay or days on the ventilator between the patients managed with the two different approaches. **Patients who received studies only when clinically indicated had less radiation exposure and had lower hospital costs.**

Bedside Ultrasound in the ICU

The advent of small, portable ultrasound machines with improved image resolution and greater depth capabilities has made bedside ultrasonography a valuable tool in the intensive care setting. In comparison to CT scans, ultrasonography does not require the transport of critically ill patients and is associated with no irradiation and no intravenous contrast exposure. It is more often available and can be repeated more easily than computed tomography. Accessibility and ease of use have made ultrasound an extension of the physical examination for the assessment of critically ill patients.

Ultrasound can be used for almost all anatomic regions. In the thorax, ultrasound assessment of pleural approximation can reliably rule out pneumothorax. Cardiac function can be evaluated in a number of ways, including estimates of ejection fraction and qualitative assessment of wall motion symmetry. In the abdomen, visualization of inferior vena cava diameter changes during the respiratory cycle can be useful to gauge a patient's central venous volume status. The Focused Assessment with Sonography for Trauma (FAST) allows for initial and serial assessments for increases in intraperitoneal fluid that can signify active hemorrhage in patients after abdominal trauma.

The Focused Assessment with Sonography for Trauma (FAST) Ultrasound can also be applied in therapeutic procedures. Real-time visualization of central venous structure during catheter insertions is associated with lower procedural-related complications and is a practice endorsed by most professional organizations. Fluid in the pericardium can be more safely sampled using ultrasound guidance for pericardiocentesis. Infectious source control can sometimes be accomplished by ultrasound-guided drainage of fluid collections in the thorax, pericardium, abdomen or soft tissues (Figures 6–1 to 6–4).

Although this method was developed to assess trauma patients in the emergency department, it offers an organized approach for assessment of the abdominal compartment in the ICU. Three of the four views taken in the FAST examination evaluate the abdomen, and the non-abdominal view evaluates the patient's pericardium.

Abdominal components of FAST examination:

1. Right upper quadrant—identifies fluid inferior to the liver

2. Left upper quadrant—identifies fluid around the spleen

3. Suprapubic region—identifies fluid around pelvis

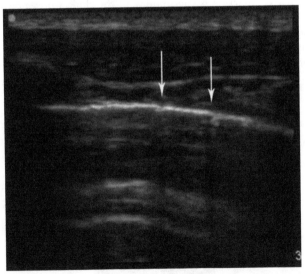

Figure 6–1. Pleural sliding to rule out pneumothorax: the bright white line represents apposition of visceral and parietal pleura. The arrows represent "comet tails" artifacts created by the interface of pleural layers. When these findings are absent, the likelihood of pneumothorax increases. (Used, with permission, from Arun Nagdev, MD, Emergency Medicien Residency Program, Alameda Health System).

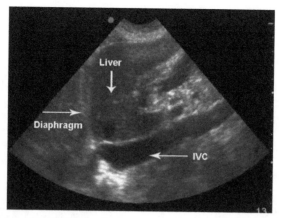

Figure 6–2. Inferior vena cava (IVC) anatomy on ultrasound. Visualization of the IVC during the respiratory cycle yields a reliable estimate of volume status. In the normovolemic state, the IVC will narrow during inspiration and distend during expiration. In severe hypovolemia, the IVC will collapse. In hypervolemia, the IVC diameter will not change throughout the respiratory cycle. (Used, with permission, from Arun Nagdev, MD, Emergency Medicien Residency Program, Alameda Health System).

Applying Echocardiography and CT Scans for the Management of Patients in the ICU

When patients in the ICU are hemodynamically unstable and ongoing resuscitative efforts do not appear to correct the patient's perfusion, one must consider whether cardiac dysfunction is contributing to the clinical presentation. Bedside echocardiography provides a real-time assessment of the patient's cardiac function. Echocardiography can be used to estimate left ventricular wall motion, ejection fractions, right-heart filling volumes, and pulmonary venous pressures. Information gleaned from such assessments can direct the initiation of inotropic agents, further volume resuscitation, or direct (or other verb?) application of vasoconstrictors.

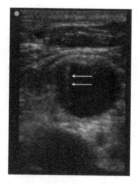

Figure 6–3. Line placement under ultrasound guidance. Real-time visualization for catheter placement: the arrows point to a needle entering the internal jugular vein for central venous access. (Used, with permission, from Arun Nagdev, MD, Emergency Medicien Residency Program, Alameda Health System).

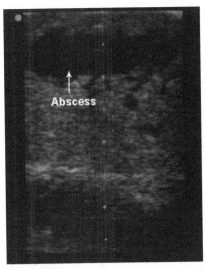

Figure 6–4. Abscess image on ultrasound. Subcutaneous abscess. (Used, with permission, from Arun Nagdev, MD, Emergency Medicien Residency Program, Alameda Health System).

Left ventricular function: Bedside echocardiography can qualitatively assess left ventricular wall motion and estimate ventricular function. These qualitative estimates can be performed with most ultrasound machines by clinicians with basic ultrasound training. More sophisticated quantitative measurements can be performed with slightly more advanced ultrasound machines that can be found in many ICUs. Such machines are able to clearly image the endocardial layer and obtain ventricular areas or volumes during the cardiac cycle. By noting the change in measured areas or volumes of the ventricle during diastole and systole, *fractional area change* or *ejection fraction* can be calculated.

$$\text{Fractional area change} = \frac{\text{End-diastolic area} - \text{End-systolic area}}{\text{End-diastolic area}}$$

$$\text{Ejection fraction} = \frac{\text{End-diastolic volume} - \text{End-systolic volume}}{\text{End-diastolic volume}}$$

Right ventricular function: The right ventricle is normally a compliant, thin-walled chamber with low pressures. In patients with critical illness, however, factors such as increased pulmonary vascular resistance, left ventricular dysfunction and marked fluid overload may alter the pressures and volume of the right ventricle. An acute increase in right ventricular pressures can contribute to right ventricular dysfunction and if severe, right ventricular failure. Just as in the assessment of the left ventricle, echocardiography can assess the right ventricle qualitatively or quantitatively. Qualitative findings of right ventricular enlargement and septal "bulging" toward the left ventricle suggest severe right ventricular dysfunction.

For quantitative measurements, image resolution must be adequate to assess chamber volumes and Doppler flow measurements (Figure 6–1).

Whether clinicians are armed with basic skills and equipment or more advanced training with slightly more sophisticated equipment, bedside echocardiography offers an accessible and non-invasive adjunct for evaluation and management of unstable or critically ill patients.

Volume status: Assessment of adequate resuscitation is crucial in the management of patients in shock. Echocardiography offers several non-invasive options for assessment of preload (ie, volume status). As mentioned previously, IVC diameter change during the respiratory cycle can reliably estimate CVP. Equipment capable of measuring doppler flow patterns can further assess preload by measuring flow across the mitral valve and within the pulmonary artery. Likewise, echocardiographic assessment of left ventricular volumes during the cardiac cycle can estimate left ventricle preload by measuring left ventricular end-diastolic volumes. Doppler technology can be used to measure flow across the left ventricular outflow tract to estimate cardiac output.

Structural pathology: In addition to wall motion abnormalities, bedside echocardiography can be used to diagnose valvular vegetations, papillary muscle rupture, and ventricular aneurysms. Defects in the ventricular or atrial septum and valvular regurgitation can be visualized with flow doppler. Increased fluid in the pericardium and its effect on filling of the ventricles during diastole will help identify tamponade physiology if preload is compromised by the amount of fluid in the pericardial space. Additionally, therapy for cardiac tamponade can be initiated with ultrasound guided pericardiocentesis and pericardial drain placement.

Computed Tomography: Computed tomography (CT) requires patient transport to radiology; however, in some instances, the information gained is worth the risk of transport. CT angiography is the study of choice for the diagnosis of pulmonary emboli. Thoracic, abdomen, and pelvic CT scans can determine sources for sepsis that are too deep for detection or obscured by artifact with bedside ultrasonography. CT scans can guide placement of percutaneous drainage catheters for source control, a key component of treatment in many septic patients.

Source Identification: When patients experience clinical decline, imaging plays a key role in identifying the source of the problem. Portable radiographs and ultrasound are generally readily accessible and do not require IV contrast and excessive radiation exposure. These studies can provide information that is nonspecific, and in the case of ultrasonography, the diagnostic accuracy is operator dependent. Additionally, there are regions of the abdomen, mediastinum, and cranium that are difficult to image with portable ultrasound due to the density of adjacent structures, especially bony structures. Computed tomography offers a more sensitive and specific way to evaluate the brain, thorax, abdomen, and retroperitoneal space. CT scans can identify fluid collections, areas of active bleeding, inflammation, and edema (Table 6–1).

When the acute decline is neurologic, non-contrast computed tomography is highly valuable to look for intracranial pathology, such as worsening traumatic brain injuries, hemorrhagic stroke, or ischemic strokes. Non-contrast CT is less sensitive in determining ischemic strokes; however, CT perfusion imaging (when available) improves accuracy in detection of irreversible cerebral ischemia. Although magnetic resonance imaging (MRI) is the most sensitive for assessment of cerebral ischemia, this study is less feasible in critically ill patients since it requires them to be isolated in the scanning cylinder for a period of time while the study is performed. Patients who require mechanical ventilation, close monitoring and frequent interventions are poor candidates for MRIs.

CLINICAL CASE CORRELATION

- See also Case 2 (Transfer of the Critically Ill Patient) and Case 4 (Hemodynamic Monitoring).

COMPREHENSION QUESTIONS

6.1 Which of the following methods provides the safest approach for placement of internal jugular central venous catheters?

   A. Using an ultrasound to mark the vein position prior to applying sterile skin prep

   B. Portable chest radiograph before and after the procedure

   C. Echocardiogram to visualize catheter in right atrium

   D. Ultrasound imaging of vein at the time of venipuncture

   E. Ultrasound of lung apices during the procedure to avoid pneumothorax

6.2 A 22-year-old woman has just arrived to the intensive care unit from an uneventful femur fixation in the operating room. During transport, her oxygen saturation dropped to 82%. The respiratory therapist reports that she became more difficult to ventilate with the ambu-bag (transport ventilation device). On your preliminary examination she has absent breath sounds on the right, her respiratory rate is 34 breaths/min and her oxygen saturation is now 87% with an increase to 100% inspired oxygen on the ventilator. The patient's blood pressure is 115/70 mm Hg and heart rate is 110 beats/min. Which of the following diagnostic test is most likely to be helpful?

   A. Ultrasound of the abdomen

   B. Computed tomography of the chest

   C. Portable chest film

   D. MRI of the chest

   E. Nuclear medicine scan of the chest

6.3 A 67-year old-man is brought to the emergency department after being found in his backyard unconscious. On initial evaluation, he is unresponsive, his skin is ashen, his extremities are cool and he is perspiring. His blood pressure is 80/65 mm Hg, his heart rate is 102 beats/min, and he has distended neck veins. He is intubated and has bilateral breath sounds. There are several trauma resuscitations on other patients occurring simultaneously, and you are given one choice of diagnostic machine to use (because all the equipments are being shared). Which instrument would you choose?

A. Portable chest radiograph machine

B. ECG machine

C. Ultrasound machine with echocardiography probe and doppler flow

D. CT Scan

E. Ultrasound with thoracic and abdomen soft tissue probe

6.4 Which of the following statements is **not** true?

A. A normal portable chest radiograph rules out a pulmonary source for oxygen desaturation.

B. Portable chest radiographs are valuable in determining the cause of acute changes in a patient's oxygenation.

C. Echocardiography can identify increased pulmonary vascular pressures.

D. Computed tomography is the study of choice to diagnose pulmonary embolus.

E. Ultrasound can be used as an extension of the physical examination.

6.5 A hospital has recently identified that transporting critically ill patients to CT imaging has inherent hazards. Which of the following patients is most appropriate to have a CT scan?

A. An 87-year-old woman, BP 110/70 mm Hg, HR 90 beats/min, RR 14 breaths/min, O_2 sat 95% with ipsilateral decreased breath sounds after central line placement.

B. A 370 lb man with a subhepatic abscess and extensive subcutaneous emphysema, fully resuscitated but on two vasopressor agents and a mean arterial pressure of 72 mm Hg.

C. A 43-year-old man on the ventilator with increased peak airway pressures, increased work of breathing, and diminished breath sounds on the left.

D. A 92-year-old woman with BP 86/48 mm Hg, HR 105 beats/min, RR 18 breaths/min, serum creatinine of 2.1 mg/dL, and distended neck veins.

E. A 22-year-old man who was stabbed with a 3-inch knife in the third intercostal space, lateral to the right nipple, BP 128/78 mm Hg, HR 82 beats/min, and RR 12 breaths/min.

ANSWERS

6.1 **D.** "Real-time" imaging of the internal jugular vein while it is being cannulated has been shown to be the safest approach when compared to the anatomic landmark technique and when compared to pre-procedure vein location marking.

6.2 **C.** Although thoracic computed tomography can give valuable information on chest pathophysiology, this patient presented with acute respiratory decompensation and signs are worrisome for right pneumothorax. Transport to the CT scanner in such a tenuous patient would invite catastrophe. Modalities such as bedside thoracic ultrasound to evaluate presence or absence of pleural sliding and portable chest radiograph (performed in a timely manner) could both identify a clinically significant pneumothorax. Right needle thoracostomy can be performed in patients for whom a high index of suspicion for pneumothorax. This procedure, when performed appropriately, is of relatively low risk and transient therapeutic benefit. Repeating auscultation once a room quiets down is quick and easy and can help confirm presence or absence of breath sounds. The important point here is if a patient is unstable and diagnosis can be made at the bedside, it is safest not to transport the patient elsewhere for diagnostics.

6.3 **C.** This patient presents in shock with no available history. Clinical findings suggest cardiac dysfunction with severe malperfusion and distended neck veins. Although an ECG can give some information that can help rule in or out a potential infarction, a bedside echocardiogram can quickly identify anatomic and functional abnormalities such as pericardial tamponade, papillary muscle rupture, severe wall motion abnormalities, septal rupture, etc. With echocardiography, the patient's volume status can also be estimated, as can the presence of increased pulmonary vascular pressures. In the instance of tamponade, echocardiography can be used real-time for a safer method of pericardiocentesis.

6.4 **A.** Patients with pulmonary emboli can have "normal" appearing chest radiographs. CT angiography of the chest is the study of choice to diagnose pulmonary emboli.

6.5 **B.** Of the patients listed, the obese man with subcutaneous emphysema will likely be technically challenging for bedside ultrasound-guided drainage of his subhepatic abscess. His body habitus and the subcutaneous air will increase artifacts and lessen the safety of the ultrasound guided technique. CT-guided abscess drainage offers a much safer route for patients who have limited ultrasound views. Patients A, C, and E all have suspected pulmonary diagnoses that can be evaluated with either portable radiographs or thoracic ultrasound. Patient D has a likely cardiac source for her symptoms and can be evaluated with bedside echocardiography.

CLINICAL PEARLS

▶ A chest radiograph after intubation can assess for the position of the endotracheal tube and also assess for pneumothorax.

▶ Previously, daily chest x-rays were done routinely on ICU patients. However, they should now only be done when clinically indicated.

▶ Ultrasound is a very useful modality in ICU patients and can assess for pleural fluid, pericardial fluid, abdominal fluid, and cardiac function.

▶ CT imaging requires transport of the ICU patient but can be critical for suspicion of pulmonary embolism.

REFERENCES

Beaulieu Y, Marik PE. Bedside ultrasound in the ICU: Part 1. *Chest.* 2005;128:881-895.

Funaki B, Lorenz JM, Navuluri R, Van Ha TG, Zangan SM. Interventional radiology. In: Hall JB, Schmidt GA, Kress JP, eds. *Principles of Critical Care.* 4th ed. New York, NY: McGraw-Hill; 2015:209-226.

Mayo P, Koenig S. ICU Ultrasonography. In: Hall JB, Schmidt GA, Kress JP, eds. Principles of Critical Care. 4th ed. New York, NY: McGraw-Hill; 2015:202-208.

Oba Y, Zaza T. Abandoning daily routine chest radiography in the intensive care unit: meta-analysis. *Radiology.* 2010;255.

Vigno P, Mucke F, Bellec F, et al. Basic critical care echocardiography: validation of a curriculum dedicated to noncardiologist residents. *Critl Care Med.* 2011;39:636-642.

A 23-year-old male organ donor in the ICU is diagnosed as brain dead after suffering a closed head trauma in a snow skiing accident. The patient is intubated and placed on a mechanical ventilator. The organ procurement team and operating room team are alerted. The patient's vital signs are as follows: blood pressure (BP) of 110/60 mm Hg, heart rate (HR) of 110 beats/minute with regular rhythm, temperature of 96°F (35.6°C), weight of 165 lb (75 kg), and height of 62 in (1.65 m). The patient's laboratory studies follow:

Laboratory Studies	
Sodium (Na^+)	150 mEq/L (136–144 mEq/L)
Potassium (K^+)	4.0 mEq/L (3.7–5.2 mEq/L)
Chloride (Cl^-)	105 mEq/L (101–111 mEq/L)
Bicarbonate (HCO_3^-)	20 mEq/L (22–26 mEq/L)
Urinary Output	150 mL/h
Arterial Blood Gas Study	
pH	7.36 (7.35–7.45)
$Paco_2$	36 mm Hg (36–44 mm Hg)
Pao_2	150 mm Hg (75–100 mm Hg)
Fio_2	35%

▶ What are the most appropriate next steps while awaiting organ transplant?
▶ What is the most important parameter that impacts organ survival?

ANSWERS TO CASE 7:
Ethics in Critical Care

Summary: This 23-year-old patient has been declared brain dead and is an organ donor. Life support should attempt to maintain his physiology and chemistries within normal limits to preserve organ integrity until procurement of the organ by the transplant team.

- **Next steps while awaiting organ transplantation:** Maintain the donor patient's physiologic parameters as close to normal values, which will include mechanical ventilation and circulation.

- **Most important criterion for organ survival:** Time is essential when attempting to maximize organ viability. As such, all paperwork should be promptly attended to, organ procurement and transplantation teams mobilized, and hematological compatibility testing should be fast-tracked to minimize unnecessary delays.

ANALYSIS

Objectives

1. To understand basic care for brain death in adult organ donor patients.
2. To understand the physiologic changes involved in organ donors.

Considerations

As this patient has identified himself as an organ and tissue donor—often noted on government-issued identification cards (eg, driver's licenses)—the transplantation team can initiate their process for organ procurement. The hospital should provide a specially trained, designated representative to initiate the proceedings by first addressing the family's emotional concerns. The hospital's designee must respect the autonomy of the family, all the while being sensitive to the bereaved family's interpretation of the donor patient's desires. However, all states have adopted legislation whereby the donor's legally established desire to donate his or her tissue (eg, donor card) supersedes that of dissenting family members. The declaration of brain death requires establishing that the patient is in an irreversible coma state with no evidence of brain stem reflexes (such as lack of breathing independently). A coordinated team approach is paramount to ensure that the transplantation process occurs in a seamless and time-sensitive manner to achieve maximum success.

APPROACH TO:

Ethical Issues of ICU Patients

Though the donor patient is clinically deceased, the critical care team should approach the patient using accepted therapies that mirror that of treating a viable person. This includes identifying any infections and treating them appropriately. The Donor Risk Index shows how these "fixed" criteria are interrelated to the variable criteria. **Donor organs are influenced by the body's physiology, which includes oxygen delivery, serum electrolytes balance, and regional and systemic cytokines.** General parameters of optimal care as well as individual factors that may affect a transplantable organ are addressed in Table 7–1.

TREATMENT TIME

It is critical that the time from organ collection to transplantation into the recipient patient is minimized. Hospitals with specialized organ transplantation programs often have streamlined practice guidelines aimed at minimizing delay and promoting more favorable outcomes with reduced complications.

Coagulopathy and Transfusion Therapy

During the interim period, the donor's organs and tissue must be adequately perfused and maintained in an appropriate media and temperature to enhance viability upon transplantation. The optimal hemoglobin and hematocrit levels for the donor patient are discussed in Table 7–1. As the patient is brain dead, the need to oxygenate the highly-consuming brain tissue is abrogated, which in turn reduces the overall oxygen demand of the body. The organs may accumulate an increase in reactive oxidant species and experience an inflammatory mediator burden and tissue damage. This can result in acute inflammatory processes, such as an acute lung injury, which will limit transplantation viability. Likewise, increased oxidative stress can promote an environment favorable for viral and bacterial overgrowth. Such infected organs pose a markedly increased chance of septicemia in the immuno-compromised recipient. Administration of packed red blood cells to the donor for perfusion of the organs and tissues has been shown to improve transplantation success. Additionally, each of the donor's organs and his tissue should have an intrinsic

Table 7–1 • RECOMMENDATIONS FOR DONOR CARE GUIDELINE PARAMETERS	
Central venous pressure 4–12 mm Hg	Glucose 70–150 mg/dL
Pulmonary artery occluded pressure 8–12 mm Hg	pH 7.40–7.45
Cardiac index >2.4 L/min/m	$Paco_2$ 30–35 mm Hg
Cardiac output >3.8 L/min	PaO_2 >80–90 mm Hg
Mean arterial pressure 60 mm Hg	Hemoglobin >10 g/dL
Systolic blood pressure >90 and <120 mm Hg	Hematocrit >30%
Urine output 1–3 mL/kg/h	

balance in anticoagulation so as to prevent uncontrolled hemorrhage and marked clotting in the organ that will limit reperfusion upon transplantation.

Body Temperature and Hormone Replacement

As a result of damage to the thermoregulatory centers of the brain, most donor bodies become hypothermic, which will reduce the metabolism of their organs. The reduced metabolism will alter the coagulation pathways and electrolyte and hormone balances, contribute to dysrhythmias, and allow for polyuria in the donor's organs and tissues. Transplantation specialists often promote a modestly increased blood glucose level in the donor patient, as there is an immunosuppressive effect induced by hyperglycemia that may benefit the recipient.

Brain death, in conjunction with the antecedent cause of death of the donor patient, may result in primary hypoadrenalism. Thus in the transplantation of the lungs, high-dose corticosteroids are often administered to promote viable transplantation. Likewise, the use of supplemental mineralocorticoids may correct any hyponatremia, especially in the context of brain death polyuria or coexisting diabetes insipidus, which will deplete sodium levels. Additional doses of corticosteroids or a steady IV infusion may be needed if donor care extends beyond 8 to 12 hours. Administration of hormones in synergistic combinations has also been shown to have a more favorable transplantation outcome than isolated hormone administration. For example, thyroid hormones can be helpful by complementing the steroids administered to treat hypotension that persists despite the use of inotropic or vasopressor agents. The recommended dose of triiodothyronine (T3) is 2 to 3 mg/h by IV.

Polyuria, which often develops after brain death, places organs at risk due to secondary hypovolemia, hypotension, and hypoperfusion. Etiologies of the polyuria include physiologic diuresis, residual effects of diuretics given for the treatment of intracranial hypertension, osmotic diuresis due to residual mannitol therapy, hyperglycemia, and diabetes insipidus (DI). Polyuria from causes other than DI usually do not produce significant hypernatremia. Hypernatremia after transplantation is associated with reduced liver function. Na^+ levels greater than 155 mEq/L are considered the maximum. IV fluid replacement with balanced salt solutions or hypotonic saline is recommended when the urine output is above 150 to 200 mL/h. Significant hyperglycemia may develop if excess dextrose and water solutions are used. Aqueous vasopressin may be administered in repeated intravenous boluses (5–10 U) or titrated as an infusion to treat polyuria. Desmopressin (DDAVP) is also effective as an intravenous bolus (0.5–2.0 μg) and is repeated as necessary to achieve the desired urine output.

Nutrition, Reperfusion, and Preconditioning

Providing adequate nutrition may facilitate glycogen deposition in the liver, which will enhance the availability of fatty acids and glutamine that is beneficial to the heart. Likewise, accumulation of omega-3 fatty acids and amino acids can promote renal protection.

Additionally, injury occurs when significant hypotension is followed by fluid resuscitation and improved tissue perfusion to the transplanted organ. An episode of controlled hypotension, however, may precondition some organs (especially the liver) before implantation, which will increase tolerance to reperfusion injury. The use of dopamine is not beneficial in preventing such injury.

Summary

The goal is to ensure viable tissue transplantation that is both compatible and functional. This is a complicated process that expands beyond the scope of critical care medicine. In the ICU setting, it is critical to consult the specialized teams of physicians and providers to ensure a successful transplantation into the recipient.

ETHICS OF RESUSCITATION AND END OF LIFE DECISIONS

In the critical care setting, physicians are often faced with complicated decisions involving cardiopulmonary resuscitation (CPR) and placement of "Do-Not-Resuscitate" (DNR) orders. The establishment of DNR orders are often achieved in conjunction with the attending physician and the patient and/or their family members as proxies. Patients should establish end-of-life desires, both in the creation of advanced directives ("living will" documents) and in conversation with family and friends. This helps simplify matters should the patient be received into the ICU in an incoherent or comatose state. These decisions should evaluate the level of resuscitation that should be enacted, such as whether more invasive procedures like CPR, advanced airways and defibrillation, and medical management of arrhythmias are permitted. Like most medical decisions, deciding whether or not to resuscitate a patient who suffers a cardiopulmonary arrest involves a careful consideration of the potential clinical benefits balanced with the patient's preferences for the intervention and its likely outcome.

If circumstances permit, all patients admitted to the ICU (or hospital for that matter), should have a discussion about their advanced directives. Patients who want full resuscitation efforts made should have their chart noted as "Full Code," indicating to all healthcare providers that efforts should be made to resuscitate in the event of cardiopulmonary failure. If a DNR order is signed by the physician and the patient or their proxy, the notation of DNR should be prominently displayed for all healthcare providers to see, preventing unwarranted invasive procedures. This should include notations on the patient (such as an alert bracelet), signage over the bed, and documentation on charts and electronic medical records.

WHEN SHOULD CPR BE ADMINISTERED?

If the patient stops breathing or cardiac arrest occurs in the hospital, the standard of care is to perform CPR so long as an overriding DNR order is not in place. Most hospitals have protocols established that dictate which personnel, equipment, and drugs are to be brought to the bedside in the instance of cardiopulmonary failure. This process is colloquially called "running a code," as most hospitals page overhead "codes" that dispatch resuscitation teams.

In the absence of advanced directives or a DNR order, most hospitals have strict policies dictating circumstances where CPR may be withheld. Often, these include situations when CPR is judged to have no medical benefit, when the patient consci-entiously voices that they do not wish to be resuscitated despite lacking the formal documentation, or when the patient is incapable of making their own decision but their health care proxy/surrogate can state the patient's intention to not receive life-saving care. **If CPR is judged to have no clinical benefit to the patient, physicians are ethically justified in withholding the resuscitation on the basis of evidence-based medicine and the principal of medical futility.** For example, a patient who is successfully resuscitated but remains in either a vegetative state or another state of terminal illness with eminent death would certainly not clinically benefit. Of concern to physicians and ethicists is the subjective definition of clinical benefit. Judging a patient's quality of life tempts prejudicial statements about patients with a chronic illness or disability. There is substantial evidence that patients with chronic conditions often rate their quality of life much higher than would healthy people. This subjective nature is best addressed by the physician establishing communication with the patient and family upon admission, especially when the patient has an end-stage illness, in order to determine their expectations and potential medical outcomes if resuscitative efforts are employed.

The reality of medicine in practice is that advanced directives and open lines of communication with patients and families are not always possible. This also includes patients and families having inappropriate expectations of medical outcomes. Often, a team approach can resolve these disagreements, where physicians can explain the medical aspects with a trained clergy person, spiritual advisor or mental health provider attending to non-medical concerns associated with death and dying. **A physician must respect the patient's autonomy with regards to medical care but is not obligated to provide life-saving measures if medical futility is clearly supported.** Individual hospitals should have protocols established jointly by physicians and medical ethicists on how to proceed in these situations. Utilization of so-called "slow codes," where resuscitation teams intentionally neglect standards of CPR and ACLS and half-heartedly attempt to revive a patient are both inappropriate and not ethically justified. Such actions undermine the patient's rights and violate the code of physician-patient trust.

In addition, another controversial subject involving end-of-life medical practice is physician-assisted suicide or euthanasia. This constitutes a physician facilitating death through the use of toxic or supratherapeutic pharmacologic interventions. In a vast majority of states in the United States, this action constitutes medical malpractice, where a physician can be legally prosecuted for charges ranging from battery to manslaughter. States that have approved such actions often involve a meticulous screening process to ensure both terminality of the patient's condition and a thorough psychological and legal review. However, this should not be confused with palliative care medicine, which may employ the ethical principle of double effect, whereby the administration of an opioid, for example, can greatly slow down the respiratory drive in a terminal patient. In the critical care setting, such patients receiving hospice palliative care must have a DNR order in place.

Advanced Directives and Surrogate Decision Makers

An advanced directive document can either be a template form or a more elaborate chronicling filled out by a patient explaining the decisions the patient would like to have made if he/she is unable to participate at the time when life-prolonging

Table 7–2 • HIERARCHY OF FAMILY RELATIONSHIPS IN SURROGATE DECISION MAKING	
1. Legal guardian with healthcare decision-making authority	4. Individual given durable power of attorney for healthcare decisions
2. Spouse	5. Adult children of patient (all in agreement)
3. Parents of the patient	6. Adult siblings of patient (all in agreement)

resuscitative efforts are being made. This document is referred to as a "living will," which should not be confused with a "last will and testament" document that outlines financial affairs and assets. Unlike the latter, an advanced directive or living will does not require an attorney or certification by a notary public. Rather, this document should be signed by the patient and two non-familial witnesses. **These documents often address the level of resuscitative efforts that should be made, including but not limited to ACLS protocols, advanced airways, nutrition, and cessation of life-prolonging interventions.** Alternatively, or in conjunction with an advanced directive, a healthcare surrogate or proxy can be established, such as a durable power of attorney. There is some controversy of how precisely living wills should be interpreted, as there is usually some ambiguity in the text or evolution of medical technology with time. Preferences expressed in a living will are most compelling when they reflect long-held, consistently stable views of the patient. This can often be determined by conversations with family members, close friends, or healthcare providers who have had a long-term relationship with the patient. In the event that a surrogate is not established in a written document, or if the document is not readily accessible upon admission to the hospital, the law generally recognizes a hierarchy of family relationships determining who the decision maker is. The unfortunate reality is that family dynamics are quite variable, which intrinsically poses a challenge when family members disagree on decisions. Table 7–2 provides the most commonly accepted surrogate hierarchy in the United States.

CONCLUSIONS

In the critical care setting, end-of-life matters are often difficult to approach if healthcare providers do not have important conversations with patients and their families. Understanding a patient's desires for CPR and life-prolonging efforts should be established while the patient has decision-making capacity and/or the family is present. If resuscitation efforts are either not desired or deemed medically futile, the establishment of DNR orders is critical. Documentation of the patient's desires is paramount. If the DNR order is in place, palliative and comfort care should be utilized to ensure minimal pain and suffering in the patient's final moments. However, such care in an overwhelming majority of states does not utilize methods of euthanasia. Emergencies do not alter the standards of medical care, but the best possible care within the patient's informed consent should be rendered under the circumstances. A patient whose organs and tissues may be viable for transplantation should be properly maintained post-mortem to ensure the greatest possible outcome for donation. In the absence of advanced directives indicating the desire to be a donor, the patient's family should be approached by the hospital's multidisciplinary team to facilitate the best mutually beneficial outcome.

CLINICAL CASE CORRELATION

- See also Case 3 (Scoring Systems and Patient Prognosis).

COMPREHENSION QUESTIONS

7.1 A 24-year-old woman sustained head trauma in a motor vehicle collision and was declared brain dead by both the attending physician and a second consulting physician. The paramedics who brought the patient to the trauma center presented her driver's license, which noted that she was an organ donor. The patient was maintained on life support to preserve the integrity of the viable organs and tissue. However, the patient's mother refused to accept her daughter's death and demanded that she remain on life support indefinitely. How should the hospital proceed?

A. Consult the hospital ethics committee for case review.

B. Consult the hospital legal council for a case review.

C. Maintain the patient on life support indefinitely per the mother's request.

D. Continue with organ and tissue procurement for donation.

E. Remove life support and suspend organ and tissue donation efforts.

7.2 A 98-year-old man is admitted to the ICU with bronchial pneumonia, end-stage renal disease, and widely metastatic prostate cancer. The patient is in a comatose state and has consistently refused to discuss end-of-life decisions with his family and physicians. The patient's 99-year-old spouse resides in a nursing home and has been declared legally incapacitated. The patient's five adult children unanimously refuse hospice care and refuse to sign a DNR certificate. While rounding in the ICU, you overhear a "code" called for the patient who has gone into cardiopulmonary failure. How should the physician and resuscitation team respond?

A. Immediately sign a DNR order and refuse CPR and ACLS protocols.

B. Enact CPR and ACLS resuscitative efforts, as per hospital guidelines.

C. Refuse CPR and ACLS protocols on the basis of medical futility.

D. Consult the patient's family immediately on how they wish to proceed.

E. Enact simulated resuscitative efforts without expediency or effort, giving the appearance to family members that all appropriate resuscitative measures are being undertaken.

ANSWERS

7.1 **D.** All fifty states in the United States have adopted legal legislation on the basis of the Uniform Anatomical Gift Act framework, which permits individuals to state their intention to donate organs or tissue through either a donor card or a government-issued identification. The donor card or identification card has legal significance and can supersede the family's refusal to donate or maintain life support when brain death has been established. Situations involving the sudden death of a younger patient are emotional events where family members struggle with the terminality of the situation. With protection by the law and a need to expeditiously procure viable organs and tissue, the organ transplantation protocol should be enacted. This should include thorough attention to the family's bereavement, but delay for ethical or legal review are not necessary considering the well-established legal precedence.

7.2 **C.** This patient has a terminal condition without the possibility of meaningful recovery or quality of life. As such, the patient would not benefit from resuscitative efforts, meeting the widely accepted standards of medical futility. A physician maintains the right to determine medical futility and can opt to withhold resuscitative efforts in the instance of cardiopulmonary failure. Use of resuscitative measures are both unlikely to have any long-term success and are likely to cause additional morbidities. This patient has consistently refused to make his end-of-life desires known to the physician and/or his family members. In his incoherent state, his proxy would ordinarily be his living spouse. However, with her being legally incapacitated and institutionalized, the closest living proxies are his adult children. Though they want full resuscitative efforts made, the physician's privilege to withhold such efforts on the basis of futility supersedes their desire. A physician ethically should not sign a DNR order in the absence of the patient's proxy's signature. As such, no formal DNR orders will be placed for this patient. Likewise, the use of half-hearted "slow codes" are unethical and are a malpractice to the physician's responsibility to the patient.

CLINICAL PEARLS

▸ A coordinated approach to the donor patient and family is crucial to address emotional and spiritual needs, optimize the physiological parameters, and work together with the transplant team.

▸ Cardiovascular instability often occurs during the evolution of brain death due to catecholamine surges, cytokine production, and neurovascular changes.

▸ Aggressive critical care interventions can correct cardiovascular instability and reverse or preserve normal organ functions, allowing transplantation to proceed.

▸ Optimally, patients should create advanced directives and in conversation with friends and family.

▸ If CPR is judged to have no clinical benefit to the patient, physicians are ethically justified in withholding the resuscitation on the basis of evidence-based medicine and the principal of medical futility.

▸ Surrogate decision making is used when there is no advanced directive, and there is a hierarchy in those family relationships.

REFERENCES

Annas GJ. Standard of care: in sickness and in health and in emergencies. *N Engl J Med.* 2010;362: 2126-2131.

Loscalzo J. *Harrison's Pulmonary and Critical Care Medicine.* New York, NY: McGraw-Hill; 2010.

Wood KE, Becker BN, McCartney JG, et al. Care of the potential organ donor. *N Engl J Med.* 2004;35:2730-2739.

A 54-year-old African-American man is evaluated in the ICU for a 24-hour history of progressive swelling of the lips. He has hoarseness and difficulty swallowing with drooling and inability to swallow his saliva. He has not had any recent insect stings, ingestion of new foods, or changes to his medications. His medical history is significant for hypertension and heart failure. Medications are carvedilol, hydrochlorothiazide, and lisinopril. On physical examination, he is awake, alert, and able to speak in short sentences with mild inspiratory stridor. Temperature is 37.0°C (98.6°F), blood pressure is 158/88 mm Hg, pulse rate is 98 beats/min, and respiration rate is 18 breaths/min. Oxygen saturation is 96% breathing ambient air. The lips are edematous, and the posterior pharynx is difficult to visualize secondary to an enlarged tongue. Inspiration is prolonged with audible stridor over the neck. The chest is clear to auscultation, but there is use of accessory respiratory muscles. No rash is noted.

Arterial Blood Gas Studies (Ambient Air)	
pH	7.34 (7.35–7.45)
$Paco_2$	72 mm Hg (36–44 mm Hg)
Pao_2	70 mm Hg (75–100 mm Hg)

▶ What is the most important initial step in the management of this patient?
▶ What are other management considerations?

ANSWERS TO CASE 8:
Airway Management/Respiratory Failure

Summary: A 54-year-old man developed upper airway obstruction and stridor due to angioedema. He is hypoxemic and hypercarbic with $Paco_2$ of 72 mm Hg.

- **Most important initial management:** The most appropriate next step in management is rapid sequence endotracheal intubation (RSI). This patient has acute respiratory acidosis indicated by his ABG and is experiencing angioedema with stridor, an indicator of impending obstruction, likely triggered by use of an ACE inhibitor. He requires immediate intubation.

- **Other considerations:** Be prepared for a bedside tracheostomy or cricothyroidotomy if endotrachial intubation is not possible. Have an anesthesiologist available to provide assistance if possible. A portable chest x-ray can evaluate the trachea and confirm correct placement of the endotracheal tube (ETT), as well as detect a potential pneumothorax. If cerebral edema is suspected, high minute ventilation with a target $Paco_2$ range of 30 to 35 mm Hg should be used to create a respiratory alkalosis, decreasing intracranial pressure (ICP), although this effect is short lived. Avoid excessive positive end-expiratory pressure (PEEP), as this may further increase ICP. Propofol may be beneficial for induction and sedation, as it lowers ICP, has anti-seizure activity, and a rapid elimination profile allowing for accurate assessment of the CNS status. A pH value less than 7.35 represents acidosis.

  The next step is to note the value of $Paco_2$ which in this case is 72 mm Hg, signifying respiratory acidosis. The patient's $Paco_2$ (72 mm Hg) – the normal value of $Paco_2$ (40 mm Hg) = $\Delta 32$. To calculate expected pH, multiply the Δ in $Paco_2$(32) by value for acute (0.008) = 0.256. Normal pH (7.40) – 0.256 = 7.144 +/– 0.02. This patient's pH of 7.34 falls into the expected range for acute respiratory acidosis. Although not given in this case, HCO_3 (normal = 24 mEq/L) would be expected to increase by 1 for every 10 increase in $Paco_2$ for appropriate compensation. Therefore, in the presence of appropriate compensation, expected HCO_3 would be approximately 27 mEq/L.

ANALYSIS

Objectives

1. Understand the indications and contraindications for endotracheal intubation (ETI).

2. Understand alternative methods for airway control.

3. Understand the most common complications of endotracheal intubation.

4. Understand the required steps and equipment for endotracheal intubation.

Considerations

The absence of signs and symptoms of an allergic reaction, such as urticaria, pruritus, bronchospasm, and hypotension, is typical of ACE inhibitor–associated angioedema. Although angioedema is most often reported within 1 week of starting or increasing the dose of the offending medication, it can also occur after years of use. The risk of recurrence with continued exposure to ACE inhibitors is substantial, and patients should be switched to an alternative medication. Methylprednisolone and epinephrine are useful in the treatment of upper airway obstruction triggered by croup and anaphylactic reactions, but they do not have a clear role in the treatment of angioedema associated with ACE inhibitors. Icatibant is a synthetic bradykinin B_2-receptor antagonist that is approved for the acute treatment of hereditary angioedema (HAE) attacks and has also been shown to be effective for the treatment of ACE inhibitor–related angioedema. This agent acts by decreasing bradykinin induced vasodilation and vascular permeability and is most effective if given within the first few hours of the angioedema attack. This patient's airway is severely compromised as evidenced by stridor, and there is insufficient time to delay intubation in order to allow a trial of therapy. Noninvasive positive pressure ventilation may decrease the patient's work of breathing and help maintain the upper airway open, but it does not adequately secure the airway and should not be used to manage upper airway obstruction, regardless of the cause. This patient exhibits inspiratory stridor, which portends possible impending airway collapse. RSI is required for the protection and control of the airway. A "wait and see" attitude in this patient would likely lead to devastating consequences. Aspiration precautions should be taken with elevation of the head of the bed to 45 degrees upright. Mechanical ventilation should be started on assist control (AC) mode of 14 breaths/minute with a tidal volume of 6 to 8 mL/kg with 100% F_{IO_2} and a PEEP of 5, keeping end-inspiratory plateau pressure under 30 cm H_2O.

APPROACH TO:

Airway Management/Ventilator Support

INTUBATION IN CRITICAL CARE SETTINGS

The **most common indications for endotracheal intubation (ETI) are hypoxic respiratory failure and hypercarbic ventilatory failure.** Treatment for hypoxia begins with the insertion of a low-flow nasal cannula and the delivery of 3 L/min of oxygen, increasing to 100% oxygen with the use of a non-rebreather mask or high-flow O_2 therapy to obtain a Sao_2 of greater than 90% to 92%. A patient with impaired consciousness and an unprotected airway may have an independent indication for ETI. It should be verified that the patient does not have an advanced directive refusing endotracheal intubation and mechanical ventilation or an existing do-not-intubate (DNI) or do not resuscitate (DNR) order. The patient's wishes or those of the family or legal guardian should be known and respected prior to invasive measures. Other secondary indications for ETI include the significant aspiration of particulate matter.

ETI may also be indicated for airway protection in patients requiring bronchoscopy and pulmonary lavage, those with neurological or traumatic injuries who require deep sedation and intubation to perform necessary imaging tests or diagnostic and therapeutic procedures, and for individuals with status epilepticus requiring deep sedation or paralysis for treatment of seizures.

Endotracheal Intubation

Endotracheal intubation (ETI) is the definitive method for control of the airway and is a common procedure for patients requiring general anesthesia. The laryngeal mask airway (LMA), a device that does not require a tube through the trachea or a laryngoscope for placement, may be an alternative for airway management in some short-duration surgeries. The LMA is a short ETT-type tube that is surrounded and held in place by a laryngeal mask. The apex of the mask, with its open end pointing downward toward the tongue, is pushed backward toward the uvula. The LMA can be effective as a short-term option and requires less technical expertise for successful placement.

Emergency situations such as cardiac or respiratory arrest require ETI. A patient with an unprotected airway, inadequate oxygenation or ventilation, or existing or impending airway obstruction may also require ETI. These indications are increasingly challenged in an era of advancing technology in oxygen delivery and noninvasive forms of ventilation. They can be further divided into three basic categories: (1) hypoxic respiratory failure (decreased Po_2), (2) hypercarbic ventilator failure, including drug overdose (elevated $Paco_2$), and (3) impaired level of consciousness, requiring airway protection to prevent aspiration. The inability of the patient to clear secretions is a more important indicator for airway protection and ETI than is absence of the gag reflex. **The lack of a gag reflex is not a sensitive predictor of the need for ETI.** Checking the gag reflex may inadvertently induce vomiting with resulting aspiration and should only be performed with suctioning equipment present and the head of the bed elevated 30 to 45 degrees. The accumulation of large amounts of secretions in the oral cavity, without ability to clear them, is an indication for ETI. If the patient can speak, is cooperative, and responds to verbal questioning, then one should consider a trial of noninvasive ventilation (NIV). The assisted ventilation provided from NIV therapy can provide additional time for the treatment of underlying medical conditions with steroids, bronchodilators, diuretics, nitrates, or other medications.

Hypoxic Respiratory Failure

Hypoxic respiratory failure, or Type 1 hypoxic respiratory failure, is defined as hypoxemia without hypercarbia. An impairment of oxygen exchange via the pulmonary alveolar capillary membrane (> A-a gradient) results in hypoxemia, leading to diminished delivery of oxygen to the cells. A quick and easy way to calculate the A-a gradient is shown below. Pao_2/Fio_2 and O_2 sat$/Fio_2$ are ratios that parallel the A-a gradient. A value <300 signifies adult respiratory distress syndrome (ARDS), whereas >300 represents non-ARDS. You should not have a negative A-a gradient as determined by the equation:

$$\text{A-a gradient} = (\text{F\textsc{io}}_2 \times 7) - \text{P\textsc{ao}}_2 - (\text{P\textsc{aco}}_2 \times 1.2),$$
$$\text{with the normal A-a gradient} < 20 \text{ mm Hg}$$

The initial treatment for all causes of hypoxemia includes: (1) ensure airway patency, (2) provide adequate ventilation, and (3) provide supplemental oxygen. A $\text{P\textsc{ao}}_2$ of 60 mm Hg or an arterial oxygen saturation of 90% to 92% are generally recognized as the minimum values acceptable. A patient with hypoxemia who improves upon delivery of increasingly higher $\text{F\textsc{io}}_2$ is suggestive of a ventilation/ perfusion (V/Q) mismatch as the cause. Hypoxemia resistant to high $\text{F\textsc{io}}_2$ concentration suggests the most likely cause is shunting (eg, ARDS). The treatment of hypoxia begins by ensuring a patent airway for adequate ventilation and oxygenation of the patient. Trials of noninvasive ventilation may be indicated, but this should not delay intubation and MV if needed. If the O_2 saturation fails to improve on 100% $\text{F\textsc{io}}_2$, then ETI and MV should be undertaken so PEEP can be administered.

Hypercarbic Ventilatory Failure ($\uparrow$ P\textsc{aco}$_2$)

Hypercarbic ventilatory failure occurs when there is an inability to remove carbon dioxide (CO_2) from the alveoli. This condition may be the result of a primary lung disorder or secondarily associated with cardiac, neurologic, or metabolic causes. The symptoms and signs of hypercarbia are explained by increased $\text{P\textsc{aco}}_2$ resulting in vasoconstriction, confusion, sedation, and acidosis. Diagnosis of hypercarbia is confirmed with an ABG with a $\text{P\textsc{aco}}_2$ >45 mm Hg and significant acidemia (pH <7.35) secondary to the elevated $\text{P\textsc{aco}}_2$. The rate of change in $\text{P\textsc{aco}}_2$ will affect the signs and symptoms. If the change in $\text{P\textsc{aco}}_2$ is gradual, then the onset of symptoms such as lethargy, headache, and confusion will also be more gradual. Rapid changes in $\text{P\textsc{aco}}_2$, however, will result in more sudden and severe symptoms. **Treatment of hypercarbic ventilatory failure includes administering supplemental oxygenation, ensuring airway patency, and increasing ventilation.** The treatment should be specifically directed toward the underlying etiology. If the patient's condition does not improve with the initial treatment, then increasing the minute ventilation is necessary to correct the acidosis. Noninvasive positive pressure ventilation should be attempted first, unless there is an obvious need for ETI. Indications requiring ETI are ventilatory failure despite CPAP and signs of impending respiratory failure such as increasing dyspnea, tachypnea, the use of accessory breathing muscles, and low tidal volume ventilation.

Impaired Consciousness and Airway Protection

Patients with Glasgow coma scale (GCS) values of 8 or less should be considered for ETI because of diminished levels of consciousness, continued hypoventilation, and a need for airway protection. Comatose patients have decreased respiratory drive, hypoventilation, and decreased ability to clear secretions. 30% of patients with subarachnoid hemorrhage and traumatic brain injury are likely to develop pulmonary edema or ARDS. When there is a concern of increased ICP and uncal herniation, hyperventilation with alkalosis has been shown to be helpful by inducing cerebral vasoconstriction, although this effect is temporary. Propofol for sedation has also been shown to reduce intracranial pressure.

Prolonged hyperventilation for prophylaxis of ICP should be avoided because of the risk for ischemic brain injury. Other indications for ETI include traumatic injury or swelling to the face or neck, or other obstructive airway processes. Nasogastric tube (NGT) insertion via the nasal route should be avoided in patients with facial trauma to avoid the risk of perforating the cribiform plate of the ethmoid bone, which separates the nasal cavity from the brain.

Contraindications to Endotracheal Intubation

With an urgent need for ventilatory support or airway control, relatively few contraindications exist for ETI. Direct laryngoscopy is contraindicated in patients with partial transection of the trachea because this can cause a complete loss of the airway. In this situation, one should consider establishing a surgical airway. If the cervical spine is unstable to manipulation as in rheumatoid arthritis (RA), then strict inline stabilization of the cervical spine is required and must be maintained during ETI to avoid cord injury and paralysis. Video-assisted ETT placement has reduced the need to hyperextend the neck during intubation.

Special Considerations

Before intubation, all the necessary equipments should be verified. This includes gloves, protective face shield, suction system, bag-valve mask attached to an oxygen source, ETT with a malleable stylet, 10 mL syringe, ETT holder, end-tidal carbon dioxide detector, stethoscope, and laryngoscope with blade or new fiberoptic technology. The fiberoptic laryngoscope allows enhanced visualization of the ETT placement past the vocal cords. The two common types of blades currently in use are the Miller straight blade and the curved MacIntosh blade. ETTs are available in different internal diameters: 7.0, 7.5, and 8 mm. In adults, the 8-mm diameter tube should be used when possible. The tracheal size is best estimated by the patient's predicted BMI and not the actual BMI of obese patients. The ETT is available both cuffed and uncuffed. The uncuffed tubes are often more appropriate for children, while cuffed tubes are indicated for older children and adults. Specialized ETTs that allow for subglottic suctioning have been proposed to reduce ventilator-associated pneumonia (VAP). Avoid cuff overinflation, as cuffs are designed as large-volume, low-pressure systems to prevent mucosal ischemia of the trachea. Pretreatment with 100% oxygen by a non-rebreather mask or a bag-valve mask is necessary to increase oxygenation in the blood. This also increases the interval before desaturation occurs.

Before initiating any invasive procedure, it must be confirmed that informed consent has been obtained, unless it is a life-threatening emergency. In any situation requiring emergent intubation, it must be ensured that there is no pre-existing "do-not-resuscitate" (DNR) or "do-not-intubate" (DNI) order. The malleable stylet is usually placed into the ETT to follow the natural curvature of the airway. IV access should already be established, and the patient's vital signs should be continuously monitored. Proper positioning of the patient prior to intubation is important. The patient's head should be in level with the lower portion of the sternum. The "sniffing position" can be accomplished by placing a pillow or folded towel beneath the patient's occiput. Axial alignment of the oral cavity, pharynx, and larynx is ideal for vocal cord visualization and can be arranged by flexing the neck and extending the head. Dentures, if present, should be removed. An assistant should perform the Sellick maneuver (applying firm pressure to the cricoid cartilage), which compresses the esophagus between the cricoid cartilage and the cervical vertebrae to avoid aspiration of the gastric content. This maneuver is performed to reduce the risk of passive aspiration of gastric contents and improve visualization of the glottis, although efficacy of this maneuver has been questioned recently.

INTRAVENOUS ACCESS AND DRUGS FOR SEDATION AND PARALYSIS

Propofol is the IV induction drug of choice for most patients because of its rapid onset and recovery, beneficial antiemetic and other properties, and relatively benign adverse side effects. Neuromuscular blocking agents and strong sedatives are used to improve visualization of the vocal cords and to reduce the likelihood of vomiting and aspiration. Midazolam and fentanyl are often used shortly before induction as a premedicant or during induction as an adjunct, respectively. Other combinations include thiopental and ketamine. A commonly used neuromuscular blocking agent is succinylcholine. Rocuronium is a substitute when there is a contraindication for succinylcholine, particularly in the presence of hyperkalemia. Succinylcholine should be avoided in hyperkalemia because of depolarization at the neuromuscular junction. Edema, obstruction, tumors, trauma, and infections can all contribute to a difficult intubation. Other situations that can make intubation more difficult are a small mandible, limited neck mobility, and an edematous tongue (angioedema, amyloidosis). *Neuromuscular blockers* used to paralyze the patient for MV are associated with neurological deficits and sequelae and should be avoided.

Confirmation

The ETT should be positioned in the mid trachea, with the ETT tip 3 to 4 cm above the carina. Bilateral breath sounds and equal expansion of the lungs should be noted. **An end-tidal carbon dioxide detector (capnography) should be connected to the ETT, and this monitor will change color within the first 6 breaths.** Lack of color change suggests that the ETT is not in the trachea; in other words, when the Pco_2 is near zero, it means the ETT is likely in the esophagus. The ETT should be repositioned until the CO_2 monitor confirms correct endotracheal placement by a change of color. A chest x-ray is needed to verify ETT placement and ensure that the ETT is not in the right or left main stem bronchus. After successful ETI, the tube should be secured via an ETT holder or adhesive tape. Facial hair should be removed if necessary to secure the ETT. Major complications of ETT placement include tracheal injury, bronchospasm, hypoxemia, hypercapnia, and death. Vomiting, bradycardia, laryngospasm, pneumonitis, and pneumonia are other potential complications. Some authorities recommend IV lidocaine prior to ETI to reduce ETI-induced bronchospasm. ETI and MV are also sometimes associated with ICU delirium.

SUMMARY

The essential goals of ETI and MV are to provide a patent airway for the delivery of oxygen and proper ventilation, which are critical to a patient's survival, as well as to allow suctioning of secretions, application of PEEP, and delivery of aerosolized medications; doses of aerosolized medications should be double the regular dose since the ETT requires saturation. The decision to proceed with invasive ETI requires an understanding of the pathologic and physiologic disorders that require its use. A qualitative colorimetric $Etco_2$ monitor is commonly used to confirm placement and is nearly 100% sensitive and specific for ETT placement in the trachea.

CLINICAL CASE CORRELATION

- See also Case 3 (Scoring Systems and Patient Prognosis), Case 9 (Ventilator Management), Case 11 (Asthmatic Management), and Case 12 (Non-invasive Methods of Ventilatory Support).

COMPREHENSION QUESTIONS

8.1 A 50-year-old man is evaluated in the ICU 1 hour after a motor vehicle accident where he was the unrestrained passenger. On examination the patient is confused, agitated, and diaphoretic. Vital signs are as follows: BP 76/50 mm Hg, HR 140 beats/minute, RR 32 breaths/minute, and Sao_2 by pulse oximetry of 72% on room air. Chest x-ray shows multiple rib fractures with an associated right pneumothorax. RSI is initiated with an 8-mm ETT and a right-sided chest tube is inserted. The patient is started on a pressure support of +10 mm Hg with 0 PEEP and Fio_2 of 100%. Additional chest x-rays and blood gas determinations are pending. Which of the following is the most reliable confirmation of proper tracheal placement of the ETT?

A. Ease of bagging with ventilation

B. Positive color changes on a CO_2 monitor attached to the endotracheal tube

C. Auscultation by stethoscope for normal breath sounds bilaterally

D. Pulse oximetry reading above 95%

E. Arterial blood gas analysis

8.2 You are called to evaluate a 19-year-old woman who was just intubated for uncontrolled seizure activity following a drug overdose. Her chest x-ray shows complete opacification of the left chest with a shift of the mediastinum also to the left. She is 5′2″ and weighs 60 kg. The front teeth are at the 32 cm mark on the ETT. Examination reveals normal breath sounds and definite expansion of the right chest, but no breath sounds and no expansion of the left chest are noted. What is the most likely etiology for this finding?

A. Tension pneumothorax

B. Barbiturate-induced lung injury

C. Adult respiratory distress syndrome

D. Esophageal placement of the endotracheal tube

E. Endotracheal tube placement in the right main stem bronchus

ANSWERS

8.1 **B.** The most reliable methods for confirming proper placement of the ETT in the trachea are direct visualization of the ETT passing through the vocal cords and confirming the change in color of a CO_2 monitor connected to the ETT. A chest x-ray is always performed for confirmation of tube placement. Sometimes, bronchoscopy may be needed to confirm proper placement or to assist in placement of the ETT. The tip of the ETT should be 3 to 4 cm above the carina. Head flexion makes the ETT tip go away from carina and can cause extubation. Head extension makes the ETT tip come closer to carina and can selectively intubate the right main stem bronchus. Other maneuvers that are usually performed include pulse oximetry and auscultation of the lung fields; however, these measures are often not as reliable predictors of accurate ETT placement, especially with the ambient noise of the ED.

8.2 **E.** The patient's ETT is placed too low, causing the right main stem bronchus to be selectively intubated. This occurs because of the direct angle into the right bronchus versus the more oblique left main stem bronchus. Proper placement of the ETT requires direct visualization beyond the cords confirmed by detection of end tidal CO_2 with capnography. A chest x-ray is performed to assure correct positioning of the ETT tip 3 to 4 cm above the carina.

CLINICAL PEARLS

▶ Clinical assessment, combined with medical experience, is the most important tool for identifying patients requiring intubation.

▶ Indications for ETI and MV are commonly divided into hypoxic respiratory failure, hypercarbic ventilatory failure, impaired consciousness, and a need for airway protection.

▶ Planned ETI in a controlled setting is always preferable to emergent airway management.

▶ Ventilation can be monitored by capnography, which noninvasively measures the partial pressure of carbon dioxide in the exhaled breath.

▶ ABG and $Paco_2$ measurements are necessary to evaluate hypercarbic ventilatory failure because pulse oximetry values can remain near normal until ventilatory collapse occurs.

▶ Unlike pulse oximetry for detecting hypoxemia, bedside monitors for detecting hypercarbia are not routinely available.

▶ Neurologic indications for ETI for impaired consciousness and presumed airway protection may account for 20% of patients intubated in the intensive care unit (ICU).

▶ Auscultation is not reliable for determining proper placement of the ETT.

▶ Patients requiring RSI usually present with increasing dyspnea, tachypnea, use of accessory breathing muscles, and low tidal volume ventilation with paradoxical breathing.

▶ ACE inhibitor–associated angioedema is characterized by the absence of signs and symptoms of an allergic reaction (such as urticaria, pruritus, bronchospasm, and hypotension); endotracheal intubation should be considered if severe upper airway edema is present.

REFERENCES

Loscalzo J. *Harrison's Pulmonary and Critical Care Medicine*. New York, NY: McGraw-Hill; 2013.

Malde B, Regalado J, Greenberger PA. Investigation of angioedema associated with the use of angiotensin-converting enzyme inhibitors and angiotensin receptor blockers. *Ann Allergy Asthma Immunol.* 2007;98(1):57-63.

Orebaugh S, Snyder JV. *Direct Laryngoscopy and Tracheal Intubation in Adults*. Waltham, MA: UpToDate; 2011.

A 33-year-old woman is admitted to the ICU after a 6-hour history of worsening asthma symptoms. Her medications include albuterol and an inhaled corticosteroid. Despite being treated with intravenous corticosteroids and high volume nebulizer with albuterol and ipratropium bromide treatments, she remains symptomatic and can speak only one to two words between breaths. On physical examination, she appears uncomfortable and tired. Temperature is 36.8°C (98.2°F), blood pressure is 150/90 mm Hg, heart rate is 124 beats/min, and respiration rate is 32 breaths/min. Oxygen saturation by pulse oximetry is 92% on 60% oxygen by face mask. Lung examination now reveals a quiet chest where diffuse expiratory wheezes were heard just hours earlier. The patient is unable to perform a peak flow maneuver. Chest x-ray shows hyperinflation and no acute infiltrates. Results of arterial blood gas studies are shown in the table below.

Arterial Blood Gas Studies	
pH	7.32 (7.35–7.45)
$Paco_2$	49 mm Hg (36–44 mm Hg)
Pao_2 (on 60% O_2)	70 mm Hg (75–100 mm Hg)
Pao_2/Fio_2 Ratio	70/0.6 = 117 (>300)
O_2 sat/Fio_2 Ratio	92/0.6 = 153 (>300)
A-a gradient	297 (<12)

▶ What is the most appropriate management for this patient?
▶ What is the best initial mode of mechanical ventilation and settings for this patient?
▶ What are the most common complications of mechanical ventilation?

ANSWERS TO CASE 9:

Ventilator Management

Summary: This is a 33-year-old woman in an acute exacerbation of asthma requiring rapid sequence intubation (RSI) and mechanical ventilation (MV) for respiratory failure.

- **Best management:** Rapid sequence intubation and mechanical ventilation.

  1. Begin with the MV parameters which will best assure an acceptable pH, $Paco_2$, and Pao_2 (eg, AC of 14, V_t 6-8 mL/kg, Fio_2 100%, PEEP 5 cm H_2O, pp <30 cm) and patient comfort.

  2. Switch off assist control (AC) to pressure support or some form of patient-controlled mode as soon as possible to increase patient comfort and reduce the need for sedation.

  3. Keep head of bed elevated at a minimum of 45 degrees as the main key to aspiration precautions and ventilator-associated pneumonia (VAP).

- **Best initial mode and mechanical ventilation settings:** Assist control (AC) mode following low-volume mechanical ventilation guidelines using 6 mL/kg as a starting tidal volume (V_t) with a goal of a plateau pressure (pp) of <30 cm H_2O and an acceptable respiratory rate (RR) favoring prolonged expiratory time would achieve the ventilatory goals of oxygenation, normal carbon dioxide, and normal pH. Other initial settings include an Fio_2 of 100% and a positive end expiratory pressure (PEEP) of 5 cm H_2O, keeping in mind that auto-PEEP with hypotension and patient distress is frequent in these cases and should be avoided.

- **Most common complications of MV:** Barotrauma, aberrant (esophageal) intubation, right main stem bronchus intubation, and ventilator-associated pneumonia.

ANALYSIS

Objectives

1. Describe the indications for mechanical ventilation.

2. Describe the various ventilator modalities and advantages and disadvantages of each.

3. Describe the complications associated with MV.

Considerations

The most appropriate management for this patient is RSI, MV, and admission to the ICU. The causes of acute ventilatory failure in patients with exacerbations of asthma are increased airway resistance and dynamic hyperinflation that reduces chest-wall compliance. Both contribute to excessive work of breathing. Bronchospasm, airway edema, and secretions, as well as excessive expiratory airway collapse, can severely reduce airway diameter, resulting in markedly prolonged expiration and high pressures. Progressive stacking of breaths can lead to an equilibration at a higher lung volume with higher positive end-expiratory alveolar pressure (auto-PEEP or intrinsic PEEP), which is associated with dynamic air trapping and hyperinflation. The associated flattening of the diaphragm decreases its function and forces greater reliance on accessory muscles, further increasing carbon dioxide production and oxygen consumption as a result of the inefficiency of these muscles compared with a properly functioning diaphragm. Severe air trapping can also cause alveolar rupture and marked elevations in intrathoracic pressure, causing reductions in venous return to the right heart, one resulting in pneumothorax and the other hypotension, respectively. Typically, patients with an asthma exacerbation initially present with respiratory alkalosis, slightly elevated or even normal $Paco_2$ levels often indicate impending respiratory failure rather than recovery, and clinical correlation is critical for interpreting arterial blood gas findings in this setting.

APPROACH TO:

Mechanical Ventilation

Continuous oximetry reading is standard in all MV patients. **The goal is to keep O_2 saturations equal to or exceeding 90%, which equals a Pao_2 of 60 mm Hg.** This is a time-tested goal of oxygenation and the elbow of the hemoglobin dissociation curve. An improving or normal neurological status is a secondary predictor of a good outcome. Increased levels of PEEP and 100% Fio_2 may be required to achieve and maintain this O_2 sat goal (Table 9–1). PEEP can prevent the collapse of small airways and alveoli by maintaining alveolar recruitment. PEEP further improves oxygenation and matching of ventilation with perfusion (VQ).

MECHANICAL VENTILATORS

The **most common reason for MV is respiratory failure due to sepsis, pneumonia, ARDS, COPD, pulmonary edema, or coma.** The objective of MV is to decrease the work of breathing and to reverse life-threatening hypoxemia, hypercarbia, and acidosis. The CO_2 from the work of breathing is redistributed back to the systemic circulation (kidneys, heart, brain, gut). MV is delivered via an endotracheal tube (ETT) or tracheostomy tube. The ETT has more dead space than a tracheostomy tube; thus the tracheostomy patient requires lower tidal volumes. The use of fiberoptic-assisted ETT is easier than direct laryngoscopy and has the added benefit of clearly seeing the ETT pass through the vocal cords into the trachea. The IV administration of lidocaine prior to intubation may decrease cardiac arrhythmia and blunt the undesired responses induced by ETT insertion into the trachea.

The MV is a machine with adjustable variations in cycling modes between inspiration (inhalation) and expiration (exhalation). Independent variables are set and monitored by microprocessors and displayed on a monitor. MV can control

Table 9-1 • GENERAL PRINCIPLES OF COMMON MECHANICAL VENTILATOR MODES	
Examples of Common MV Modes	General Principles of MV Modes
Airway pressure release ventilation (APRV)	• Positive pressure breath delivery, positive intrathoracic pressure during inspiration
Assist control (AC) ventilation	• Breaths can be triggered by patient, set by MV, or both
Continuous pressure airway pressure ventilation (CPAP)	• FIO_2, V_t, flow rates, PEEP, PS, IPAP, EPAP can be delivered, measured, and monitored by the MV
Controlled mandatory ventilation (CMV)	
JET ventilation and high-frequency ventilation (HFOV)	
Pressure support ventilation (PSV), pressure-controlled ventilation (PCV)	
Synchronized intermittent ventilation (SIMV, IMV)	

many different means of delivering a positive pressure breath to the patient. This inspiration under positive pressure created by the MV totally reverses the normally negative inspiratory cycle in the spontaneously breathing patient. Some of the more common ventilator modes include: assist control (AC), synchronized intermittent ventilation (SIMV), pressure support ventilation (PSV), controlled mechanical ventilation (CMV), and pressure release ventilation (PRV).

Tidal volume (V_t), fractional inspired concentration of oxygen (FIO_2), respiratory rate (RR), positive end-expiratory pressure (PEEP), peak inspiratory pressure (PIP), humidification, and warming of inspired air can all be controlled by the MV.

The different MV settings provide a predetermined mixture of patient-initiated (spontaneous) and MV-delivered controlled breaths (see Table 9-1 for common MV modes). **The best choice is the one that delivers and meets the physiologic needs for oxygenation and ventilation while maintaining patient comfort and decreasing the need for sedation.**

MVs have sensors that must be activated to deliver an MV breath. Inside the MV tubing, an artificial nose humidifies the respiratory circuit. The artificial nose reduces contamination by respiratory water-borne pathogens by eliminating water reservoirs. Upper airway heat and humidification is also achieved with the patient's own respiratory system. The respiratory circuit tubing should not be changed unless there is a good reason (eg, leak). Reduced manipulation of the MV circuitry has decreased patient infection rates and contamination by resistant organisms. MV circuits are equipped with a built-in reusable suction catheter. This is a clean, closed system in which a collapsible plastic cover built in to the suction catheter allows for its reuse as needed. MV also has the flexibility to allow for the in-line delivery of aerosolized medications without disconnecting the patient from the MV.

Medications commonly used in MV include β_2 agonists, ipratropium bromide, steroids, antibiotics, and mucolytics. Invasive ventilation with MV is needed when noninvasive ventilation (NIV) fails or in situations requiring better airway control. Patients intubated for respiratory failure develop respiratory muscle fatigue and thinning of the diaphragm, and muscle retraining is required. Muscular dysfunction must be reversed. Anxiety, which is the most common treatable side effect of MV, can be minimized with pressure support MV and the use of patient-driven MV modes (SIMV, PSV, CPAP). SIMV is associated with improved synchronization between the patient's natural breathing pattern and the MV. The respiratory demand and the amount of required ventilator support determines the mode of ventilation.

Assist control ventilation is usually the initial MV mode since delivery of a backup respiratory rate and minute ventilation is assured regardless of patient contribution. SIMV or IMV are equivalent since all IMV devices are synchronized. The main goal of MV is to supply needed ventilation and oxygenation by retraining and strengthening the respiratory system and resting the fatigued respiratory muscles. An eventual goal is to exercise the rested muscle to allow successful extubation. Extubation is considered successful when reintubation is not required within the next 48 hours. NIV (ie, CPAP, BIPAP) may be useful following extubation, especially in patients with underlying lung disease like chronic obstructive pulmonary disease (COPD).

Daily portable chest x-rays are advised for all MV patients during the **acute** course of the disease. This aids not only in evaluating the placement of ETT, the recognition of new infiltrates, the development of barotrauma, and the placement of central venous lines, but also in detecting abnormalities of nasogastric tubes (NGT) or feeding tubes. The extension of the chin away from the chest can move the ETT down and selectively intubate the right main stem bronchus. In contrast, flexion of the chin toward the chest can pull the ETT up and extubate the patient if the ETT is not properly placed. The recommended placement of the tip of the ETT is 3 to 4 cm above the carina (T_4 level) to avoid these changes due to chin motion.

ASSIST CONTROL VENTILATION

In **AC, MV breaths are delivered at a preset rate and tidal volume.** If a spontaneous breath is not generated within a specified time, a mechanical breath will be delivered at a scheduled time period depending on the rate set. For example, the MV will cycle a breath every 3 seconds for set rate of 20 breaths/min, even if no spontaneous breath occurs within that minute. The patient can only breathe and receive MV breaths above the set rate, but never below it. Lack of coordination between the patient's breathing and the MV breaths may cause significant patient discomfort and an increase in the work of breathing (Figure 9–1).

The goals of MV are to provide adequate minute ventilation (V_m = rate × V_t) and minimize the risk of barotrauma. In an AC mode, if the patient breathes above the set MV respiratory rate, the machine will deliver another full MV breath, which can lead to an acute respiratory alkalosis. Tachypnea on the AC MV mode can lead to the stacking of MV breaths with trapping of air as the expiratory time decreases. This results in auto-PEEP. Intrinsic and auto-PEEP are

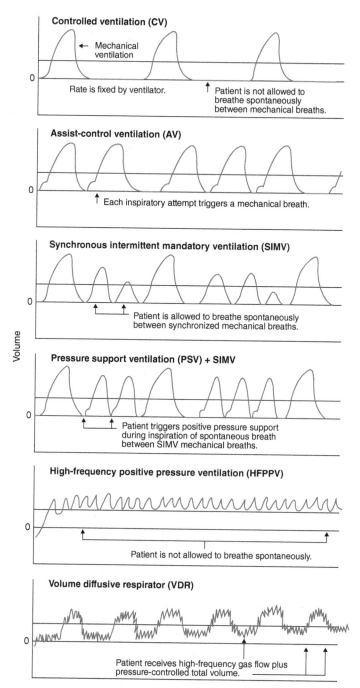

Figure 9–1. Mechanical ventilator modes. Waveforms of various mechanical ventilator modes demonstrating volume versus time. (Reproduced, with permission, from Gomella LG, Haist SA. *Clinician's Pocket reference*. 11th ed. New York: McGraw-Hill Education, 2007. Figure 20-20).

factors of fast respiratory rates and shorter exhalation times (reverse I-E ratios). If during exhalation the pressure does not return to baseline (0), this intrinsic PEEP increases the inspiratory effort; the patient's next inspiratory effort must overcome this new baseline pressure to initiate the next spontaneous breath. Lengthening the expiratory time by decreasing the volume or rate alleviates this problem and decreases the intrinsic PEEP/auto-PEEP. Disconnecting a patient from the MV circuit eliminates the PEEP and the alveoli that has been recruited. These alveoli will then collapse and are difficult to re-expand. Should this auto-PEEP be the cause of hemodynamic deterioration, the disconnecting maneuver to reduce the PEEP can be lifesaving. Intravascular volume should be increased with fluids since PEEP decreases venous return (preload) and affects pulmonary capillary wedge pressure (PCWP) readings if pulmonary artery catheterization (PAC) is present.

SYNCHRONIZED INTERMITTENT MANDATORY VENTILATION

SIMV is similar to AC, except that **breaths that are spontaneously generated by the patient occur without activating an MV breath.** Breaths initiated by the patient are only in the V_t amount generated by the patient and not by the MV. Both ventilator breaths and spontaneous breaths generated by the patient can be assisted with PSV. SIMV should not be used without PSV since this actually increases the work of breathing. With SIMV, at least 5 cm H_2O of pressure support (PS) should be applied. All IMV are synchronized to keep a ventilator breath from pushing against a patient's natural or forced exhalation. This will avoid possible barotrauma and pneumothorax (PTX) secondary to increased intrabronchial pressures.

PRESSURE SUPPORT/CONTROLLED VENTILATION

Pressure support ventilation (PSV) and pressure-controlled ventilation (PCV) were originally designed for weaning or liberating the patient from MV. These modalities should be used in combination when SIMV is used, since SIMV needs a support mode. In PSV, the patient is spontaneously breathing and each patient breath is assisted by a preset amount of "pressure support" measured in centimeter H_2O. Pressures can be set for inhalation and exhalation, as well as for continuous or intermittent application. With increased inhalation pressure, V_t increases. This effect usually reaches a maximum at pressures of 25 to 30 cm H_2O. PSV acts as an assist device that allows the patient to establish the V_t and respiratory rate at levels which are most comfortable. This mode delivers maximum patient comfort and thus requires the least amount of sedation.

PCV is the same as PSV except there is a preset pressure that **must** be reached with every patient-initiated breath. PCV activates itself only if the preset pressure is not reached by the patient's own efforts. It is technically referred to as a series of ventilations that are time-triggered, time-cycled, and pressure-limited. PSV and PCV are ideally used when low airway pressure is required, as in patients with a pneumothorax, and when there are concerns of barotraumas.

CONTINUOUS POSITIVE AIRWAY PRESSURE

CPAP/BiPAP are commonly used as a spontaneous breathing trial (SBT) to reduce the need of or liberate a patient from MV. In CPAP, there is a continuous pressure so that each inspiration is assisted by a preset amount of pressure. Since CPAP is continuous, it acts as PEEP during exhalation. Ventilation on CPAP occurs on spontaneous breaths by the patient. No preset mechanical breaths occur, which leads to more patient comfort and a decreased need for sedation.

AIRWAY PRESSURE RELEASE VENTILATION

Airway pressure release ventilation (APRV) is another form of MV that allows patients to breathe spontaneously over intermittent and variable levels of CPAP. APRV may be thought of as alternating levels of CPAP with or without pressure support. APRV allows patients to breathe spontaneously over intermittent and alternating levels of CPAP. These alternating levels of CPAP are called P_{high} and P_{low}; the higher level (P_{high}) is a recruiting maneuver, and an alternating lower set pressure (P_{low}), or PEEP, maintains patency of the recruited airways. In an APRV, the inspiratory cycle is set by the length of the inspiratory time. For example, a cycle time of 6 seconds = RR of 10 breaths/minute (60 sec/6 sec = 10 cycles). *APRV works best at respiratory rates of <15 breaths/min, preferably near 12 breaths/min or less.* Alveoli are recruited, preventing their collapse, by the continuous pressure set and maintained by APRV.

JET VENTILATION AND HIGH-FREQUENCY VENTILATION

Jet ventilation is rarely used in routine practice. Bronchopleural fistula is one condition in which high-frequency ventilation (HFOV) may assist healing by having low inflation pressures. For HFOV, *the patient must be temporarily paralyzed since oxygenation is controlled by diffusion and CO_2 by ventilation.* The use of paralytic agents had significant neurological sequelae in patients who eventually recovered. A small V_t is delivered at very high respiratory rates in the range of 180 to 600 breaths/min. The HFOV or jet ventilation is an alternative mode of MV that protects the lungs. Most clinical trials on HFOV have been performed on neonates. Awareness of the injurious effects of mechanical ventilation has led to a renewed interest and advances in using **HFOV in adult ALI/ARDS patients. HFOV is characterized by rapid oscillations** of a diaphragm (at frequencies of 3-10 Hz, ie, 180-600 breaths/min) driven by a piston pump.

The pressure swings become more attenuated as they move distally from the airways to the alveoli, resulting in a very small V_t. Use of HFOV in inhalation injuries has been an effective treatment. Alsaghir and colleagues demonstrated that placing the patient in the prone position may improve oxygenation and reduce mortality in patients with ARDS or more severe illnesses. Notably, the prone position makes nursing care much more difficult.

VOLUMETRIC DIFFUSIVE RESPIRATION

Volumetric diffusive respiration (VDR), a form of **high-frequency ventilation,** is very effective in cystic fibrosis and smoke inhalation patients due to the copious secretions.

VDR requires a high degree of respiratory therapy education and time. VDR acts as a high-frequency percussive ventilator, enabling the ability to clear copious secretions.

SEDATION AND OTHER RELATED MV ISSUES

In order to reduce potential complications in MV patients, a series of steps can be taken which may be referred to as the "ventilator bundle." This includes **elevation of the head of the bed at 45 degrees, daily sedative interruption, deep vein thrombosis (DVT) and GI hemorrhage prophylaxis, and a daily readiness assessment with a spontaneous breathing trial.** The major goal of sedation in MV is to control anxiety and provide better coordination between the patients' own breathing efforts and the MV. Propofol is a frequently used agent for this purpose. Propofol is a short-acting, *intravenously* administered *hypnotic* agent. Its uses include induction and maintenance of *general anesthesia*, sedation for *mechanically ventilated* adults, and *sedation for procedures*. It is an extremely short-acting agent, which often causes vasodilation with hypotension; the hypotension usually responds to increased fluids or discontinuation of the drug. *In critically ill patients, propofol is superior to lorazepam both in effectiveness and overall cost.* Propofol is a favorite agent of neurologists and neurosurgeons; it decreases intracranial pressure and is cleared rapidly, enabling quick evaluation of the patient's mental status merely by discontinuing infusion. *It has no analgesic properties.*

A **propofol syndrome** has been described in about 1% of patients, consisting of **rhabdomyolysis and metabolic acidosis.** Propofol produces sedation first without causing respiratory depression until higher doses are reached; this makes MV easier to deliver. Paralytic agents should be avoided unless absolutely necessary because of their frequent neurological sequelae.

Acid suppression with a proton pump inhibitor (PPI) or H_2 antagonist is recommended to prevent GI bleeding from gastric sources; the main drawback is bacterial overgrowth because of the acid suppression, leading to aspiration pneumonia with potentially antibiotic-resistant pathogens. H_2 antagonists may have an advantage over PPI in this instance. **DVT prophylaxis** is standard practice in patients expected to have a prolonged hospital stay. As MV patients tend to fall in this category, it is important to consider treating those predisposed to DVT formation prophylactically. The **daily readiness assessment** is used to determine if the patient is ready to be weaned off of mechanical ventilation.

The dose and delivery of aerosolized medications such as β_2 agonist and ipratropium bromide should be doubled above the standard dose (2 U dose vials) for MV patients with an ETT. The ETT increases the area of aerosol deposition, thus requiring larger volume of medication to reach the airways. 90% of the volume of aerosolized medications remains in the tubing of the aerosol delivery equipment.

CLINICAL CASE CORRELATION

- See also Case 8 (Airway Management), Case 10 (Respiratory Weaning), Case 11 (Asthmatic Management), and Case 12 (Non-invasive Methods of Ventilatory Support).

COMPREHENSION QUESTIONS

9.1 A septic patient in the ICU with ARDS and severe hypoxia on 90% FIO_2 is in respiratory distress requiring low-volume ventilation. The chest x-ray shows bilateral infiltrates with a normal heart size, a typical x-ray presentation in ARDS. The patient's ideal body weight is 80 kg. Initially, what amount of tidal volume should be used for the mechanical ventilator in this patient?

A. 750 mL

B. 480 mL

C. 300 mL

D. 550 mL

E. 250 mL

9.2 A 67-year-old woman with advanced lung disease is in respiratory distress in the ICU. Rapid sequence intubation and mechanical ventilation is started. The mechanical ventilator's current settings are a rate of 20 breaths/min, V_t of 800 mL, a PEEP of 5 mm Hg, PS of 10 mm Hg, and an FIO_2 of 40%. On ABG, the pH is noted to be 7.53. Which of the following actions can you take to avoid worsening the patient's alkalemia?

A. Increase PEEP

B. Increase the rate

C. Increase the V_t

D. Choose pressure support with synchronized intermittent mandatory ventilation (SIMV)

E. Choose assist control ventilation (ACV)

ANSWERS

9.1 **B.** Previously, it was thought that tidal volumes (V_t) of 10 to 15 mL/kg were required to prevent atelectasis during MV; however, these higher volumes are no longer used. The Surviving Sepsis Guidelines recommend a strategy of low-volume ventilation using a V_t of 6 to 8 mL/kg with a plateau pressure <30 mm Hg H_2O. This method is referred to as low-volume ventilation and is very effective in supporting patients with sepsis and ARDS. The best initial V_t is approximately 480 mL, using 6 mL/kg. The arterial pH should be kept at 7.20 or higher. Bicarbonate treatment should only be considered when the pH is below 7.20. This low-volume ventilation method is effective in preventing and treating ARDS. Sedation will be needed for patient comfort with this method.

9.2 **D.** In ACV mode, breaths are delivered at a preset rate and tidal volume. The ventilator delivers breaths regardless of spontaneous breathing by the patient, potentially leading to increased ventilation and an acute respiratory alkalosis. To prevent this, AC should be avoided, and an alternate patient-driven MV mode should be chosen as soon as possible and the patient is stable. PSV with or without SIMV acts as an assist device that allows the patient to establish the V_t and respiratory rate at levels which are most comfortable. This mode delivers maximum patient comfort and thus requires the least amount of sedation.

CLINICAL PEARLS

▶ Low-volume ventilation is the key in patients with ARDS to prevent alveolar barotrauma.

▶ PEEP can prevent the collapse of small airways and alveoli by increasing alveolar recruitment.

▶ Ventilated patients benefit from a MV "bundle" of orders aimed at reducing complications.

▶ PSV increases patient comfort, as well as resistance to spontaneous respiration by patient, and also helps reduce the need for sedation.

▶ PSV is also helpful when used as a bridge of support post-ETT.

▶ Avoid neuromuscular blockade since it is associated with long-term neurological defects.

▶ Do not change the plastic circuitry of MV unless needed. Unnecessary changing of tubing increases the rate of infection.

▶ The use of artificial noses for humidification in MV circuitry reduces the risk of waterborne respiratory infections compared with the use of in-line humidifiers.

▶ Volumetric diffusive percussive respiration (VDR) enables clearance of copious secretions in patients with smoke inhalation and patients with cystic fibrosis.

▶ Respiratory acidosis, hypoxemia, and fatigue are indications for intubation and mechanical ventilation in patients with an acute exacerbation of asthma.

REFERENCES

Alsaghir Ah, Martin CM. Effect of prone positioning in patients with acute respiratory distress syndrome: a meta-analysis. *Crit Care Med.* 2008;36(2):603-609.

Gomella LG, Haist SA. *Clinician's Pocket Reference.* 11th ed. New York, NY: McGraw-Hill Education; 2007; Figure 20-20.

Loscalzo J. *Harrison's Pulmonary and Critical Care Medicine.* New York, NY: McGraw-Hill; 2013.

Malhotra A. Clinical therapeutics, low-tidal-volume ventilation in the acute respiratory distress syndrome. *N Engl J Med.* 2007;357:1113-1120.

A 56-year-old, 70 kg man with a history of HIV presents with pneumocystis pneumonia requiring intubation. On ICU day five he is still on mechanical ventilation, and his oxygen saturation is now 92% on Fio_2 of 30% on pressure support (PS) of 10 cm H_2O. He has a spontaneous respirations of 14 breaths/ minute and a positive end expiratory pressure (PEEP) of 5 cm H_2O. He demonstrates spontaneous respiratory efforts of an average tidal volume of 450 mL and a negative inspiratory pressure of –30 cm H_2O. An arterial blood gas (ABG) shows pH of 7.40, $Paco_2$ 38 mm Hg, and a Pao_2 of 100 mm Hg. His vitals are within normal limits, and the patient has remained afebrile with a normal white cell count for the past 2 days. On physical examination the patient responds appropriately to questions by shaking his head. Upon auscultation, he demonstrates bilateral air movement throughout. Chest radiographs demonstrate clearance of upper lobe pulmonary infiltrate present on admission x-ray.

▶ What is the next best step in management?
▶ Can the patient be liberated from the mechanical ventilator?

ANSWERS TO CASE 10:

Respiratory Weaning

Summary: This 56-year-old man has significantly improved from his pneumonia and respiratory failure. His spontaneous respiratory efforts point to a successful extubation. Mechanical ventilation (MV) is no longer needed and should be removed. After conducting a successful spontaneous breathing trial (SBT), the patient should be liberated from MV.

- **Next best management step:** A spontaneous breathing trial should be performed since the weaning parameters are acceptable. If the SBT is successful, the next step would be extubation and liberation from MV.

- **Liberation from mechanical ventilation: The patient can come off the ventilator depending on certain criteria.** The patient should be prepared for the extubation process by elevating the head of the bed to minimize aspiration risk. He should be closely monitored postextubation; difficult cases can be extubated to BiPAP as a bridge to unassisted spontaneous breathing. It is important to clinically assess vital signs to make sure they are stable and to ensure that the patient maintains adequate mentation, has minimal secretions, and has an adequate cough.

ANALYSIS

Objectives

1. To understand the clinical and the objective parameters that predict a successful liberation from mechanical ventilation.

2. To understand the predictors of weaning failure.

3. To understand a logical approach to weaning.

Considerations

This 56-year-old man with pneumocystis pneumonia required intubation for respiratory failure and was treated for 5 days in the ICU. The patient is generally alert and responsive. Weaning parameters are favorable, with a Pao_2 of 60 mm Hg or greater, an Fio_2 <60%, and a PEEP <5 mm H_2O present. When the MV patient reaches these criteria, it is safe to proceed to spontaneous breathing trials; if these trials are successful, the next step is extubation and liberation from MV. Pressure support ventilation (PSV) or continuous positive airway pressure (CPAP) would be the best way to wean this patient. Many patients are still extubated successfully with mixed criteria. Post extubation patients should be watched closely for signs of early deterioration.

APPROACH TO:
Respiratory Weaning

DEFINITIONS

BiPAP (bilevel positive airway pressure): A noninvasive form of ventilation in which the upper airways of the lungs are kept open by providing a flow of air through a face mask and a lower pressure upon exhalation is provided.

CPAP (Continuous positive airway pressure): A type of therapy that applies a small amount of positive pressure at all times to keep the airways and alveoli open.

Spontaneous breathing test (SBT): This is a temporary cessation of mechanical ventilation while the patient remains intubated, usually with a T tube in place to assess for safety of extubation.

INTRODUCTION

Appropriate care of the ventilated patient is imperative to accelerate extubation and prevent infections. While the patient is intubated, there are several interventions that may reduce infection. These include minimizing manipulation of an endotracheal tube and ventilator tubing and performing meticulous hand hygiene before and after any contact with the system. Furthermore, following weaning protocols can facilitate timely extubation and reduce the risk of infection, particularly the risk for ventilator-associated pneumonia (VAP). Patients should have daily "sedation vacations" and be assessed for extubation readiness. While intubated, patients should be in a semi-upright or upright position, as this decreases aspiration of upper airway secretions, and mouth care should be performed, as this may also reduce the risk of infection. Although ventilator circuits do not need to be changed regularly, any accumulating condensate should be drained carefully into a patient-specific drainage container. Continuous aspiration of subglottic secretions using a specially designed endotracheal tube attached to a suction device may reduce the risk for aspiration, but data for this procedure are inconclusive. Selective decontamination of the oropharynx (using topical gentamicin, colistin, or vancomycin) or of the entire gastrointestinal tract is controversial and not uniformly recommended.

Weaning or liberation from invasive or noninvasive mechanical ventilation is the process of freeing the patient from positive pressure mechanical ventilation (see Case 11 for more information on noninvasive mechanical ventilation [NIV]). Because of the significant morbidity and mortality associated with prolonged mechanical ventilation, it is generally accepted that all mechanically ventilated ICU patients should be assessed on a daily basis for their readiness to wean. This assessment should include the cessation of sedation and a reevaluation of its need. Weaning started after the first formal assessment of the patient's respiratory condition indicates that weaning could be successful. Nearly 50% of patients with unexpected self-extubation during the weaning process do not require reintubation. It is important to be aware of the frequency of weaning failures and predictors of such failures.

TABLE 10–1 • STEPS TO BE CONSIDERED FOR WEANING PROCESS	
1. Treatment of acute respiratory failure	4. A spontaneous breathing trial
2. Clinical judgment that weaning may be possible[*]	5. Extubation (BIPAP bridge)
3. Assessment of the readiness to wean[†]	6. Possible reintubation

[*]Usually requires Pao_2 > 60 mm Hg, an Fio_2 < 60 cm H_2O, and RR < 25/min
[†]f/V_t<105 (frequency/Tidal volume (L) = rapid shallow breathing index RSBI can assist)

APPROACH TO WEANING

Liberation from MV is a central component in the care of the critically ill patient. To start weaning a patient from MV, one must begin with a patient who is ready for the process and who has a good possibility of success (Table 10–1).

Underlying disease should be treated since its persistence can contribute to requiring continued MV. Successful weaning depends on many variables, including adequate mental status, muscle strength to maintain spontaneous breathing, and hemodynamic stability. Other questions to be answered before weaning include: "Are the ABG values acceptable?" and "Are electrolyte values normal, including Mg^+, K, Ca_2^+, and PO_4?" Additionally, adequate nutrition must be maintained. However, overfeeding should be avoided, especially with carbohydrates; increased CO_2 production may result and may require increased minute ventilation (Ve). Fatty meals are advised since fat produces more energy than carbohydrates (8 kcal for each gram of fat versus 4 kcal for every gram of carbohydrates) with much less CO_2 production. Some basic weaning goals should be attained: Pao_2 of 60 mm Hg or more with an Fio_2 <60% and a PEEP <5 cm H_2O. When the MV patient reaches these criteria, it is safe to proceed to spontaneous breathing trials and if successful, to move to extubation and liberation from MV.

WEANING PREDICTORS

Weaning is the progressive reduction in the amount of support provided by a mechanical ventilator. The term **weaning** is frequently used to describe the transition from intubation and full mechanical support to spontaneous breathing by the patient with a protected airway. Weaning predictors act as guidelines to identify those patients who qualify for spontaneous breathing trials and liberation from MV with successful extubation. These predictors are based on measurements of the work of breathing, that help determine whether the patient's respiratory system can adjust to spontaneous unassisted respiration.

A negative inspiratory force (NIF) greater than −25 cm H_2O is predictive of successful weaning from MV. This confirms that the patient's respiratory muscle strength is suitable and that the patient's own respiratory system is conditioned to breathe without MV support. Stable vital signs with an improving clinical picture **during the weaning process** is critical. Stable vital signs can be used to predict the stability of the ABG, reducing the need for repetitive ABG analyses. ABG studies are costly, painful, and not free of possible complications, including distal arterial occlusion or dissection of the artery. Achievement of a spontaneous minute ventilation

(V_e) <10 L/min (maintaining oxygenation without excessive work) is also an excellent predictor of successful liberation from MV.

WEANING TECHNIQUES

A successful trial of spontaneous breathing has become the gold standard for weaning. Every intubated patient on MV should be evaluated daily with a trial of some form of spontaneous breathing. A sedation holiday should also be attempted; if sedation is still required, it can be restarted at half the previous dose. The patient should be on a minimal sedation dose to avoid depression of respiratory functions. Trials of spontaneous breathing can be performed with or without MV assistance. Weaning trials with MV assistance increase the safety of the procedure since respiratory parameters are more precisely monitored and patient deterioration can be diagnosed earlier (Table 10-2). So-called traditional T-piece trial with $FIO_2\%$ delivery only via plastic tubing without the aid of MV gives a realistic evaluation of the patient's breathing without MV help or the resistance of MV sensor valves. Surveys of respiratory departments have shown that SIMV with or without PS assistance was the most common method of MV weaning. This was closely followed by T-piece trials and by PS weaning. Use of the rapid shallow breathing index RR/V_t of <105 as shown by Yang and Tobin has an excellent predictive value of extubation failure. Various weaning parameters are better predictors in specific diseases.

T-Piece Trials

T-piece trials are conducted in a spontaneously breathing patient via an ETT connected to an FIO_2 source (thus the T) with the open end of the FIO_2 hose open to ambient air. This method is the oldest and still most effective method of ventilator weaning techniques. Sequentially increasing the amount of time the patient spends on the T-piece will enhance the prospect of complete liberation from MV. A spontaneous breathing trial daily is as efficient and effective as multiple short trials and is less labor intensive. If needed, PEEP can always be added to the circuit by an expiratory valve or possibly be better accomplished with the patient breathing spontaneously on the MV with the desired PEEP level and a CPAP setting of 0 cm H_2O. These measures are not needed if the patient is on PEEP <5 cm H_2O. The FIO_2 source should be humidified, creating a mist at the open end of the T-piece. If this fine aerosol disappears completely during inspiration, the patient's inspiratory flow is overcoming the inspiratory FIO_2 flow and inhaling 21% room air via the open end of the tube. This circumstance causes a lower actual FIO_2 versus the set FIO_2, affecting the ABG values because of a decrease in FIO_2 reflected in the lower PaO_2.

Table 10–2 • APPROACH TO FAILURES OF THE SPONTANEOUS BREATHING TEST
If the patient fails a spontaneous breathing test, the clinician should:
(1) Address all contributory causes of failure to wean
(2) Not perform or repeat a spontaneous breathing trial for 24 h
(3) Support the patient with a nonfatiguing mode of ventilation (most commonly PSV)
(4) Consider NIV, if appropriate
(5) Consider tracheostomy

Noninvasive Ventilation

Noninvasive ventilation (NIV) is a useful tool in the difficult-to-wean patient. It avoids the complications of intubation and sedation and reduces the total time of invasive MV. The goal of NIV in weaning can be separated into two parts: to prevent extubation failure and to provide a rescue therapy for postextubation respiratory distress. NIV permits early extubation in patients who fail to meet standard extubation criteria.

Pressure Support Ventilation Weaning

Pressure support ventilation (PSV) allows the patient to determine the most comfortable depth, length, flow, and rate of breathing. It is used as a weaning tool by gradually reducing pressure support by 2 to 4 cm H_2O as long as the patient is successfully tolerating these decreases. This results in a progressive reduction in ventilatory support over hours or days. PSV is superior to SIMV in reducing the duration of mechanical ventilation in difficult-to-wean patients. PSV weaning compared to T-piece weaning revealed T-piece weaning to be superior. However, one small prospective trial has recently suggested that PSV weaning is superior to T-piece weaning in patients with chronic obstructive pulmonary disease (COPD).

Intermittent Mandatory Volume Weaning

SIMV is a poor weaning mode (unless associated with PS) and should not be used in isolation as a weaning tool. SIMV with PS weaning involves a progressive reduction of the respiratory rate in steps of 1 to 3 breaths/minute. SIMV may actually contribute to respiratory muscle fatigue because of the increased work of breathing due to ventilator factors (increased effort to activate the SIMV demand valve, inspiratory and expiratory dyssynchrony). SIMV with T-piece spontaneous breathing resulted in a longer duration of MV compared to PSV. SIMV had higher rates of weaning failure. SIMV-based weaning strategies resulted in a longer duration of MV (5 days) compared with a PSV-based strategy (4 days) and T-piece ventilation (3 days).

The Endotracheal Tube

The largest endotracheal tube (ETT) that can be safely inserted should be used (≥ 8 mm). A larger caliber facilitates the removal of secretions by suction catheter and decreases in airflow resistance. Reducing high plateau pressures to <30 cm H_2O with V_t volumes of 6 to 8 mL/kg will avoid barotrauma. **The mere presence of an ETT in the trachea can induce significant bronchospasm.** This is often noticed in the operative room postintubation. The presence of the ETT may cause bronchospasm or "rock bag" ventilation, as it is sometimes described when this occurs during the anesthetic period. The administration of IV lidocaine prior to intubation may prevent ETT-associated bronchospasm. Intravenous corticosteroids may be used even though most volatile anesthetics are excellent bronchodilators. Additionally, aerosolized β_2 agonists may also be used; these are easily delivered to the patient.

Role of Tracheostomy in Weaning

Tracheostomies can be important in weaning difficult patients. **A tracheostomy is usually far less irritating to the patient than an endotracheal tube, and the reduced need for sedation usually facilitates weaning.** Tracheostomy provides a secure airway, which reduces the work of breathing and minimizes the risk of pneumonia associated with MV (ventilator-associated pneumonia [VAP]). Studies have not determined whether early or late tracheostomy is superior.

MANAGEMENT OF THE DIFFICULT TO WEAN PATIENT

A difficult-to-wean patient is defined as one who has already failed at least one spontaneous breathing trial or has required reintubation within 48 hours of extubation. The failure of a spontaneous breathing trial may be accompanied by a significantly increased inspiratory effort with respiratory muscle fatigue. This may induce short-lasting, high-frequency fatigue. Failure of either a spontaneous breathing trial or extubation demands an identification of the exacerbating factors that caused the failure. Adjustments must be made that will increase the success of weaning and provide adequate ventilatory support. The clinician should conduct a careful physical examination and review the patient's diagnostic tests to uncover and treat any reversible contributory factors leading to weaning failure.

The most widely used modes of ventilation are assist control ventilation (ACV), synchronized intermittent mechanical ventilation (SIMV), and pressure support ventilation (PSV). One classification system divides ICU patients into those simple to wean and those difficult to wean (also called prolonged weaning) groups.

- **Simple-to-wean patients** are those who are successfully extubated on the first attempt. This group consists of approximately 70% of intubated patients in the ICU, and they have a low mortality rate (about 5%).

- The **difficult-to-wean or prolonged-weaning patients** (requiring up to three attempts or up to 7 days from the onset of weaning efforts) require greater efforts for successful liberation from mechanical ventilation.

These difficult-to-wean, or prolonged-weaning patients, have a mortality rate of 25%. Longer duration of MV is associated with an increased mortality and expense (mechanical ventilation costs more than $2000/d), and it has been estimated that the 6% of patients who require prolonged MV consume 37% of ICU resources. More severely ill patients usually require longer periods of MV. Overall, 40% to 50% of the time spent on mechanical ventilation occurs after the weaning process has started. Most critically ill patients require a period of rest after intubation. The weaning process should begin very soon after intubation.

Reintubation rates are higher in patients with advanced age, pre-existing comorbidities such as chronic respiratory and cardiovascular disorders, and severe illnesses. Studies have shown reintubation to be associated with a high mortality rate.

WEANING PROTOCOLS

A lack of attention to the screening process to determine the ability of a patient to pass through the weaning process or unnecessary delays in progression through the weaning steps are associated with increased patient morbidity and mortality. The proper use of weaning protocols has reduced ventilator-associated pneumonia, lowered self-extubation rates, lowered tracheostomy rates, and minimized hospital costs. To be effective, these weaning protocols should include an interdisciplinary team approach with nursing and respiratory therapy personnel in association with physicians, all of whom are experienced in the use of MV and weaning procedures.

> ## CLINICAL CASE CORRELATION
>
> - See also Case 8 (Airway Management/Respiratory Failure), Case 9 (Ventilator Management), Case 11 (Asthmatic Management), and Case 12 (Non-invasive Methods of Ventilatory Support).

COMPREHENSION QUESTIONS

10.1 You are called to assess a 39-year-old, 60 kg woman who is on day 2 in the ICU on mechanical ventilation for acute respiratory distress (ARDS) secondary to pancreatitis. This morning her ABG values with sedation are: pH 7.33, $Paco_2$ 55 mm Hg and PaO_2 91 mm Hg on assist control (AC) with settings of tidal volume of 500 mm Hg, FIO_2 60%, respiratory rate of 13 breaths/min, and a positive end-expiratory pressure (PEEP) of 8 cm H_2O and plateau pressure of 40 cm H_2O. What is the next best step in management of this patient?

A. Increase respiratory rate and increase tidal volume

B. Change to noninvasive positive pressure ventilation

C. Switch to low tidal volume ventilation with plateau pressure <30 cm H_2O

D. Increase PEEP to 10 cm H_2O

E. Stop mechanical ventilation and place patient on O_2 nasal cannula

10.2 An 88-year-old man has been on mechanical ventilation for 2 days. He has been suffering from respiratory failure secondary to a COPD exacerbation. Today the patient's ABG shows pH 7.38, $Paco_2$ 38 mm Hg and PaO_2 100 mm Hg on CPAP mode of 5 H_2O, PEEP of 5 cm H_2O, tidal volume of 450 mL, and FIO_2 of 25%. The patient is alert and awake. His spontaneous weaning parameters are a negative inspiratory force (NIF) of −35 cm H_2O, respiratory rate of 17 breaths/min, and tidal volume of 400 mL. You decide to extubate the patient because he meets the criteria for weaning. However, as soon as the patient is extubated he becomes hypotensive and hemodynamically unstable. What's the next best step?

A. Leave the patient intubated and give him a vasopressor

B. Leave the patient intubated and give him an aerosol treatment

C. Leave the patient intubated on present settings

D. Put patient on noninvasive ventilation

E. Leave the patient extubated and wait for 30 minutes

ANSWERS

10.1 **C.** This patient does not meet the criteria to wean from the ventilator, as her F_{IO_2} is 60%, her PEEP is not below 5, and her ABG indicates a level of acidosis. Her MV settings should be adjusted to comply with low tidal volume ventilation with a goal plateau pressure of 30 cm H_2O or less.

10.2 **D.** This patient meets the criteria to wean or liberate from MV since his numbers and his clinical presentation of mentation are acceptable. The improving clinical status indicates a key fulfillment of weaning parameters. Good weaning parameters tend to be positive predictors of successful extubation. This patient, though he meets the criteria to wean, develops hemodynamic instability post-extubation. In some patients with advanced age, pre-existing comorbidities such as chronic respiratory and cardiovascular disorders, and severe illnesses, reintubation rates are higher. Studies have shown reintubation to be associated with a high mortality rate. Patients at risk for reintubation, such as this 88-year-old man with COPD, can benefit from noninvasive ventilation after extubation as a bridge.

CLINICAL PEARLS

▶ Pressure support ventilation (PSV) is the simplest and most effective method of weaning patients from MV.

▶ Weaning increases the patient's respiratory effort and increases myocardial oxygen (O_2) demand, making it a cardiopulmonary stress test.

▶ Assessment of the readiness to wean and reductions in sedative infusions should be considered early and frequently in critically ill patients receiving mechanical ventilation.

▶ After the acute insult has improved or resolved, clinicians should have a low threshold for conducting a spontaneous breathing trial in all critically ill patients.

▶ A V_d/V_t ratio of >105 is an excellent predictor of weaning success, especially when combined with an NIF exceeding −25 cm H_2O and a stable clinical picture.

▶ Weaning protocols are not a replacement for expert clinical opinion and management.

REFERENCES

Brochard L. Pressure support is the preferred weaning method. Paper presented at the 5th International Consensus Conference in Intensive Care Medicine: Weaning from Mechanical Ventilation. 2005 April 28-29.

Loscalzo J. *Harrison's Pulmonary and Critical Care Medicine.* New York, NY: McGraw-Hill; 2013.

A 45-year-old man is admitted to the ICU for acute onset dyspnea, wheezing, and severe respiratory distress. The patient had a previous admission that required intubation. His medications include a high-dose inhaled corticosteroid salmeterol combination and albuterol as needed. He has not responded to aggressive bronchodilation therapy and intravenous corticosteroids in the ICU. He is in marked distress and is anxious. Temperature is 37.0°C (99.6°F), blood pressure is 150/95 mm Hg, pulse rate is 130 beats/min, and respiration rate is 30 breaths/min; Body Mass Index (BMI) is 35. Cardiac examination reveals a rapid and regular rhythm with no murmurs. Pulmonary examination reveals a quiet chest. Chest radiograph shows hyperinflation but no infiltrates. The patient undergoes rapid sequence induction and intubation and is started on mechanical ventilation (MV). Arterial blood gas (ABG) values are as follows.

Arterial Blood Gas Studies (Normal Reference Range)			
pH	7.28 (7.35-7.45)	Pao_2 / Fio_2 ratio	80 (> 350)
$Paco_2$	50 mm Hg (36-45 mm Hg)	HCO_3	26 (22-26 mEq/L)
Pao_2	80 mm Hg (> 80 mm Hg)	Hemoglobin	18.0 g/dL (13.8-17.2 g/dL)
Fio_2	100% with PEEP 5		

► What is the most important next step in the management of this patient?
► What other treatment options should be undertaken simultaneously?
► What additional predictors indicate a high likelihood of intubation?

ANSWERS TO CASE 11:
Asthmatic Exacerbation

Summary: A 45-year-old man with a severe asthma exacerbation requiring intubation and MV is admitted to the ICU. A patient on asthmatic rescue medications without improvement and a prior history of an ICU admission with MV are important risk factors for developing status asthmaticus. Aside from tachypnea, there is an ominous sign of a quiet chest on physical examination. A quiet chest indicates that the patient may have a very severe airway obstruction or is so fatigued that he is unable to generate enough airflow to wheeze. This patient's severe respiratory distress is confirmed with an ABG showing an acute respiratory acidosis.

- **Most important next management step:** Rapid-sequence intubation (RSI) and mechanical ventilation.

- **Other treatment options:** High dose and frequent use of aerosolized bronchodilators with albuterol and ipratropium bromide. IV corticosteroids and magnesium infusion should be started. Low-volume mechanical ventilation is likely ideal. Sedation should be used for anxiety, improving coordination with MV, and decreasing the compliance of the chest wall.

- **Predictors of high likelihood of intubation:** Prior severe asthmatic episode requiring intubation, quiet chest, overuse of rescue agents, frequent nighttime exacerbations, and respiratory acidosis.

ANALYSIS

Objectives

1. To understand the pathophysiology of an acute asthma exacerbation.

2. To describe the classical findings and their correlation with an exacerbation of acute asthma.

3. To understand the correct stepwise treatment of an acute exacerbation of asthma.

Considerations

This patient has a severe airflow obstruction caused by status asthmaticus and should be managed quickly with MV. The mechanical ventilation settings should be set with parameters for a prolonged expiratory time and low tidal volumes at 6 mL/kg. Ventilation in patients with severe airway obstruction may result in breath stacking and auto–positive end-expiratory pressure (auto-PEEP) when the preceding breath is unable to be completely emptied. The goal is to maximize ventilation by allowing adequate time for exhalation and to avoid increasing auto-PEEP. Increased auto-PEEP will result in increases in end-expiratory pressures, decreased venous return, hypotension, and barotrauma. Strategies that increase expiratory time include decreasing the tidal volume and respiration rate, increasing inspiratory flow rates, and judicious use of sedation and analgesia. Clinical suspicion of hemodynamic compromise caused by auto-PEEP can be immediately diagnosed and treated by disconnecting the ventilatory circuit at the endotracheal tube. This will allow trapped intrathoracic air and pressure to escape, causing the venous return to improve by allowing passive hypercapnia. Attempts to increase minute ventilation (through increases in respiration rate and/or tidal volume) increase the risk for development of auto-PEEP and hemodynamic compromise. A large-bore (≥ 8 mm) endotracheal tube (ETT) should be used to facilitate the suctioning of secretions and to decrease resistance to airflow during MV of asthmatic patients. Bronchodilator agents, corticosteroids, and magnesium sulfate should be started immediately. Noninvasive ventilation (NIV) would be useful in more stable patients.

APPROACH TO:
Asthmatic Patient

Overall, the national asthma prevalence rate is 10% and has risen by 61% in the last 20 years. Patients are predisposed to severe exacerbations from many different sources: allergens, exercise, infections (both viral and bacterial), cold air, emotional stress, gastroesophageal reflux (GERD), sinusitis, and postnasal drip. Asthma accounts for about 2 million ED visits, 500,000 admissions, and 5000 deaths per year in the United States, and it is the third leading cause of preventable admission. Asthma is responsible for 10 million lost school days each year, at a cost of >$12 billion/y. The mortality from asthma has not decreased over the last 20 years, even with advancements in treatment. The underlying cause of asthma still remains unknown. However, it is known that an inflammatory process leads to airway obstruction, increased mucus production, and smooth muscle hypertrophy; these changes lead to airway narrowing and airflow obstruction during the expiratory phase. If uncontrolled, airway remodeling and irreversible airway obstruction develops. The early and late phases of an allergic response contribute to airway inflammation and increased mucus production. The **early-phase response**, occurring within 1 hour of allergen exposure, is marked by histamines and other mediators released and allergic symptoms such as sneezing, itchy eyes, runny nose, and respiratory symptoms such as wheezing, coughing, and shortness of breath. The **late-phase response**, occurring 3 to 10 hours after exposure, can last for as long as 24 hours and prolongs the asthma attack and results in more severe congestion and inflammation. There is still evidence of inflammation of the airways 6 months after an acute attack, even with successful treatment. Patients with vocal cord dysfunction (VCD) have inspiratory and expiratory wheezing, respiratory distress, and anxiety. During attacks, VCD can be difficult to distinguish from asthma. Potential clues that suggest VCD include sudden onset and abrupt termination of the attacks, lack of response to asthma therapy, prominent neck discomfort, lack of hypoxemia, lack of hyperinflation on chest radiography and immediate relief of wheezing and bronchospasm upon intubation.

ICU admissions for refractory asthma range from 2% to 20%, affected somewhat by adherence to best practice protocols. When protocol therapies are used, ICU admissions fall by 41%; in contrast, when a new group of physicians assumes responsibilities for the ED or ICU, admissions generally increase. Aggressive bronchodilation with inhaled short-acting β_2-adrenergic agonists (SABA), such as albuterol and recently added ipratropium bromide, are indicated. They can be given either in high-volume aerosolized form or via frequent aerosol treatments. IV corticosteroids are also used for the relief of inflammation and bronchodilation. Steroids increase the number of β_2 receptor sites available, thereby enhancing the effectiveness of β_2 agonists and avoiding tachyphylaxis to these agents. **Aerosol treatments in intubated patients should be with double the amount normally recommended; this overcomes the increased deposition in the ETT.** Sedation with IV propofol via intermittent IV bolus as needed dosing is recommended rather than continuous infusion; this protocol enables patients to be comfortable and reduces the ventilator pressure needed. Propofol causes relaxation of the respiratory muscles, increasing the compliance of the chest wall; it also decreases cardiac output and causes vasodilation, which can lower the BP. This requires increased fluid administration. The use of safe pressures for MV may require an acceptance of a passive hypercapnia. Sedation helps the patient tolerate the feeling of the elevated $Paco_2$. Intravenous magnesium sulfate may also help in relaxing the airways. In order to avoid barotrauma and pneumothorax, it is necessary to pay careful attention to MV and ventilate the patient with safe airways pressures. Low-volume MV with a tidal volume (V_t) of 6 to 8 mL/kg of ideal body weight is needed to avoid unsafe high pressures. The pH should be maintained above 7.20, regardless of the $Paco_2$ level, as long as there is no hypoxia.

RISK FACTORS

Attention should be paid to factors associated with an increased risk of death from asthma, such as previous intubation or admission to an ICU, two or more hospitalizations for asthma during the past year, low socioeconomic status, and various coexisting illnesses.

MANAGEMENT

All patients should be treated with inhaled SABAs, systemic corticosteroids, and oxygen to achieve an arterial O_2 sat exceeding 90%. High-dose ipratropium bromide given in combination with SABAs has shown to **increase** bronchodilation.

Oxygen, Compressed Air, and Heliox

Oxygen should be administered. Patients with chronic severe asthma and chronic hypercarbia should be carefully monitored since excessive oxygen may lead to increasing hypercarbia due to hypoventilation. The **elbow of the oxyhemoglobin dissociation curve lies at 90% saturation, equivalent to a Pao_2 of 60 mm Hg. Small decreases below this point lead to a dramatic fall in oxygen delivery. High PEEP, which is already increased intrinsically because of the reduced expiratory time, should be avoided.** Heliox, which is a mixture of helium and oxygen with a density about one-third that of air, can also be used to reduce airflow resistance in the bronchial tree where turbulent flow predominates. **Heliox reduces airway flow resistance,** eases the work of breathing, and improves the delivery of aerosolized medications. A heliox mixture can be used in severe cases. Heliox may affect digital readouts in MV calibrated for oxygen, and these readouts may not be correct.

Adrenergic Agents

SABAs should be administered immediately to a patient with an asthmatic exacerbation. The administration of SABAs can be repeated up to three times every 20 minutes via aerosols or high-volume continuous nebulizer treatment. Rescue inhaler use of a SABA agent, such as albuterol, is the drug of choice. Levalbuterol, the R-isomer of albuterol, is effective at half the dose of albuterol, but trials have not consistently shown an advantage over racemic albuterol. Continuous high-dose inhalation of SABAs for acute rescue bronchodilation with the addition of ipratropium bromide provides a second but different short-acting bronchodilator option. Should the patient need intubation, doubling the normal recommended dose of inhaled albuterol and ipratropium is advised because of the increased deposition of these drugs in the ETT. Oral or parenteral administration of β_2-adrenergic agonists is not recommended and is associated with an increased frequency of side effects. In severe cases, parenteral use of a β_2 agonist such as epinephrine (1/1000 solution) subcutaneously (SC) can be used with as many as three doses every 20 minutes apart. This is generally reserved for younger patients with severe anaphylaxis with upper airway obstruction. Brethine in SC form or epinephrine IV may have a better side effect profile in these cases.

Anticholinergic Agents

When added to an inhaled β_2-adrenergic agonist, **ipratropium bromide** improved symptoms and lung function equivalent to the addition of salmeterol, a long-acting inhaled β_2-adrenergic agonist (LABA). In poorly controlled asthmatics, the addition of tiotropium in once-a-day metered dose inhaler (MDI) form was superior to doubling of the dose of an inhaled glucocorticoid and was equivalent to the addition of inhaled salmeterol, a LABA. Ipratropium or tiotropium added to a SABA caused a greater and longer lasting bronchodilator effect. The use of ipratropium together with a SABA in severe airflow obstruction, compared with a SABA alone, reduced the rate of hospitalization by 25%.

Glucocorticoids

Systemic corticosteroids are a **cornerstone** to successful treatment of most individuals with asthmatic exacerbations. Their use is associated with a faster improvement in lung function, fewer hospitalizations, and a lower rate of relapse after ED discharge. Although the optimal dose of corticosteroids is unknown, clinical trials have shown no added efficacy in doses of prednisolone exceeding 100 mg/d. The most recent guidelines recommend the use of 40 to 80 mg of prednisolone each day in the morning for 5 to 7 days.

Inhaled Corticosteroids, Hydration

Evidence does not support the use of inhaled corticosteroids (ICS) for acute exacerbations of asthma. Dehydration should be avoided, but **aggressive hydration or mucolytic agents are not recommended in asthmatic exacerbations.** Autopsy of asthmatics show impacted mucous in the airways. Elevation of the head of the bed at 45 degree is important to prevent aspiration pneumonia and ventilator-associated pneumonia (VAP).

Leukotriene Antagonists

The efficacy of leukotriene antagonists (LTAs) in the acute setting is unclear. They are excellent agents with a favorable safe side effect profile in moderate and mild cases of asthma. A 20% improvement in PFTs and PEFR, which is the same response expected due to the normal diurnal rhythm, may be accentuated in asthmatics. It should not be used alone without steroids since it improves symptoms but does not control underlying inflammation.

Magnesium

Magnesium (Mg$^+$) plays a role in neuromuscular function and is more effective in relieving **severe** asthmatic exacerbations than mild to moderate instances. **Magnesium decreases muscle constriction via competition with calcium and prevents acetylcholine release, thereby decreasing cyclic GMP.** Histamine release is also reduced. There is evidence that IV magnesium can induce bronchodilation and reduce the neutrophilic burst of the inflammatory response. The effects of IV magnesium are rapid, within 5 to 10 minutes, but the duration of action is also short. It has an excellent therapeutic-to-toxicity ratio at dosages of 2 to 4 grams per hour as a continuous IV drip, and it is widely used in asthmatics refractory to standard treatment. In **children, intravenous magnesium sulfate has been shown to significantly improve lung function and reduce rates of hospital admission.** A beneficial effect of nebulized magnesium sulfate is less substantiated.

Methylxathines and Antibiotics

Methylxanthines, once a standard treatment for asthma in the ED and ICU, are now rarely used because of their adverse effects (narrow therapeutic-to-toxic ratio) and lack of proven efficacy. These agents (theophylline, aminophylline) are no longer recommended for routine use. Theophylline is still used in the most severe cases where any improvement is welcome. The main side effects of methylxanthines include tachycardia, cardiac arrhythmias, and nausea and vomiting. Serum levels should be targeted to about 8 µg/dL since this level is associated with maximum bronchodilator effect and minimum side effects. Theophylline blocks the effect of adenosine and its effect on SVT.

Antimicrobial Agents

Antibiotics should not be used routinely but rather reserved for patients in whom a bacterial infection (eg, pneumonia or sinusitis) seems likely. The majority of asthmatic exacerbations are caused by viral infections, which can lead to a secondary bacterial superinfection. The antibiotic chosen should be based on the most likely pathogens as well as healthcare versus non healthcare exposure.

Volatile Anesthetics

Volatile anesthetics are potent bronchodilators. Conventional tests of airway resistance demonstrate little difference between halothane, isoflurane, or enflurane (Ethrane).

Halothane appeared to be a more potent bronchodilator than isoflurane. Endotracheal intubation (ETI) by itself can induce severe bronchospasm. Volatile anesthetics are useful in treating severe status asthmaticus when the patient is unresponsive to conventional treatments. **Isoflurane may be the most appropriate choice of volatile anesthetics due to its minimal depressive influence on cardiovascular and arrhythmogenic potential.** Increased cerebral flow, cerebral edema, and increased intracranial pressure may be associated with the use of volatile agents in hypercapnic patients who may have suffered a degree of hypoxic brain injury.

Other agents

Omalizumab is recommended for patients with severe asthma who have evidence of allergies, have an elevated IgE level, and remain symptomatic despite optimizing therapy with combination therapy of high-dose inhaled corticosteroids and a LABA. This therapy can be associated with serious anaphylactoid reactions and should only be begun by providers who are skilled at monitoring and treating these complications. Please refer to Case 12 on noninvasive ventilation.

Intubation and Mechanical Ventilation

The use of invasive ventilatory support can be lifesaving in patients with an asthmatic exacerbation. **About 30% (range 2%-70%) of such individuals admitted to the ICU require intubation.** The decision for mechanical ventilation (MV) is based on clinical judgment. **Progressive hypercapnia, deterioration of mental status, exhaustion, and impending cardiopulmonary arrest** strongly suggest the need for ventilatory support. Authorities agree that intubation should be considered before these signs develop. A physician who has experience with intubation and airway management should ideally be managing the MV. The high pressures encountered by MV should be mitigated with low tidal volumes of 6 to 8 mL/kg of ideal body weight and started in the assist control mode at a low rate of 8 to 10 breaths/min to avoid high plateau pressures and auto—positive end-expiratory pressure (auto-PEEP). Plateau pressures should be kept at <30 cm H_2O when possible to avoid barotrauma. Passive hypercapnia with a pH of 7.20 or greater may be needed to attain safe ventilation pressures. Sedation with short-acting agents like propofol will assist the patient in tolerating this treatment. Bicarbonate therapy should be reserved for patients with arterial pH lower than 7.20. Permissive hypercapnia is not uniformly effective, and consultation with or comanagement by physicians who have expertise in ventilator management is appropriate to avoid risks.

Quick access to chest tube placement in the case of pneumothorax should be available. Strategies to reduce auto-PEEP often result in hypoventilation. The ensuing hypercapnia, termed *permissive hypercapnia*, is well tolerated as long as it develops slowly and the carbon dioxide tension remains at 90 mm Hg or less. When necessary, the pH can be managed pharmacologically. Daily ABGs and chest x-rays should be performed. Sedation may be needed to keep the patient comfortable and breathing in synchrony with the MV. This can usually be achieved with benzodiazepines combined with opioids or propofol. **Ketamine is an attractive agent because of its bronchodilating properties; however, its CNS effects, tachycardia, and**

hypertension limit its use. Switching to CPAP with PSV when possible will help the patient tolerate MV via better coordination with the MV. Patients should be kept with the head of bed elevated at 45 degrees to avoid aspiration pneumonia and VAP. Auto-PEEP is a common problem in patients receiving full or partial ventilatory support, especially those needing high pressures for ventilation or having short expiratory times.

The clinician needs to understand fully the physiology of auto-PEEP to choose the appropriate ventilator settings. The recommended settings for initial ventilation are as follows: tidal volume of 6 to 8 mL/kg, respiratory rate of 11 to 14 breaths/min, flow rate of 100 L/min, and PEEP of 5. Allow the maximum possible time for exhalation by combining small tidal volumes with slow respiratory rates and short inspiratory times. Static end-inspiratory pressure (plateau pressure) levels of 30 cm H_2O or greater correlate with hyperinflation and auto-PEEP. Auto-PEEP rises directly with minute ventilation. The lungs and chest walls become less elastic, and work of breathing rises. Venous return, BP, and cardiac output fall. Paralyzing agents are associated with myopathy, which prolongs hospitalization by 1 day, and intubation increases this time to 4.5 days. Fatalities due to asthma in the ICU averaged 2.7%. In intubated patients, the rate rises to 8.1%. Deaths from acute exacerbations of asthma in general are reported in <0.5% of patients. Pulmonary lavage via flexible bronchoscope is used to remove mucous plugs frequently found in patients with severe asthma. This procedure carries some risk.

CONCLUSION

Physicians have proven to be poor judges of the severity of an asthma attack, and it is essential to use objective criteria when triaging a patient to an unmonitored bed versus an ICU bed. SABAs and early administration of systemic corticosteroids are the mainstays of treatment now, along with the additional benefit of an anticholinergic agent. When ventilatory support is needed, noninvasive ventilation can be attempted but must not delay intubation and MV. Status asthmaticus carries significant complications, including death. Any history of severe attacks, including those with the need for rapid sequence intubation (RSI) and MV, should raise a red flag and lead to observing the patient closely.

CLINICAL CASE CORRELATION

- See also Case 9 (Ventilator Management), Case 10 (Respiratory Weaning), and Case 12 (Noninvasive Methods of Ventilatory Support).

COMPREHENSION QUESTIONS

11.1 A 35-year-old woman is admitted in an ICU for an acute asthma exacerbation. She has a history of frequent asthma exacerbations that occur suddenly without warning symptoms and require unscheduled visits; however, between these exacerbations, her examination and pulmonary function studies have been unremarkable. Her current medications are inhaled budesonide and inhaled albuterol. On physical examination, she is in moderate distress with audible inspiratory and expiratory wheezing. Temperature is 37.0°C (98.6°F), pulse rate is 110 beats/min, and respiration rate is 26 breaths/min. Monophonic inspiratory and expiratory wheezing is heard predominantly in the central lung fields. Other than tachycardia, the cardiac examination and remainder of the physical examination are normal. She receives intravenous methylprednisolone and three nebulized albuterol-ipratropium bromide treatments. On follow-up evaluation one hour later, she still has wheezing, tachycardia, and tachypnea and is in moderate respiratory distress. Oxygen saturation is 96% breathing ambient air. Which of the following is the most appropriate next step in management?

A. A combination of aerosolized steroids and LABA

B. Intravenous (IV) corticosteroids

C. Laryngoscopy

D. Magnesium infusion

E. Ceftriaxone/Azithromycin

11.2 A 42-year-old man has had lifelong asthma with significant environmental allergies and frequent exacerbations. Over the past year he has had daily symptoms with frequent nighttime awakenings requiring the use of rescue therapy. His current medications are high-dose inhaled corticosteroids with a LABA and an as-needed SABA by metered-dose inhaler. He has required three extended courses of prednisone therapy for exacerbations over the past year. He is allergic to house dust mites, cats, molds, and trees. Allergen avoidance and desensitization have been attempted but have not been effective. Pulmonary examination discloses scattered wheezing. Laboratory studies reveal a leukocyte count of 8200/µL (8.2×10^9/L) with 8% eosinophils and an IgE level of 320 international units/mL (320 kilounits/L) (normal range, 0-90 international units/mL). Spirometry shows an FEV_1 of 65% of predicted. Chest radiograph is normal. Which of the following is the most appropriate treatment?

A. Azathioprine

B. Methotrexate

C. Omalizumab

D. Tumor necrosis factor α inhibitor

E. Corticosteroids

ANSWERS

11.1 **C.** The most appropriate next step in management is laryngoscopy. Patients with vocal cord dysfunction (VCD) have inspiratory and expiratory wheezing, respiratory distress, and anxiety. During attacks, VCD can be difficult to distinguish from asthma. Potential clues include sudden onset and abrupt termination of the attacks, lack of response to asthma therapy, prominent neck discomfort, lack of hypoxemia, and lack of hyperinflation on chest radiography. The distinction between the two conditions can be more difficult when patients have asthma as well as VCD. Laryngoscopy in symptomatic patients can reveal characteristic adduction of the vocal cords during inspiration. Recognizing VCD is essential to avoid treating patients with repeat courses of systemic corticosteroids and other therapies for severe asthma while delaying the start of therapies targeted at VCD. These include speech therapy, relaxation techniques, and treatment of underlying causes such as anxiety, postnasal drip, and gastroesophageal reflux. Intravenous magnesium sulfate can be considered in acute asthma exacerbations, but it has no role in treating VCD.

11.2 **C.** The most appropriate treatment is to initiate omalizumab. This patient has severe asthma that appears to be refractory to high-dose inhaled corticosteroid and LABA therapy. Omalizumab is recommended for patients with severe asthma who have evidence of allergies, have an elevated IgE level, and remain symptomatic despite optimizing therapy with combination therapy of high-dose inhaled corticosteroids and a LABA. This therapy can be associated with serious anaphylactoid reactions and should only be begun by providers who are skilled at monitoring and treating these complications. The cost of omalizumab can exceed several thousand dollars per month. Because response to this treatment is highly variable, continued treatment may not be justified if there is no clear improvement after 6 months of initiating omalizumab.

CLINICAL PEARLS

▶ An ETT should be greater than or equal to 8 mm to allow for suctioning and to decrease resistance during the MV of asthmatics.

▶ V_t of 6 to 8 mL/kg of ideal body weight should be used in MV to avoid barotrauma.

▶ Heliox and general anesthesia are beneficial in patients unresponsive to initial treatments.

▶ A quiet chest in an asthmatic exacerbation is a bad prognostic sign with decreased ventilation.

▶ Previous intubation, overuse of rescue medications, and frequent night-time awakenings are all high-risk signs of asthmatic exacerbation, need for admission, and aggressive treatment.

▶ Continuous high-dose inhalation of SABAs and ipratropium bromide is of great value for bronchodilation in the acute treatment regimen.

▶ Intravenous magnesium and heliox can be used as adjunctive therapy in severe asthma.

▶ Barotrauma from positive-pressure ventilation is common in asthmatic patients.

▶ The primary ventilator strategy for patients with severe obstructive lung disease is to allow adequate time for exhalation before the next delivered breath and to minimize auto–positive end-expiratory pressure.

▶ Omalizumab is recommended for patients with severe asthma who have evidence of allergies, have an elevated IgE level, and remain symptomatic despite optimizing therapy with high-dose inhaled corticosteroids and a LABA.

REFERENCES

Benninger C, Parsons JP, Mastronarde JG. Vocal cord dysfunction and asthma. *Curr Opin Pulm Med*. 2011;17(1):45-49. PMID: 21330824.

Lazarus SC. Emergency treatment of asthma. *N Engl J Med*. 2010;363:755-764.

Oddo M, Feihl F, Schaller MD, Perret C. Management of mechanical ventilation in acute severe asthma: practical aspects. *Int Care Med*. 2006;32(4):501-510.

A 55-year-old man is hospitalized in the ICU with acute onset of respiratory distress. He has a long history of chronic obstructive pulmonary disease (COPD) with frequent exacerbations leading to multiple hospitalizations. He has never been intubated before for any of these exacerbations. On physical examination, he is afebrile, blood pressure is 170/100 mm Hg, and heart rate is 123 beats/min. There is jugular venous distention. Although the patient is in apparent respiratory distress, he is still able to answer questions and follow directions. Decreased breath sounds are heard in both lungs. There is 1+ lower extremity edema. A chest radiograph shows hyperinflation without infiltrates or pneumothorax. The remainder of the physical examination is normal. Laboratory results are below:

Arterial Blood Gas Studies (Normal Reference Range)	
pH	7.48 (7.35-7.45)
$Paco_2$	30 mm Hg (36-45 mm Hg)
PaO_2	60 mm Hg (> 80 mm Hg)
Fio_2	100% with PEEP 5
PaO_2/Fio_2 ratio	60 (> 350)
HCO_3	26 mEq/L (22-26 mEq/L)
Hemoglobin	18.0 g/dL (13.8-17.2 g/dL)

▶ What is the next best step in managing this patient's respiratory status?
▶ What other treatment options should be considered concurrently?

ANSWERS TO CASE 12:

Noninvasive Ventilator (NIV) Support for Hypoxic Respiratory Failure

Summary: This 55-year-old man is in hypoxic respiratory failure secondary to an exacerbation of COPD. He is cooperative, awake, and spontaneously breathing. He has never been intubated before.

- **Next step in management:** This patient is in need of ventilatory support before rapid sequence intubation (RSI). Noninvasive positive-pressure ventilation (NIPPV) via high flow oxygen (HFO) should be delivered by way of a special nasal cannula at 50 lpm of 100% Fio_2. In this patient's case, improvement in the patient's respiratory distress followed, and the patient was successfully discharged from the ICU 48 hours later without need for intubation and mechanical ventilation (MV). In patients with hypoxic respiratory failure, HFO has been shown to be equally or more effective than BiPAP. A recent study comparing HFO, BiPAP and high O_2 facemask demonstrated that patients using HFO had more ventilator-free days, a higher probability of survival, and a lower likelihood of intubation in patients with a PaO_2/Fio_2 ratio <200.

- **Other considerations:** Inhaled β_2 agonists, ipratropium bromide, IV corticosteroids and antibiotics are also indicated in this acute COPD exacerbation.

ANALYSIS

Objectives

1. Be familiar with different methods of noninvasive methods of ventilatory support (NIV, HFO, NIPPV).

2. Learn the indications for the use of different modes of noninvasive methods of ventilatory support.

3. Understand and know the settings for the different modes of noninvasive methods of ventilatory support.

4. Understand how to liberate the patient from noninvasive methods of ventilatory support.

Considerations

The best approach to this awake and cooperative patient is to initially use some form of NIV in the form of HFO or noninvasive positive-pressure ventilation (NIPPV) to relieve the respiratory failure. **If improvement is not rapidly seen after NIV use, intubation and mechanical ventilation (MV) should not be delayed.** NIV reduces the need for endotracheal intubation and mortality among patients with acute exacerbations of COPD or severe cardiogenic pulmonary edema and possibly reintubation rates. The physiological effects of noninvasive ventilation include a decrease in the work of breathing and improvement in gas exchange.

HFO therapy through a special high-flow-capable nasal cannula delivers heated and humidified oxygen to the nose at high flow rates. This generates low levels of positive pressure in the upper airways, and the fraction of inspired oxygen (FIO_2) can be adjusted. It may also decrease physiological dead space by removing expired CO_2 from the upper airways, possibly explaining the observed decrease in work of breathing. In patients with acute respiratory failure of various origins, HFO has been shown to result in better comfort and oxygenation than standard oxygen therapy delivered through a face mask. Respiratory failure increases the work of breathing; accordingly, respiratory-related cardiac output requirements are increased from 1% to >20% of the total cardiac output. If not treated quickly, RSI and MV may be required. NIV and NIPPV serve to decrease the work of breathing, decrease anxiety, and improve the status of the pulmonary edema by decreasing cardiac and pulmonary preload and afterload, thereby improving cardiac output and decreasing the need for sedation.

APPROACH TO:

Noninvasive Positive-Pressure Ventilation and Noninvasive Ventilation

INTRODUCTION

Noninvasive positive-pressure ventilation which can include NiPAP, NIPPV or HFO, and noninvasive ventilation (NIV) are terms that can be used interchangeably. NIV is an effective treatment for the common multiple causes of respiratory failure: (1) exacerbations of COPD, (2) exacerbations of congestive heart failure (CHF), (3) hypoxic respiratory failure, and (4) post extubation support. Successful use of NIV avoids the higher risk of endotracheal intubation (ETI) and MV. With NIPPV, the positive pressure increases intrathoracic pressure and decreases venous return, causing a decrease in preload and acting as immediate treatment of CHF. NIV delivers relief from respiratory distress by improving ventilation and oxygenation. **NIPPV use may also reduce mortality in these diseases.** BiPAP is the most common mode of NIPPV. It delivers a preset amount of inspiratory positive airway pressure (IPAP) and expiratory positive airway pressure (EPAP) via face mask. The difference between the IPAP and EPAP is the actual PSV provided to the patient, decreasing venous return (preload).

INITIAL INTERVENTIONS

Supplemental oxygen is used to deliver the desired FIO_2 via BiPAP through a tight-fitting facemask. This has become the predominant method of providing NIPPV. Successful NIPPV support leads to a decrease in respiratory rate (RR), increase in tidal volume (V_t), and decrease in dyspnea. NIPPV support has markedly increased over the past two decades and has become an integral tool in the management of both acute and chronic respiratory failure in the acute care, critical care, and chronic care settings.

INDICATIONS FOR NIPPV

Selection of patients for NIPPV must be considered carefully. Preferred patient inclusion criteria consist of a spontaneously breathing and cooperative patient, moderate to severe dyspnea short of respiratory failure requiring intubation, tachypnea (>24 breaths/min, RSI >105), increased work of breathing (accessory muscle use, pursed-lips breathing), hypercapnic respiratory acidosis (pH range 7.10-7.35, $Paco_2$ >42 mm Hg), and hypoxemic respiratory failure (Pao_2/Fio_2 <200 mm Hg, Pao_2 <60 mm Hg on room air with HFO).

APPLICATION OF NONINVASIVE VENTILATION

The experience and expertise of healthcare providers, specifically nursing and respiratory therapy staff, cannot be underestimated. NIPPV implementation is dependent on the staff learning curve and the time demands of nursing and respiratory therapy. Another important consideration is the potential for delay in definitive therapy. NIV can also assist in mild community-acquired pneumonia (CAP), mild *Pneumocystis jiroveci* pneumonia, mild bacterial pneumonia, cystic fibrosis, asthmatic exacerbation, mild acute respiratory distress syndrome, the immunocompromised state with respiratory distress, "do not intubate" status, neuromuscular respiratory failure, postoperative respiratory distress and respiratory failure, and decompensated obstructive sleep apnea or cor pulmonale.

Patient Interfaces and Mask Devices

NIPPV differs from invasive ventilation by nature of the interface between the patient and the ventilator. Invasive ventilatory support (IMV) is provided via either an ETT or tracheostomy tube. NIPPV support uses a variety of interfaces, and these have continued to evolve with modifications based on patient comfort and efficacy. **Nasal masks and orofacial masks** were the earliest interfaces, followed by the subsequent development and use of **full-face masks, mouthpieces, and nasal pillows.** Nasal masks and orofacial masks are still the most commonly used devices. Orofacial masks are used almost twice as frequently as nasal masks. Proper fitting of the mask is a key component to successful NIV. Typically, the smallest mask providing a proper fit is the most effective. Straps hold the mask in place. Care must be taken to minimize excess pressure on the face or nose, which would otherwise create pressure ulcers. Any cuff used in these interfaces should be kept below 25 mm Hg to prevent tissue necrosis.

NIV Following Extubation

NIV can be used in various ways to facilitate weaning from MV. One randomized study of patients with COPD in whom a ventilator weaning trial was unsuccessful found that extubation directly to NIV shortened ICU stay. Taken together, the evidence suggests that the use of NIV in patients in whom a trial of extubation has failed should be limited primarily to those with chronic lung disease and hypercapnia. Most patients treated with NIPPV receive PSV with CPAP, which is the most basic level of support. BiPAP is the most common mode of support and requires provision and control in the amount of both IPAP and EPAP. The difference between IPAP and EPAP is the amount of pressure support provided to the patient by the ventilator. EPAP is equivalent to positive end-expiratory pressure (PEEP). While volume ventilators can be used to provide NIPPV support, the previously described dedicated models are the best. Less sedation is needed because of increased patient comfort with the use of NIPPV.

Initial Ventilator Settings and Adjustments

The primary goals of NIPPV are: (1) adequate ventilation and oxygenation, (2) correction of respiratory failure, and (3) an acceptable level of patient tolerance and comfort. Adjustments are often necessary to achieve these endpoints. The initial settings should focus on achieving adequate tidal volumes, usually in the range of 6 to 8 mL/kg. Enough support should be provided to reduce the respiratory rate to <25 breaths/min. F_{IO_2} is adjusted to achieve adequate oxygenation with a minimum pulse oximetry level of 90% to 92%. Serial ABG measurements are essential to monitor the response to therapy and guide further adjustments.

Providers should start at 10 cm H_2O IPAP and 5 cm H_2O EPAP; pressures <8 cm H_2O IPAP/4 cm H_2O EPAP are not advised, as this may be inadequate. Adjustments should be made as needed to achieve a tidal volume of 6 to 8 mL/kg of ideal body weight (IPAP and/or EPAP).

Subsequent Adjustments Based on Arterial Blood Gas Values

- Increase IPAP by 2 cm H_2O increments if persistent hypercapnia exists.
- Increase IPAP and EPAP by 2 cm H_2O if persistent hypoxemia exists.
- IPAP is usually limited to 20 to 25 cm H_2O (increased gastric distention, worsens patient comfort).
- Maximal EPAP should be limited to 10 to 15 cm H_2O.
- Begin F_{IO_2} of 100% and adjust to the lowest level with an acceptable pulse oximetry value >90%.
- Set the back up respiratory rate to 12 to 16 breaths/min by using adaptive BiPAP.

Predictors of success include a good response to a trial of NIPPV for 1 to 2 hours with a decrease in $Paco_2$ >8 mm Hg from baseline and an improvement in pH >0.06 units. Predictors of failure include an increased severity of illness and acidosis (pH <7.25), especially if due to hypercapnia ($Paco_2$ >80). NIPPV trials may be as short as a few minutes in patients with immediate failure and probably should not exceed two hours if patients fail to improve. Follow intubation criteria when NIPPV fails. Never let NIV delay intubation if indicated.

COMPLICATIONS OF NIPPV

Complications common to both NIPPV and invasive ventilation occur less frequently in patients undergoing NIPPV. When compared to CPAP, BiPAP has less morbidity, lower mortality, fewer adverse events, and lower medical utilization in adults with COPD and acute respiratory failure. NIPPV is also effective in the perioperative and posttransplantation settings. **Facial and nasal pressure sores and**

air leaks are the main complications of NIPPV. This pressure can be minimized by intermittent NIPPV application at scheduled breaks of 30 to 90 minutes. Rebalancing of strap tension to minimize mask leaks without excessive mask pressures is also helpful. Early wound care is important. Gastric distention can be avoided by limiting peak inspiratory pressures to <25 cm of H_2O. Nasogastric tubes can be placed but can increase leaks from the mask. The use of nasogastric tubes also bypasses the lower esophageal sphincter and permits reflux to occur with more ease. Aspiration of gastric contents, especially with emesis, can also occur during NIPPV. NIPPV should be avoided in patients with ongoing emesis or hematemesis.

Barotrauma complicates both NIPPV and invasive ventilation but occurs much less frequently with NIV and NIPPV. Hypotension related to increased positive intrathoracic pressure can be reversed with increased intravenous fluids. NIV increases patient breathing comfort, requiring less sedation. Increase in the usage of NIPPV helps avoid the risks and costs of endotracheal intubation and mechanical ventilation, provides shorter ICU and hospital stays, and reduces costs associated with infectious complications. **Episodes of ventilator-associated pneumonia are reduced by half or more when NIPPV is used.**

CONCLUSIONS

NIV/NIPPV are most effective in patients with moderate to severe disease and multiple causes of respiratory failure, including COPD and CHF. Those with hypercapnic respiratory acidosis are generally the best responders (pH 7.20-7.30). The greatest benefits are realized in the relief of symptoms and dyspnea. NIPPV is also effective as a bridge support to freely breathing patients after early extubation. Secretions may be a limiting factor to the use of NIPPV. NIPPV is also effective in patients with muscular dystrophy, kyphoscoliosis, and postpolio syndrome, as well as in cases of obesity-hypoventilation or obstructive sleep apnea (OSA). In OSA, NIPPV corrects hypercapnia, facilitates diuresis, and provides an opportunity for restorative rapid eye movement (REM) sleep. NIPPV should be avoided in upper airway obstruction. NIPPV can also be used during invasive procedures such as bronchoscopy and percutaneous gastrostomy to maintain oxygenation and ventilation.

> ## CLINICAL CASE CORRELATION
>
> - See also Case 8 (Airway Management/Respiratory Failure), Case 9 (Ventilator Management), Case 10 (Respiratory Weaning), and Case 11 (Asthmatic Exacerbation).

COMPREHENSION QUESTIONS

12.1 A 65-year-old woman is evaluated in the ICU for rapidly progressive dyspnea. She was admitted with angina, coronary artery disease, and chronic heart failure. Her home medications include aspirin, lisinopril, metoprolol, rosuvastatin, and furosemide. On physical examination, she is alert and in moderate respiratory distress. Temperature is 37.0°C (98.6°F), blood pressure is 155/95 mm Hg, pulse rate is 100 beats/min and regular, and respiration rate is 30 breaths/min. Oxygen saturation is 87% breathing ambient air and increases to 95% breathing 3 L/min of oxygen by nasal cannula. Jugular venous distention is present. Cardiac examination reveals an S3. Pulmonary examination reveals crackles bilaterally. A chest radiograph shows small bilateral pleural effusion. Which of the following is the most appropriate management?

A. Begin intravenous furosemide infusion

B. Initiate intubation and mechanical ventilation

C. Initiate noninvasive positive pressure ventilation

D. Initiate ultrafiltration

12.2 A 61-year-old man is admitted to the hospital for a COPD exacerbation requiring intubation and mechanical ventilation. He receives intravenous glucocorticoids, antibiotics, and supportive care. He is a former smoker and is moderately deconditioned. After five days of mechanical ventilation, his condition has improved, but a spontaneous ventilation trial fails, with increased respiration rate and work of breathing after 20 minutes. On physical examination, he is afebrile, blood pressure is 132/85 mm Hg, and pulse rate is 75 beats/min. Breath sounds are decreased throughout both lung fields. At the end of his spontaneous breathing trial, he appears fatigued but is awake and alert. The remainder of the examination is unremarkable. Which of the following is the most appropriate management?

A. Extubate now and initiate bilevel noninvasive positive pressure ventilation immediately

B. Extubate now and provide supplemental oxygen via nasal cannula

C. Recommend tracheostomy placement

D. Repeat spontaneous breathing trial in one hour

ANSWERS

12.1 **C.** In patients with respiratory failure due to heart failure or COPD exacerbation, noninvasive positive pressure ventilation decreases the need for mechanical ventilation, improves respiratory parameters, and may decrease mortality. The most appropriate management is noninvasive positive pressure ventilation (NIPPV) and supplemental oxygen. This patient has developed respiratory insufficiency due to heart failure with pulmonary edema and pleural effusions. Intubation and mechanical ventilation could be used to deliver positive pressure support, but this process is invasive, requiring intubation and often sedation, and is associated with an increased risk of hospital-acquired pneumonia. Intubation and mechanical ventilation are options if this patient does not respond to NIPPV. Ultrafiltration is an option for fluid removal and can be performed in the setting of diuretic failure before overt need for kidney replacement therapy.

12.2 **A.** Extubation followed by noninvasive positive pressure ventilation support may decrease the ICU length of stay and improve survival in COPD patients. The most appropriate management is to extubate the patient now and initiate bilevel NIPPV. This patient's condition is improving after intubation for a COPD exacerbation with hypercapnic respiratory failure. For patients on invasive ventilatory support, the use of NIPPV after extubation to facilitate weaning has been shown to have improved outcomes. This strategy has been shown in some studies to decrease the ICU length of stay and improve survival. These patients require careful follow-up and observation for reintubation if they do not remain stable on NIPPV. Extubating this patient without immediate NIPPV support could be considered, but there are indications that he may not be ready for unsupported breathing yet. Tracheostomy is a good option for patients who have been intubated for an extended period of time. This patient's condition is improving, and he is unlikely to need mechanical ventilation for an extended period of time.

CLINICAL PEARLS

▶ In hypoxic respiratory failure, high flow nasal oxygen seems to be the superior mode of NIV.

▶ NIPPV is best used for patients with moderate exacerbations of chronic obstructive pulmonary disease, cardiogenic pulmonary edema and/or hypoxic respiratory failure.

▶ BiPAP is the most commonly used NIPPV.

▶ NIV works best in patients in **moderate** distress and should be avoided in patients with decreased mental status.

▶ The complications of NIV occur less often than with invasive (intubated) mechanical ventilation.

▶ Rates of intubation and mechanical ventilation have decreased with the increased use of NIV.

REFERENCES

Berg KM, Clardy P, Donnino MW. Noninvasive ventilation for acute respiratory failure: a review of the literature and current guidelines. *Intern Emerg Med.* 2012 Dec;7(6):539-545.

Burns KEA, Meade MO, Premji A, Adhikari NKJ. Noninvasive ventilation as a weaning strategy for mechanical ventilation in adults with respiratory failure: a Cochrane systematic review. *CMAJ.* 2014;186(3):E112-E122.

Frat JP, Thille AW, Mercat A, et al. High-flow oxygen through nasal cannula in acute hypoxemic respiratory failure. *N Engl J Med.* 2015;372:2185-2196.

Kelly CR, Higgins AR, Chandra S. Videos in clinical medicine, noninvasive positive-pressure ventilation. *N Engl J Med.* 2015;372:e30.

A 43-year-old woman was struck by an automobile while crossing the street. She sustained bi-frontal cerebral contusions, a right tibial plateau fracture, left-sided rib fractures, and a grade II splenic laceration. Her brain, chest, and abdominal injuries are being managed non-operatively. On hospital day four, the patient develops respiratory distress and is transferred to the ICU. On examination, her BP is 130/80 mm Hg, pulse is 110 beats/min, respirations are 32 breaths/min, and GCS is 15. Her chest radiograph is normal.

▶ What are priorities in this patient's management?
▶ What are the possible causes of the patient's current condition?
▶ What are the risk factors for this patient's condition?

ANSWERS TO CASE 13:
DVT/Pulmonary Embolism

Summary: A 43-year-old woman with multiple injuries following blunt trauma develops acute respiratory distress requiring transfer to the ICU on hospital day four.

- **Priorities in management:** The initial priority is to determine the adequacy of oxygenation and ventilation. In this case, we must determine her ability to maintain airway patency and capacity to handle the work of breathing; she should be placed on high-flow oxygen. The patient's mental status, level of pain, oxygenation and acid/base status must also be taken into account as we determine whether intubation and/or mechanical ventilation is needed. Given her recent history of major multisystem trauma, she is at high risk for venous thromboembolic complications. A contrast enhanced helical CT scan pulmonary embolism (PE) protocol should be obtained to confirm or exclude the diagnosis. Documenting the presence of a deep venous thrombosis (DVT)/PE would be important prior to starting anticoagulation, given the bleeding risks associated with her brain and splenic injuries. In patients with a low risk of bleeding and/or if a long delay is expected before CT scan evaluation can be obtained, immediate anticoagulation therapy is appropriate when a PE is suspected.

- **Possible causes:** The possible causes include pneumonia, mucus plugging, pneumothorax, acute lung injury, fluid overload, pulmonary embolism, and cardiac ischemia.

- **Risk factors for pulmonary embolism:** Risk factors for venous thromboembolic diseases include *stasis* (bed rest, immobilization), *hypercoagulability* (trauma, estrogen), and *endothelial injury* (trauma, surgery). Factors associated with increased risk of PE after trauma include age ≥ 40, pelvic fracture, lower extremity fracture, shock, spinal cord injury, and brain injury. Variables associated with very high risk for PE are major operative procedure, venous injury, >3 ventilator days, and having two or more high-risk factors.

ANALYSIS

Objectives

1. Learn the risk factors and preventive strategies for DVT/PE in the critical care setting.

2. Learn the diagnostic strategies for patients with suspected DVT/PE.

3. Learn the treatment strategies for patients with PE.

Considerations

This woman who is a victim with multiple trauma including traumatic brain injury, chest injury, splenic injury, and orthopedic injuries develops acute respiratory distress on hospital day four. Immediately following the stabilization of this life-threatening condition, we need to determine the cause responsible for her sudden clinical deterioration. A chest x-ray, ECG, and serum troponin levels are helpful to identify causes such as primary cardiac process, acute lung injury, and pulmonary infections. A CT angiography of the chest would help determine if pulmonary embolic disease is the cause of her problem. Systemic anticoagulation would be indicated if PE is identified.

APPROACH TO:
Venous Thromboembolism

DEEP VENOUS THROMBOSIS

Deep venous thrombosis refers to clot formation in the deep veins of the body located predominantly in the lower extremities and pelvis, though upper extremities veins can also be involved. A **deep vein** is defined as any vein paired with a named artery. The majority of deep venous thrombosis occurs when clots form in the valve cusps of the calf. Once developed, 20% of distal lower extremity (tibial level) DVTs will propagate proximally, resulting in the potential for PE. Rudolph Virchow, a 19th century German physician, first described the triad of circulatory stasis, hypercoagulability, and endothelial injury as factors that contribute to venous thromboembolic diseases. **Circulatory stasis** refers to stagnation of normal blood flow in the veins. Stagnation of blood allows time for the cross-linking of fibrin polymers and clot formation. Conditions associated with stasis are bed rest, travel (eg, long airline flight), immobility (eg, casting a lower extremity in extension), limb paralysis, spinal cord injury, and obesity.

Under usual circumstances the coagulation/fibrinolytic systems maintain a delicate balance between thrombogenesis and thrombolysis. A **hypercoagulable state** implies an imbalance in coagulation homeostasis usually associated with a derangement of a protein or protein receptor involved in the clotting cascade. Clinical examples of hypercoagulable states include malignancy, trauma, pregnancy, and inflammatory conditions.

Deficiency of Protein S, Protein C, and Antithrombin III are host conditions producing hypercoagulable states. Protein S and C deficiency leads to an overabundance of factors Va and VIIIa causing thrombosis. Antithrombin III deficiency results in the activation of factors XIIa, XIa, and IXa, leading to thrombosis. Factor V Leiden mutation renders factor V resistant to Protein C, and this mutation is the most common genetic cause of hypercoagulability, occurring in 5% to 8% of the population; heterozygotes with factor V Leiden mutation carry a seven-fold increased risk of thrombosis, and homozygotes have an eighty-fold increased risk in comparison to the general population.

Endothelial injury may occur as the result of surgery or traumatic injury, which then activates the extrinsic pathway of the coagulation cascade. Activation of the extrinsic pathway leads to the activation of factor VIIa; tissue factor/factor VIIa/calcium complex then activates factor Xa and joins the common pathway of the coagulation cascade.

DVT/PE Prevention (Thromboprophylaxis) Strategies

Prevention strategies should be implemented for all hospitalized patients, especially those with **moderate** and **high** risk. Low-risk patients are minor surgery patients and medical patients who are fully mobile, and these individuals are generally not encountered in the ICU setting. Moderate risk patients include most general surgery, open gynecological surgery, and urological surgery patients, as well as severely ill and bedridden medical patients. High-risk patients include those patients following hip or knee arthroplasty, hip fracture surgery, major trauma, and spinal cord injury. With this risk-stratification scheme, **the estimated DVT risk without prophylaxis is <10% for low-risk patients, 10% to 40% for moderate-risk patients, and 40% to 80% for high-risk patients.** The recommended prophylaxis strategy for the low-risk group is early and frequent ambulation. The recommendations for the moderate-risk group include low molecular weight heparin (LMWH), low-dose unfractionated heparin (LDUH), or fondaparinux; however, if the patient has a high bleeding risk, then mechanical thromboprophylaxis should be implemented instead. For high-risk patient, prophylaxis with LMWH, fondaparinux, or oral vitamin K antagonist (INR 2-3) is recommended; for high-risk patients with a high bleeding risk, temporary mechanical thromboprophylaxis is recommended.

Diagnosis of DVT

The diagnosis of deep venous thrombosis can be made by a combination of clinical, laboratory and imaging data. Imaging studies provide the most sensitive and specific diagnostic information. The Wells score consists of a list of clinical criteria with a single point awarded per criteria (Table 13–1) and calculates the clinical probability of the diagnosis of DVT in hospitalized patients. Wells scores ≥3 are associated with a high probability of DVT, scores 1 to 2 are associated with a moderate probability of DVT, and scores of 0 represent a low probability of DVT. The Wells score has correlated with imaging confirmation of DVT in 76%, 21%, and 10% of patients in the high, medium, and low probability groups, respectively. The Homan's sign, or pain in the calf with ankle flexion, is not reliable for DVT diagnosis, as it is only present in one third of cases of DVT.

The fibrin degradation product D-dimer can be elevated with DVT. The most common method of D-dimer quantification is the ELISA test. D-dimer screening

Table 13–1 • WELLS SCORE CRITERIA FOR PREDICTION OF DVT
One point per criteria. Scores ≥3 have a high probability of DVT, scores 1-2 have a moderate probability of DVT and scores of 0 have a low probability of DVT.
Malignancy
Bed rest for >3 days
Pain along the course of a deep vein
Paralysis
Swelling of the entire leg
Calf circumference >3 cm compared with the asymptomatic leg
Pitting edema in the affected leg
Collateral superficial veins—not varicose veins

is a good method for the evaluation of asymptomatic medical patient and outpatients for the presence of a DVT. In the ICU patient population, D-dimer elevations can occur as the result of medical interventions, surgeries, or traumatic injuries, thus making this an unreliable test in this population.

The diagnosis of DVT is generally confirmed with imaging studies. **Duplex ultrasound** is a noninvasive, reproducible examination that can demonstrate the flow characteristics and compressibility of the popliteal and femoral veins. It should be the first imaging study ordered. Ultrasound of the popliteal and femoral veins has a sensitivity and specificity for proximal DVT of 100% and 99% respectively. It is less sensitive and specific (70% and 60%, respectively) for DVT of the calf. If two negative ultrasounds are performed one week apart, the diagnosis of DVT is essentially excluded.

Treatment of DVT

Systemic anticoagulation is the standard treatment of DVT. Anticoagulation options include subcutaneous low molecular weight heparin (SC LMWH), intravenous unfractionated heparin (IV UFH), monitored subcutaneous unfractionated heparin (SC UFH), fixed-dose SC UFH, or subcutaneous fondaparinux. When possible, an oral vitamin K antagonist (warfarin) should be initiated concurrently with heparin or LMWH. When administering IV UFH, a bolus of 80 units/kg should be given, followed by a continuous infusion of 18 units/kg/h titrated to a target PTT >1.5 times normal. In adults, 150 to 200 units/kg of SC LMWH once a day is as effective as 100 units/kg of SC LMWH twice a day and continuous IV UFH titrated to a PTT >1.5 times normal. Daily LMWH has the advantage of a stable dose-response curve thus obviating the need for frequent laboratory monitoring. In comparison to a heparin drip, LMWH has the advantages of being associated with a lower risk of heparin-induced thrombocytopenia (HIT) and lower cost.

To prevent recurrence, patients with DVT and DVT/PE require an extended period of anticoagulation with either LMWH or warfarin. The duration of anticoagulation therapy depends on the circumstances of clot formation. DVT that occurs after a reversible inciting event (eg, surgery, trauma, pregnancy) requires a minimum of three months of treatment. Unprovoked DVT formation in patients with no risk factors for bleeding requires a minimum of three months of treatment and possibly indefinite treatment for some patients. Isolated distal DVT formation may be treated with three months of anticoagulation therapy.

Systemic fibrinolysis is rarely recommended for DVT treatment. Compared to heparin therapy, systemic fibrinolytic therapy results in increased thrombolysis, lower risk of post-phlebitic syndrome; however, this treatment is associated with significantly increased risk of bleeding complications. There is no significant difference in the risk of death or DVT recurrence between systemic fibrinolysis and continuous heparin infusion. Catheter-directed fibrinolysis has had moderate success when used to treat DVT, with total clot dissolution in 31% and partial dissolution in 52% of the treated patients. Catheter-based treatment with fibrinolytics has evolved and may be combined with percutaneous mechanical thrombectomy. Several case series have reported this combination therapy as being 82% to 100%

successful, and catheter-directed thrombolysis is associated with 1% incidence of PE and no increase in deaths or strokes. Catheter site bleeding is a potential complication requiring blood transfusions in 4% to 14% of the treated patients. Percutaneous mechanical thrombectomy appears safe, but there is insufficient evidence to support routine use at the present time.

Vena Cava Filters

Vena caval filters are mechanical devices placed to prevent pulmonary embolism from venous thrombi. The indications for inferior vena cava (IVC) filters are: (1) evidence of PE or ileofemoral DVT with either a contraindication to anticoagulation, complication from anticoagulation, or a failure of anticoagulation, (2) massive PE with evidence of ongoing DVT, (3) free floating ileofemoral or IVC thrombus, (4) DVT in the setting of severe cardiopulmonary disease, and (5) poor compliance with anticoagulation. Although rarely applied, the relative indications for IVC filter placement are prophylactic IVC filter placement for: (1) Trauma patients and (2) very high-risk patients (eg, immobilized, hypercoagulable patients).

The PREPIC study is the only randomized controlled trial to evaluate the efficacy of IVC filter placement for the prevention of PE in patients with proximal DVT. The study found that PE occurred in 1.1% of patients with an IVC filter and 4.8% of patients without an IVC filter in place. At 2 years, recurrent DVT was found in 20.8% of the IVC filter patients compared with 11.6% of the patients without a filter. At eight-year follow-ups, symptomatic PE was found in 6.2% of the IVC filter patients and 15.1% of patients without a filter. The incidence of post thrombotic syndrome and death were the same in both groups. The study concluded that IVC filters are only beneficial in high-risk patients and that widespread use of filters is not recommended. Long-term studies show that vena caval filters are associated with filter fragmentation, caval thrombosis, and filter erosion. Given the questionable benefits and filter-related complications, vena caval filters should be applied with great caution.

Thromboembolism After Trauma

Factors associated with a high risk of PE after trauma include age ≥ 40 years, pelvic fracture, lower extremity fracture, shock, spinal cord injury, and head trauma. High-risk variables associated with major operations include venous injury, >3 days on the ventilator, and two or more high-risk factors. The highest-risk trauma patients are those with a spinal cord injury, with reported DVT rates of 80% and PE rates of 5%. **Pulmonary embolism is the most common cause of death in spinal cord injury patients.**

The authors of a National Trauma Data Bank study have proposed a thromboprophylaxis strategy for trauma patients at risk for DVT/PE. Patients at high-risk for DVT/PE and without contraindications for heparin should receive prophylactic doses of LMWH. Those patients with a contraindication for heparin should have mechanical compression stockings in place at all times. Those patients at very high risk for DVT/PE without contraindications for heparin should be treated with a prophylactic dose of LMWH combined with mechanical compression. If the very high-risk patient has a contraindication for heparin, mechanical compression stockings should be worn and serial color-flow Doppler studies performed to monitor for DVT.

PULMONARY EMBOLISM

Most pulmonary embolisms (PEs) occur when a thrombus breaks free from the endothelial wall, travels through the right heart, and lodges in the pulmonary artery. PE causes ventilation/perfusion mismatching, increases pulmonary vascular resistance, and induces cytokine-mediated pulmonary vasoconstriction. Symptoms depend on the degree of pulmonary arterial obstruction, severity of the inflammatory response, and the patient's physiological reserve. Most patients with PE have dyspnea (79% of patients in PIOPED II study), some patients have hypoxemia, and most have an increased A-a gradient. At times, extravasation of blood into the alveoli can produce pleuritic chest pain, cough, or hemoptysis.

Large PEs can present as acute right heart failure and cardiac arrest. Patients with larger PEs may experience right-heart strain. **T-wave inversions in lead V1 and II may be present on ECG and are 99% specific for PE.** Echocardiography is a useful adjunct in the evaluation of patients with suspected PE, with sensitivity and specificity reported at 51% and 87%, respectively. Echocardiography has been reported to have 97% sensitivity and 98% specificity in patients with massive PEs. CT angiography (CTA) is the diagnostic image of choice for the majority of ICU patients, with 82% to 100% sensitivity and 89% to 98% specificity. It is important to keep in mind that the sensitivity and specificity of CTA are affected by the pretest probability of disease in the given patient; thus, in high-risk patients, the negative predictive value of CTA is only 60%. For high-risk patients, the combination of a CTA and CTV (CT venography of the upper thigh and pelvis) helps improve the negative predictive value to 82%.

Empiric anticoagulation should be considered in high-risk patients without significant bleeding risks. Treatment with either unfractionated heparin or LMWH is acceptable, and treatment principles for PE are similar to those for the treatment of DVT. Hemodynamically unstable patients with large central PEs can be considered for catheter-directed therapy, such as catheter-directed thrombolytic therapy or catheter-directed mechanical clot disruption therapy.

COMPREHENSION QUESTIONS

13.1 A 24-year-old woman is brought in by ambulance to the emergency department as a Level I trauma after crashing into a tree at 75 kmph. The paramedics found the patient ejected from the automobile, semi-conscious with an open left femur fracture. The patient's initial systolic blood pressure in the ED was 80 mm Hg. After a blood transfusion, the patient's mental status improved, and her blood pressure increased to 96/40 mm Hg. Upon reviewing the pelvic film, you notice a diastasis of the right sacroiliac joint and pubic symphysis. The patient gives no history of prior medical conditions. She is currently taking oral contraceptive pills. All of the following are risk factors for venous thromboembolism in this patient EXCEPT:

A. Age

B. Lower extremity fracture

C. Hypotension

D. Pelvic fractures

E. Oral contraceptive pills

13.2 After placement of a pelvic binder and rapid splinting of the left femur fracture, the above patient went to the CT scanner and was found to have a 4 cm cerebral contusion in the right frontal lobe, three right-sided rib fractures, a grade II splenic laceration, and an extra-peritoneal pelvic hematoma with no active extravasation. Which of the following thrombosis prophylaxis measures should be **avoided** in this patient?

A. Bilateral sequential compression devices

B. Immediately start prophylactic SC UFH upon arrival in the ICU

C. Graduated compression stockings

D. Start SC UFH after 48 hours in the ICU if there is no enlargement of the cerebral contusion

13.3 This same patient is taken to the ICU for continuous monitoring and hourly neurological examinations. What is the best test to screen for DVT?

A. D-dimers

B. Platelets

C. CT scan

D. Ultrasound

E. Coagulation profile

13.4 By hospital day 4 the patient has been started on LMWH and her pelvis and femur fractures stabilized with external fixation devices. She has been hemodynamically stable. She has now developed swelling and pain in her right thigh and calf. What is the best diagnostic approach for her at this time?

A. CT angiography

B. CT venography

C. Duplex ultrasonography

D. Echocardiography

E. Venography

13.5 In the absence of contraindications for anticoagulation, the most appropriate therapy for femoral DVT with associated PE is:

A. Inferior vena caval filter

B. SC UFH upon arrival in the ICU

C. SC LMWH 150 to 200 units/d followed by transition to warfarin

D. Unmonitored IV UFH drip followed by transition to warfarin

E. Aspirin 325 mg PO daily

ANSWERS

13.1 **A.** The patient is at very high risk for DVT/PE because she has two or more high-risk factors for DVT/PE. Her risk factors are pelvic fractures, a lower extremity fracture, and shock. Oral contraceptive pills contribute to an increased estrogen state, which is also a risk factor for DVT/PE. Her age in this case is not a contributing risk factor because only age > 45 is generally considered a risk factor.

13.2 **B.** The patient is at very high risk for a DVT/PE given her long-bone fracture, pelvic fractures, and hypotension; however, she has multiple contraindications to systemic anticoagulation therapy at this time, namely intracerebral hemorrhage and splenic injury. In the initial 48 hours the patient should have graduated compression stockings and sequential compression devices on both lower extremities. The patient should *not* be started on SC UFH immediately due to the risk of bleeding. If the patient's head injury and splenic injury remain stable, she should be started on prophylactic dosing of SC UFH after 48 hours.

13.3 **D.** Bedside ultrasound is the standard for screening for DVT. CT venography is not an appropriate screening examination for DVT. A platelet count and coagulation profile do not diagnose the presence of DVT. The patient will have elevated D-dimer levels due to continuous clot formation and degradation occurring in the trauma patient. Although screening duplex examinations are done at a number of trauma centers, the 2008 American College of Chest Physicians Evidence Based Clinical Practice Guidelines specifically recommend against screening studies for asymptomatic patients.

13.4 **C.** The concern at this time should be DVT involving the proximal veins. This can be diagnosed by CT venography, venography, or duplex sonography. Venography has the disadvantage of being invasive and requiring the administration of intravenous contrast. CT venography is a study that requires contrast administration; therefore, the duplex is the preferred diagnostic study for DVT diagnosis. CT angiography is useful only if the patient has a pulmonary embolism. Echocardiography would not be useful for DVT diagnosis.

13.5 **C.** The patient should be started on a full anticoagulation regimen starting with a LMWH, monitored IV UFH, fixed-dose SC UFH, or SC fondaparinux. The LMWH is dosed at 150 to 200 units/kg/d or 100 units/kg/twice daily. To initiate a heparin drip, give an 80 unit/kg bolus and titrate the PTT to 1.5 times normal starting with 18 units/kg/h. Regardless of which anticoagulation regimen is started, warfarin should be started simultaneously and titrated to an INR of between 2.5 and 3.0. IVC filter would only be considered if the patient develops PE while on appropriate DVT treatment or if anticoagulation is contraindicated.

CLINICAL PEARLS

▶ DVT prophylaxis is variable depending on the patient's risk for thromboembolism development.

▶ The combination of CTA and CTV has greater negative predictive value than CTA alone in the high-risk patient population.

▶ Dyspnea is the most common presenting symptom in patients with PE.

▶ Venous Doppler studies of the lower extremities is considered the first-line diagnostic test to assess for venous thromboembolism.

REFERENCES

Karthikesalingam A, et al. A systematic review of percutaneous mechanical thrombectomy in the treatment of deep venous thrombosis. *Euro J Vasc Endovasc Surg.* 2011;41(4):554-565.

Kearon C, Aki AE, Orneals J, et al. Antithrombotic therapy for VTE disease: CHEST Guidelines and expert panel report. *Chest.* 2016;149(2):315-352.

Knudson MM, Ikossi DG, Khaw L, et al. Thromboembolism after trauma: an analysis of 1602 episodes from the American College of Surgeons National Trauma Data Bank. *Ann Surg.* 2004;240(3): 490-496; 496-498.

Velopulos CG, Haut ER. Venous thromboembolism: prevention, diagnosis, and treatment. In: Cameron JL, Cameron AM, eds. *Current Surgical Therapy.* 11th ed. Philadelphia, PA: Elsevier Saunders; 2014:958-963.

Wells PS, et al. Application of a diagnostic clinical model for the management of hospitalized patients with suspected deep-vein thrombosis. *Thrombosis Haemostasis.* 1999;81(4):493-497.

A 55-year-old man presents to the ED with sudden onset of chest pain described as crushing pressure, shortness of breath, and diaphoresis. He was shoveling snow from his driveway two hours ago. The ECG shows a heart rate of 65 beats/min and ST-segment elevations of 3 mm in leads II, III, and aVF. Troponin levels are elevated, and blood pressure is 134/86 mm Hg. He continued to have chest pain after three doses of sublingual nitroglycerin and has required nitroglycerin 10 mcg/min IV to keep him free of chest pain. The patient was immediately transferred to the ICU. The patient was given aspirin (ASA) 325 mg and clopidogrel, and low molecular weight heparin (LMWH) was started. ECG changes persist after one hour but are now only 1-mm elevations of the ST segments. Mild Jugular venous distention (JVD) is noted on physical examination. The lungs have minimal rales at both lung bases. The heart sounds are normal without murmurs, and there are no S3 and S4 sounds heard. There is no lower extremity edema. The patient is breathing at 18 breaths/min without labor. He states he smokes 1 pack per day (PPD) for the last 20 years. He has a history of dyslipidemia but is not compliant with statin therapy.

▶ What is the most likely diagnosis?
▶ What immediate therapeutic steps are indicated?
▶ What is the preferred treatment option for his condition?

ANSWERS TO CASE 14:

Acute Coronary Syndrome

Summary: A 55-year-old man presents with an acute ST-elevation myocardial infarction (STEMI).

- **Most likely diagnosis:** Inferior wall ST-segment elevation MI (STEMI). ST elevations present in II, III, and aVF with elevated cardiac biomarkers confirm diagnosis of STEMI.

- **Immediate steps in treatment:** Administer aspirin 325 mg, clopidrogel, pain control with nitroglycerin and morphine, low flow oxygen via nasal cannula, β-blockade (if not in heart failure), prepare patient for percutaneous coronary intervention (PCI) and activate the cardiology and catheterization team.

- **Treatment option:** Differs depending upon whether the MI is a STEMI or a non-STEMI (NSTEMI), with **PCI being the preferred treatment** for STEMI and thrombolytic therapy (TPA) an option when PCI is not possible. Bypass surgery backup should be available.

ANALYSIS

Objectives

1. To understand the typical presentation/risk factors and initial management in the ICU.

2. To understand the criteria for diagnosing STEMI/NSTEMI.

3. To understand the differences between and treatments of STEMI and NSTEMI.

4. To understand the prognosis associated with acute coronary syndrome (ACS).

Considerations

This 55-year-old man presents with the acute onset of chest pain after exertion two hours ago. The patient has ST elevation in ECG leads II, III, and aVF, which is consistent with inferior leads. The elevated cardiac markers are consistent with an acute MI. The most important therapeutic considerations include oxygen, aspirin, pain control, and nitroglycerin beta-blockade to reduce the myocardial oxygen consumption. The patient required IV nitroglycerin to resolve the pain. The patient is noted to have minimal JVD and minimal rales in the lungs. The patient should be considered for acute reperfusion, either via thrombolytic therapy or percutaneous coronary intervention. The patient is a smoker and should be instructed to quit; he also has dyslipidemia and is not compliant with statin therapy and should be counseled regarding restarting.

APPROACH TO:

Acute Coronary Syndrome

The typical presentation of ACS is chest pain. It is the goal of the physician to determine whether the pain is non-cardiac or cardiac and initiate prompt management. There are other life-threatening conditions which must be ruled out that can mimic ACS (ie, aortic dissection, tension pneumothorax, pulmonary embolism esophageal rupture, perforating peptic ulcer, and pancreatitis). A pertinent history and physical must be conducted in a timely manner to rule out or in the possible diagnoses.

The mnemonic OPQRSTA is a simple tool to use when evaluating patients.

Onset: Ischemic chest pain can present typically or atypically and comes on due to ischemia and destruction of myocardial tissue. It can also present with other symptoms such as shortness of breath (SOB), fatigue, or new left bundle branch block (LBBB).

Palliative/Provocation: Ischemic pain is exacerbated with activity due to increased cardiac oxygen demand. The pain is not relieved with changing position.

Quality: The terms crushing, squeezing, tight, and pressure are typically used. In some cases, the patient cannot qualify the nature of the discomfort but places their clenched fist in the center of the chest, known as the "Levine sign" or feeling "impending doom."

Radiation: Ischemic pain usually radiates to the upper extremities, upper abdomen, or jaw but rarely to the back as in aortic dissection.

Site: Ischemic pain is diffuse and usually unable to be pinpointed to an exact origin.

Timing: Ischemic pain typically occurs after exertion and may persist even if resting, depending upon the degree of coronary artery blockage present.

Associated symptoms: Ischemic pain is often associated with other symptoms. The most common symptom is shortness of breath, which may be due to mild pulmonary congestion from ischemia-mediated diastolic dysfunction. Other symptoms may include nausea, indigestion, vomiting, diaphoresis, dizziness, lightheadedness, and fatigue.

Atypical Symptoms: Roughly **25% of patients** with ACS present with atypical symptoms rather than typical chest pain. **They are more likely to be older, diabetic, and women.**

RISK FACTORS

Coronary heart disease (CHD) is the most common type of heart disease, killing over 370,000 people annually. Every year roughly 735,000 Americans have a heart attack. Out of these, 525,000 are first-time heart attacks. **There are four modifiable risk factors for CHD: (1) hypertension, (2) smoking, (3) dyslipidemia, and (4) diabetes.** Non-modifiable risk factors include gender (male > female), prior myocardial infarction (MI), family history of early CHD, and age.

Smoking is the most important, easily modifiable risk factor. People who smoke >20 cigarettes a day have a two- to three-fold increased risk of dying from CHD compared to nonsmokers. Hypertension is only diagnosed in two out of three patients, and only one in three are adequately controlled with medication. Even high normal pressures, systolic blood pressure (SBP) 130 to 139 mm Hg and diastolic blood presure (DBP) 85 to 89 mm Hg increase risk compared with lower levels. Diabetic patients have impaired epithelial and smooth muscle function with increased leukocyte adhesion, which promotes atherosclerosis. These patients have a four-fold increase of CHD compared to people who do not have diabetes.

Dyslipidemia, including elevated LDL cholesterol, triglycerides and decreased HDL, are all independent factors associated with increased risk of atherosclerosis. Family history of first-degree male relative <55 years of age or female family member <65 is a risk factor for developing CHD in the future. This factor can be modified by utilizing appropriate intensive statin therapy.

INITIAL WORKUP/TREATMENT

A brief preliminary history and examination should be obtained. 12-lead ECG should be performed and interpreted. The initial ECG is often *not* diagnostic in patients with ACS. The ECG should be repeated often if the initial study is not diagnostic but the patient remains symptomatic and high clinical suspicion for ACS persists. Resuscitation equipment should be brought to the bedside, that is, defibrillator and equipment for intubation. A continuous cardiac monitor should be attached to the patient and oxygen given as necessary to maintain O_2 sat above 90%. IV access and blood work should be obtained, including electrolytes, renal function, coagulation panel, and cardiac biomarkers.

Aspirin 325 mg should be given to all patients; if there is a history of anaphylaxis due to aspirin, clopidogrel (Plavix) can be given.

Nitrates. Sublingual nitroglycerin should be administered at a dose of 0.4 mg every 5 minutes for a total of three doses, after which an assessment of blood pressure and pain relief should guide the need for intravenous nitroglycerin. Reduction of the infarct size has been shown in experimental animal studies with the administration of nitroglycerin. Patients should be asked if they have recently used **phosphodiesterase-5 inhibitors for erectile dysfunction (ED)**, which may cause severe hypotension if combined with nitroglycerin. Caution must be used in an **inferior wall MI with involvement of the right ventricle.** In this setting, patients are dependent on preload to maintain cardiac output. Nitroglycerin causes vasodilation and may cause severe hypotension. This should respond to fluid administration, and a high normal range central venous pressure (CVP) in the 10 to 12 mm Hg range should be maintained.

Morphine. IV morphine sulfate should be given at an initial dose of 2 to 4 mg, with increments of 2 to 8 mg, repeated at 5 to 15 minutes to relieve chest pain and anxiety. Morphine can reduce sympathetic stimulation caused by pain and anxiety, thereby decreasing cardiac workload and risks associated with excess catecholamines.

STEMI VS NSTEMI

Myocardial infarction (MI) is defined as a clinical or pathological event caused by ischemia of myocardial tissue with evidence of myocardial injury or necrosis. Criteria are met when there is a trend of rise and/or fall of cardiac biomarkers, along with supportive evidence of typical symptoms, suggestive ECG changes, or imaging evidence of new loss of viable myocardium or new regional wall motion abnormality.

The term ACS is used to describe patients in whom there is a suspicion of myocardial ischemia. There are three types of ACS: STEMI, NSTEMI, and unstable angina (UA). The first two are characterized by typical rise and/or fall in biomarkers after myocardial injury. Criteria for diagnosis of MI depends upon the detection of a rise and/or fall of cardiac biomarkers, typically cardiac troponin [cTn] with at least one value above the 99th percentile upper reference limit and with at least one of the following:

- Symptoms of ischemia (such as chest pain or pressure)

- Development of pathologic Q waves in the ECG

- New or presumed new significant ST-segment-T wave (ST-T) changes or new left bundle branch block (LBBB)

- Identification of an intracoronary thrombus by angiography or autopsy

- Imaging evidence of new loss of viable myocardial tissue or a new regional wall motion abnormality.

Unstable angina is diagnosed in patients with ischemic symptoms suggestive of ACS without elevation in biomarkers with or without ECG changes indicative of ischemia even at rest. Due to the insensitivity of creatine kinase MB (CK-MB) compared to troponin, the finding of a normal CK-MB does not exclude the diagnosis of MI using the current definition. Elevations of troponin typically take 2 to 3 hours, while elevations for CK-MB take longer and drop faster. Newer troponin markers that can be detected within one hour of injury are being evaluated.

ECG. The ECG is the mainstay for the initial diagnosis of patients with suspected ACS. It allows initial categorization of the patient with a suspected MI to be grouped into one of three groups based on the pattern:

- STEMI; ST elevation or new LBBB

- Non-ST elevation ACS, with either NSTEMI or unstable angina (ST-depression, T wave inversions, or transient ST-elevation)

- Undifferentiated chest pain syndrome (non-diagnostic ECG)

ST elevation MI. The ECG evolves through a typical sequence for patients experiencing a STEMI. Although not frequently seen, the earliest change in a STEMI is the development of a peaked T wave that reflects localized hyperkalemia. Thereafter, the ST segment elevates in the leads recording electrical activity of the involved region of the myocardial tissue.

- Initially, there is elevation of the J-point, and the ST segment retains its concave appearance.

- Over time, the ST-segment elevation becomes more pronounced and the ST segment becomes more convex or rounded upward.

- The ST segment may eventually become indistinguishable from the T wave; the QRS-T complex can actually resemble a monophasic action potential.

ECG CRITERIA FOR THE DIAGNOSIS OF STEMI

Diagnostic criteria are as follows: new ST-segment elevation at the J point in two contiguous leads: >0.1 mV in all leads other than leads V2-V3; for leads V2-V3, the following parameters apply: ≥0.2 mV in men ≥40 years, ≥0.25 mV in men <40 years, or ≥0.15 mV in women.

Over time, there is further evolution of the ECG changes. The ST segment gradually returns to baseline, the R wave amplitude becomes substantially reduced, and the Q wave deepens. In addition, the T wave becomes inverted. These changes generally occur within the first two weeks after myocardial injury but may progress more rapidly, within several hours of presentation.

Bundle branch block or paced rhythm. Both LBBB, which is present in approximately 7% of patients with STEMI, and pacing can interfere with the ECG diagnosis of STEMI. Approximately one-half of patients with LBBB and an acute MI do not have chest pain. New right bundle branch block, though generally not interfering with the ECG, suggests an adverse prognosis similar in degree to LBBB. Patients with LBBB, compared to those without, are much less likely to receive aspirin, beta blockers, and reperfusion therapy, particularly if they present without chest pain. Similar observations have been made in patients with a paced rhythm. Careful evaluation of the ECG may show evidence of ischemia in patients with LBBB or a paced rhythm. However, the clinical history and cardiac enzymes are of primary importance in diagnosing MI in this setting.

BIOMARKERS

A variety of biomarkers have been used to evaluate patients with symptoms of acute MI (Figure 14–1). The cardiac troponins I and T as well as the MB isoenzyme of creatine kinase (CK-MB) are most frequently used. Values ≥99th percentile of the upper reference limit should be used to consider a value abnormal. This value for troponin and CK-MB will vary depending on the assay and lab used. An elevation in the concentration of troponin alone or concomitant elevated CK-MB is required for the diagnosis of acute MI. **If both are collected and the troponin value is normal but the CK-MB is elevated, the elevation is most likely due to release from non-myocardial tissue. At least one-third of patients with ACS have elevated troponins but have normal values for CK-MB.**

Troponin is the preferred marker for the diagnosis of MI because of its increased specificity and sensitivity compared to CK-MB. However, an elevation in cardiac troponins must be interpreted in context of the clinical presentation and ECG findings because it can be elevated in a variety of clinical settings. Guidelines recommend that if there are elevations of cardiac troponin (cTn) in a clinical situation

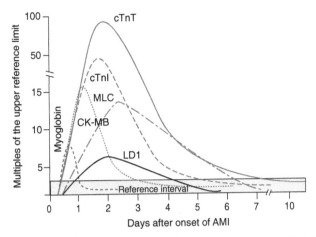

Figure 14–1. Serum markers after acute myocardial infarction. AMI, acute myocardial infarction; CK-MB, MB fraction of creatine kinase; cTnI, cardiac troponin I; cTnT, cardiac troponin T; LD1, lactate dehydrogenase isoenzyme 1; MLC, myosin light chain. (Reproduced, with permission, from Tintinalli JE, Stapczynski S, Cline DM, et al. *Tintinalli's Emergency Medicine.* 7th ed. New York: McGraw-Hill Education, 2011. Figure 52–1).

where ischemia is not present, the term cardiac injury should be used. Three points should be considered when using troponin to diagnose acute MI:

1. With contemporary troponin assays, most patients can be diagnosed within 2 to 3 hours of presentation.

2. A negative test at the time of presentation, especially if the patient presents early, does not exclude myocardial injury.

3. Acute MI can be excluded in most patients by 6 hours, but the guidelines suggest that if there is a high degree of suspicion of an ACS, a 12-hour sample should be obtained. However, very few patients become positive after eight hours.

Other causes of biomarker elevation: Other mechanisms for cardiac injury must be considered when ACS has been ruled out (eg, heart failure, rapid atrial fibrillation, myocarditis, sepsis, etc). Small amounts of cardiac injury can occur in critically ill patients, which may or may not represent an acute MI. Troponin elevations also occur in chronic kidney disease. In the ICU, life-threatening causes of chest pain with troponin elevation not due to coronary artery disease are acute pulmonary embolism, in which troponin release may result from acute right-sided heart overload, myocarditis, and stress-induced cardiomyopathy.

ACS TREATMENT

STEMI: The first step in the management of the patient with an acute STEMI is prompt recognition, since the beneficial effects of therapy with reperfusion are greatest when performed early in the presentation. Once the diagnosis of STEMI is made, early management involves several goals: ASA, time to PCI, TPA, and medical management.

Reperfusion: Prompt restoration of myocardial blood flow is critical to minimize myocardial ischemia and to reduce mortality. A decision must be made quickly to initiate reperfusion with fibrinolytic agents or PCI.

Percutaneous coronary intervention (PCI): Prompt PCI is the gold standard for treatment of a STEMI. The 2013 American College of Cardiology Foundation/ American Heart Association guideline for the management of STEMI recommends PCI for any patient with an acute STEMI who can undergo the procedure **within 90 minutes or less for patients transported to a PCI-capable hospital or 120 minutes or less for patients who initially arrive at a non-PCI capable hospital and are transported to a PCI-capable hospital.**

Patients with typical and persistent symptoms in the presence of a new or presumably new LBBB are also considered eligible for PCI. For patients presenting 12 hours or more after symptom onset, the performance of PCI is reasonable if the patient has severe heart failure, hemodynamic or electrical instability, or persistent ischemic symptoms.

Fibrinolysis: The 2013 American College of Cardiology Foundation/American Heart Association guideline for the management of STEMI recommends the use of fibrinolytic therapy in patients with symptom onset within 12 hours who cannot receive PCI within 120 minutes of first medical contact. The time interval from hospital arrival to initiation of fibrinolytic drug infusion should be less than 30 minutes.

Fibrinolytic therapy generally does not improve outcomes in patients presenting 12 hours or later and is not indicated in those who are stable and asymptomatic. However, fibrinolysis can be considered up to 24 hours after symptom onset if the patient has ongoing chest pain and PCI is not available. Patients receiving fibrinolytic therapy benefit from pretreatment with clopidogrel but not from a glycoprotein (GP) IIb/IIIa inhibitor.

Bypass surgery: Coronary artery bypass graft surgery (CABG) is rarely performed in patients with STEMI. The main indications are failure of fibrinolysis or PCI, or hemodynamically important mechanical complications. The benefit of revascularization must be weighed against the increased mortality associated with CABG in the first three to seven days after STEMI. Therefore, if the patient is stabilized, surgery should be delayed to allow myocardial recovery. Patients with critical anatomy should undergo CABG during the initial hospitalization.

Anticoagulation therapy: Anticoagulation therapy includes the use of ASA, clopidogrel and low molecular weight heparin (LMWH). Glycoprotein IIb/IIIa antagonists should be considered in addition to ASA and heparin in patients with non-STEMI and as adjunctive therapy in patients with STEMI undergoing angioplasty.

Beta blockers: Oral beta blockers are administered universally to all patients without contraindications who experience an acute STEMI. Contraindications include heart failure, evidence of a low cardiac output, risk for cardiogenic shock, bradycardia, heart block, or reactive airway disease. β-blockers decrease heart rate and decrease oxygen demand of myocardial muscle. β-blockers also prevent recurrent ischemia and life-threatening ventricular arrhythmias.

ACE inhibitors (ACEI): ACEI should be administered early in the course of ACS for most patients. ACE inhibitor therapy can prevent ventricular remodeling, resulting in a reduction in the development of heart failure and death. ACE inhibitor therapy reduces the risk of recurrent MI and other vascular events. In patients who cannot tolerate an ACE inhibitor due to coughing, an angiotensin-receptor blocker (ARB) is an alternative.

Statin therapy: Intensive statin therapy should be initiated as early as possible in all patients with STEMI. Atorvastatin 80 mg/day should be initiated, rather than gradual dose titration upward. The goal of intensive high-dose intensive statin therapy is to stabilize coronary artery plaques, reverse endothelial dysfunction, decrease thrombogenicity, and reduce inflammation.

NSTEMI and unstable angina: Patients with unstable angina (UA) or NSTEMI should be treated with an early medical regimen similar to that used to treat STEMI with one exception: there is no evidence of benefit (and possible harm) from fibrinolysis. Initial therapy should in initiated within 20 minutes of presentation.

PROGNOSIS

Survivors of a first-time MI face substantial risk of further cardiovascular events, including death, recurrent MI, heart failure, arrhythmias, angina, and stroke. Short-term (in-hospital or 30-day) mortality has been decreasing over the past 30 years due to the increasing use of reperfusion strategies and proven preventative therapies such as beta blockers, aspirin, and statins. The current 30-day mortality after all acute coronary syndromes (STEMI, NSTEMI, and unstable angina) is around 2% to 3%. Similar to short-term outcomes, long-term mortality rates after MI have declined significantly. Short-term mortality is lower in patients with NSTEMI (2%-4%) compared to patients with STEMI (3%-8%) treated with PCI within 2 hours of hospital arrival. The risk of re-infarction or stroke at three years was approximately 6% to 7% and 1.5% to 2%, respectively.

CLINICAL CASE CORRELATION

- See also Case 4 (Hemodynamic Monitoring), Case 15 (Cardiac Arrhythmias), and Case 16 (Acute Cardiac Failure).

COMPREHENSION QUESTIONS

14.1 A 73-year-old woman is evaluated in the ED and transferred to the ICU because of chest pain of 4 hours' duration. Her medical history includes a 20-year history of hypertension and Type II diabetes mellitus. Her medications include metformin, atenolol, and ASA. On physical examination, her blood pressure is 130/84 mm Hg, and her heart rate is 87 beats/min and regular. Her jugular vein is distended to 5 cm while the patient is upright. She has a faint left carotid bruit and bibasilar crackles to one quarter up from the lung bases. A normal S1 and S2 is heard, with a grade II/VI holosystolic murmur heard best at the apex to the axilla. An electrocardiogram from six months ago was normal. The ECG in Figure 14–2 was seen during the chest pain. The initial serum troponin measurement is elevated. She is now admitted to the ICU for an MI. She is free of chest pain while on IV nitroglycerin, and her vital signs are stable. Which of the following is the most likely ECG diagnosis?

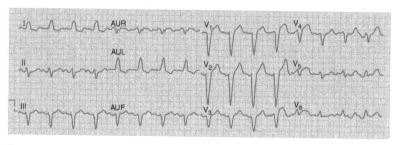

Figure 14–2. 12-lead ECG.

A. Left bundle branch block with normal sinus rhythm
B. Idioventricular tachycardia
C. Right bundle branch block
D. Third-degree atrioventricular block (complete heart block)
E. Mobitztype II second-degree atrioventricular block

14.2 A 55-year-old man in the ICU has ACS, with 2 mm of ST elevation on the leads II, III, and aVF. The troponins are positive. The blood pressure is 130/70 mm Hg on a nitroglycerin drip at 5 μg/kg/min keeping the patient chest pain free, but ECG changes persist and only 1 mm of ST elevation is seen. There is no lower extremity edema. The patient was given ASA upon entry into the ED. What is/are the next best steps in the management of this patient?

    A. Anticoagulation, IV β-blocker, ACE inhibitor, nitroglycerin, and alert catheterization lab

    B. Give tissue plasminogen activator (TPA)

    C. Increase nitroglycerin to 10 μg/kg/min

    D. Get β-natriuretic peptide (BNP) level

    E. Call cardiac surgeon for stat CABG post-PCI

ANSWERS

14.1 **A.** LBBB is associated with absent Q waves in leads I, aVL, and V6; a large, wide, and positive R wave in leads I, aVL, and V6 ("tombstone" R waves); and prolongation of the QRS complex to >0.12 seconds. The chest pain, elevated cardiac biomarkers, and new-onset left bundle branch block are considered equivalent to having an ST-elevation myocardial infarction (STEMI). Repolarization abnormalities are present, consisting of ST segment and T wave vectors directed opposite to the QRS complex. The presentation of ACS with new left bundle branch block should be considered equivalent to a STEMI and true posterior wall MI, with management including early coronary intervention. The maximum benefit is provided by reperfusion within 12 hours of the onset of symptoms. The QRS complex is >0.12 seconds in BBB.

14.2 **A.** This patient is having a STEMI. Antithrombotic (heparin) therapy is indicated. The combination of heparin and ASA reduces the incidence of MI. When administered immediately, ASA reduces mortality in patients with unstable angina or acute infarction by diminishing platelet aggregation. Clopidogrel should be considered in patients with ACS who are unable to take ASA and in high-risk patients in whom percutaneous transluminal coronary angioplasty (PTCA) is planned. Clopidogrel provides additional antiplatelet activity when added to ASA. It should be withheld if CABG is a possibility due to the increased risk of perioperative bleeding. Glycoprotein IIb/IIIa receptor antagonists inhibit the cross-bridging of platelets secondary to binding fibrinogen. Early intravenous β-blocker therapy reduces infarct size, decreases the frequency of recurrent myocardial ischemia, and improves survival. β-Blockers diminish myocardial oxygen demand by reducing heart rate, systemic arterial pressure, and myocardial contractility. An ACE inhibitor should be administered early in the course of ACS in most patients. ACE inhibitor therapy may also reduce the risk of recurrent infarction. In patients who cannot tolerate an ACE inhibitor, an ARB is an alternative. Statin therapy appears to improve endothelial function and reduce the risk of future ACS.

CLINICAL PEARLS

▶ ACS include STEMI, unstable angina, and non-ST elevation MI (non-STEMI).

▶ Atypical symptoms are found in 25% of ACS patients, especially women, diabetics, and the elderly.

▶ Non-STEMI is associated with elevated cardiac biomarkers, while unstable angina is not.

▶ ICU patients, comorbidities, and instability usually preclude acute CABG or PCI.

▶ Therapy of MI includes β-blockade, statins, ASA, and ACE inhibitors.

▶ Negative cardiac biomarkers at time of presentation, especially if the patient presents early, do not exclude myocardial injury.

▶ Troponin elevations are common in ICU patients. Although not always due to myocardial ischemia or infarction, these elevations are associated with poor outcomes.

▶ Other life-threatening condition that mimic ACS must be ruled out.

▶ CHD modifiable risk factors include hypertension, smoking, dyslipidemia and diabetes.

▶ Non-modifiable risk factors for CHD include gender, prior MI, family history of MI and age.

▶ Combined use of PDE-5 inhibitors and nitroglycerin can cause severe hypotension.

REFERENCES

Goodman SG, Menon V, Cannon CP, et al. Acute ST-segment elevation myocardial infarction: American College of Chest Physicians Evidence-Based Clinical Practice Guidelines (8th Edition). *Chest.* 2008;133:708S.

Hamm CW, Bassand JP, Agewall S, et al. ESC Guidelines for the management of acute coronary syndromes in patients presenting without persistent ST-segment elevation: the task force for the management of acute coronary syndromes (ACS) in patients presenting without persistent ST-segment elevation of the European Society of Cardiology (ESC). *Eur Heart J.* 2011;32:2999.

O'Gara PT, Kushner FG, Ascheim DD, et al. 2013 ACCF/AHA guideline for the management of ST-elevation myocardial infarction: executive summary: a report of the American College of Cardiology Foundation/American Heart Association Task Force on Practice Guidelines. *Circulation.* 2013;127:529.

Papadakis MA, McPhee SJ, pp 320-430 *Current Medical Diagnosis and Treatment.* New York, NY: McGraw Hill; 2015.

A 44-year-old man presents to the emergency department with a 1-hour history of palpitations. The patient states that he felt "lightheaded" and that his heart felt like it was "racing." He denies shortness of breath, chest pain, dyspnea, and syncope. His medical history is unremarkable, and there is no family history of sudden cardiac death. He takes no medication. On physical examination, he is afebrile, blood pressure is 115/63 mm Hg, and pulse rate is 150 beats/min. The patient is in mild acute distress. Cardiac examination reveals a tachycardia with a regular rhythm. The remainder of the examination shows no abnormalities. Baseline electrocardiogram is shown in Figure 15–1.

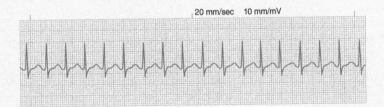

Figure 15–1. ECG tracing.

▶ What is the most likely diagnosis?
▶ What is the appropriate treatment for this patient?

ANSWERS TO CASE 15:

Supraventricular Tachycardia (SVT)

Summary: A 44-year-old man presents to the ICU with acute onset of palpitations, lightheadedness, tachycardia with a heart rate (HR) of 150 beats/min, and an ECG showing atrial tachycardia/ SVT with narrow QRS with visible retrograde P waves (AVRNT).

- **Most likely diagnosis:** Atrial tachycardia. The classic finding of SVT will show a tachycardic rhythm (>100 beats/min) and a narrow QRS complex (<12 ms) as well as retrograde P waves.

- **Treatment:** The drug of choice for SVT is adenosine. If pushed rapidly through an intravenous line, adenosine can be used to diagnose and treat supraventricular tachycardia, as well as AV nodal reentrant tachycardia (AVNRT) and AV reciprocating tachycardia (AVRT). Ninety-five percent of these arrhythmias will terminate properly. Theophylline blocks the effect of adenosine. Adenosine transiently blocks the atrioventricular (AV) nodal conduction and interrupts the reentrant circuit, thereby terminating AVRNT and AVRT but not other supraventricular arrhythmias. Adenosine given in the presence of other supraventricular arrhythmias, including atrial tachycardia, should only slow the ventricular rate or have no effect. If the patient is stable, carotid massage or vagal maneuvers may be helpful. If there is any concern for underlying Wolff-Parkinson-White (WPW), which is another form of AVRNT, adenosine may also be used; however, adenosine is contraindicated when WPW is associated with **atrial fibrillation.**

ANALYSIS

Objectives

1. To develop an approach to diagnose the different types of cardiac arrhythmias.

2. To recognize the most common types of supraventricular and ventricular arrhythmias.

3. To be familiar with a rational workup and treatment of the cardiac arrhythmia.

Considerations

Continuous monitoring of vital signs and ECG should be employed immediately. Replacement of intravascular volume, usually with intravenous (IV) normal saline (NS), will increase the preload and ventricular volume, blood pressure (BP), and cardiac output (CO). The electrolyte levels should be assessed and corrected if abnormal. Continuous infusion of antiarrhythmic drugs may be employed in order to maintain normal sinus rhythm (NSR). The next priority is to determine the etiology of the cardiac arrhythmia. Cardiac electrical activity occurs before mechanical activity in the heart; P waves occur before atrial contractions; the QRS

Table 15–1 • NORMAL ECG INTERVALS AND DURATIONS		
Interval	Time in Seconds	1 Small ECG Box = 0.04 second(s); 1 Large ECG Box = 0.20 seconds
PR interval	0.12-0.20	3-5 small ECG boxes or 1 large box of ECG
QRS	<0.12	3 small ECG boxes
QTc	<0.44	Variable length, depending on HR; half the HR or R to R interval

complex occurs prior to each ventricular contraction, and T waves occur prior to each ventricular repolarization. The accepted duration or interval time of these waves is seen in Table 15–1.

The morphology of P waves, such as P mitrale, can also suggest certain atrial diseases. Abnormal P-wave morphology may be seen in mitral valve regurgitation, or the peak in the second half of the P wave seen in left atrial enlargement. The early, tall notch in the first half of the P wave is seen in right atrial enlargement, or P pulmonale. The morphology of the P wave can be upright, biphasic, or inverted in the inferior leads (II, III, aVF) and is best seen in those leads. The inferior leads look directly at the atria. A large negative P wave seen in lead V1 is also indicative of left atrial enlargement.

Drugs such as digoxin, β-blockers (BBs), and calcium channel blockers (CCBs) are used to treat the more common supraventricular arrhythmias (SVTs). These agents block the AV node and are contraindicated in WPW. **The drugs of choice for treating WPW are adenosine (if patient is not in atrial fibrillation), procainamide, or amiodarone,** which prolong conduction in the aberrant track and slow repolarization. In unstable patients, immediate electrocardioversion should be used. Hypoxemia and any electrolyte imbalances, especially of K^+ and Mg^+, should be corrected. Atrial tachycardia may arise from any area of the right or left atrium, and the most common arrhythmic pathway is reentry.

APPROACH TO:

Cardiac Arrhythmias

Arrhythmias can be classified according to their origin. Supraventricular arrhythmias (SVTs) usually have a narrow QRS with visible retrograde P waves (P waves seen after the QRS complex) and originate above the AV node. P waves may also appear to be absent because they can become buried in the QRS complex. Ventricular arrhythmias generally have a wide QRS complex (>0.12 ms) similar to a bundle branch block pattern with AV dissociation and can be monomorphic or polymorphic. Arrhythmias are also classified according to rate. Tachycardia is defined as a rate ≥100 beats/min. Bradycardia is classified as a rate <60 beats/min. Common signs and symptoms of these arrhythmias are palpitations, lightheadedness, dyspnea, chest pain, syncope or presyncope, and fatigue. Syncope requires a loss of blood flow to both cerebral hemispheres at the same time. Evaluation of an arrhythmia is based on a recent ECG, an old ECG if available for comparison, a CBC, electrolyte determinations, TSH, ABG or O_2 sat, glucose, BUN, and creatinine levels. ECD is indicated for hemodynamically unstable patients regardless of the rhythm.

SUPRAVENTRICULAR ARRHYTHMIAS

Tachyarrhythmias (>100 beats/min)

- **SINUS TACHYCARDIA:** Normal sinus rhythm (NSR) is defined as an SA nodal rhythm with a frequency of 60 to 100 beats/min. Heart rates >100 beats/min originating in the SA node are defined as a sinus tachycardia (ST). ST is associated with anxiety, pain, fever, dehydration, stress, and drugs both therapeutic and recreational. Atrial tachycardias arise from ectopic atrial foci and/or the pulmonary veins. Valsalva maneuvers and/or carotid massage can terminate the SVTs. ST, as in multifocal atrial tachycardia (MAT), is defined as an ectopic atrial rhythm with more than two different P-wave morphologies at a rate >100 beats/min. MAT is typically seen in patients with COPD or other pulmonary disease processes. MAT responds to treatment of the underlying COPD, especially hypoxia with hypercapnia. Antiarrhythmic therapy is usually unnecessary since MAT is self-limiting and responds to treatment of the underlying cause and may worsen arrhythmia if used.

- **SUPRAVENTRICULAR TACHYCARDIA (SVT):** SVT is a regular and rapid rhythm with a narrow QRS, with rates between 160 and 180 beats/min. The most common type, atrioventricular nodal reentry tachycardia (AVNRT), involves reentry electrical activity within the atrioventricular node (AVN). A late P wave can be seen in the final portion of the QRS complex, which is consistent with retrograde P-wave conduction via the AVN. SVT is a benign rhythm in the absence of structural disease. A true SVT should respond to treatment with IV adenosine if it is unresponsive to vagal maneuvers. Adenosine breaks the arrhythmia and causes a long pause in the electrical activity, which resets the AV node for normal AVN conduction (Figure 15–2). Adenosine is contraindicated in the presence of bronchospasm, COPD, and asthma.

- **ATRIAL FLUTTER:** Atrial flutter is recognized by sawtooth P waves with a regular R to R pattern. All P waves have the same morphology and are conducted at regular rates. The P-wave rate and pulse rate varies from 240 to 350 beats/min. Conduction of P waves to QRS varies from 2 to 1 or 3 to 1 P waves for every QRS complex conduction leading to a heart rate of 100 to 150 beats/min. Flutter may turn into atrial fibrillation (AF) over time. One must rule out secondary noncardiac causes of atrial flutter such as hyperthyroidism, high caffeine intake, overuse of vasoconstricting nasal sprays, β_2 agonists, theophylline, and substance abuse with alcohol, cocaine, or amphetamines.

- **ATRIAL FIBRILLATION:** AF is the **most common sustained ectopic atrial tachyarrhythmia.** AF is an **irregularly irregular rhythm** on ECG without any discernible P waves being recognized (chaotic pattern as atria fibrillate).

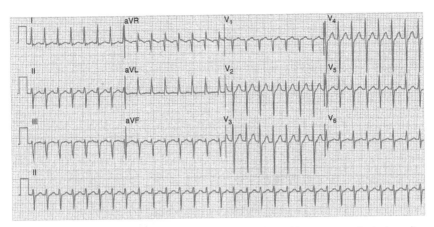

Figure 15–2. AV nodal reentrant tachycardia. HR of 150 beats/min with narrow complex tachycardia. (Reproduced, with permission, from Longo DL, Fauci AS, Kasper DL, et al. *Harrison's Principles of Internal Medicine.* 18th ed. New York: McGraw-Hill Education, 2012. Figure e30–13).

Regularization of the R-R interval (becomes less irregular) in AF at heart rates of <60 can be a sign of digoxin toxicity. AF can be classified as:

1. Acute <48 hours

2. Chronic AF persisting for >48 hours

3. Paroxysmal AF

4. Indeterminate AF

This classification helps choose treatment options. Treatment of AF requires anticoagulation in the short-term and long-term with warfarin (Coumadin) or dabigatran to reduce stroke rates in patients who have a CHADS2 score >2. In patients whose CHADS2 score is <2, treatment with ASA is recommended. Stools should be checked for occult blood or any signs of active bleeding before starting heparin or warfarin (Coumadin). **Dabigatran,** a new oral direct thrombin inhibitor, can be used as an alternative to warfarin in nonvalvular AF. Dabigatran does not require frequent blood tests for international normalized ratio (INR) or prothrombin time (PT) monitoring. Now that an antidote for it is available, increased used of these new oral novel anticoagulants should increase.

An **echocardiogram or a transesophageal echo study is excellent for the evaluation of valvular disease causing AF.** The identification of **intracardiac thrombi** must be excluded prior to cardioversion. Clots in the left atrial appendage are commonly found. To determine whether the risk of stroke is high enough to warrant chronic anticoagulation in AF, risk stratification scores have been developed. One such stratification scheme is known as CHADS2 score, with one point each for the presence of the following, with a maximum score of 6 (Table 15–2). When clots are present, anticoagulation is needed for a period of 4 weeks prior to performing elective ECD. Over 80% of patients with AF have some form of underlying heart

Table 15–2 • CHADS2 Scoring	
Congestive Heart Failure	1 point
Hypertension	1 point
Age (>75 years)	1 point
Diabetes	1 point
Stroke OR TIA	2 points

After calculating the CHADS2 Score, anticoagulation, aspirin and or clopidrogel can be recommended

disease; frequently, atrial septal defects are found. In the elderly, the primary underlying cause is hypertension. To treat AF or any SVT, Valsalva maneuvers or carotid massage should be attempted to increase vagal tone, to slow AVN conduction, and to cause increased refractoriness. ECD is used in all unstable patients regardless of tachyarrhythmia. IV heparin should be given for any AF of unknown duration, and an evaluation for intracardiac thrombi should be done before attempting ECD to NSR. Anticoagulation should continue for 1 month post ECD in AF patients. ECD is an alternative to pharmacological cardioversion of AF of any duration. AF treatment requires anticoagulation, no matter whether treated with rhythm control or conversion to NSR. If the heart rate exceeds 110 beats/min, the patient may need additional AVN blockade. A recommended INR range of 2.0 to 3.0 is optimal for patients with a CHADS2 score >2.

The risk of stroke is the lowest in patients with a CHADS2 score of 0 (1.2%). The risk is 18% per year for a CHADS2 score of 6 (maximum score). Patients with a CHADS2 score of ≥3 and patients with a history of stroke are at high risk and should be considered for chronic anticoagulation dosing with warfarin or dabigatran. Patients with a CHADS2 score of 1 or 2 should be assessed on an individual basis for ASA versus warfarin therapy. Cerebrovascular accident (CVA) rate in nonrheumatic AF is 5%. Risk factors for stroke are a history of previous TIA or CVA, an MI, hypertension, age >65 years, diabetes, left atrial enlargement, and left ventricular dysfunction.

In nonvalvular AF, the use of warfarin with a target INR of 2 to 3 reduces the stroke risk by 68%, which usually outweighs the bleeding risk. In patients without risk factors, ASA may be sufficient and will decrease the stroke rate by 42%. In patients older than 65, heart rate control may be the best, especially when compared to the expected side effects of antiarrhythmic drugs used to maintain rhythm control. The goal is to maintain a heart rate <100 beats/min. Beta blockers (BBs) and calcium channel blockers (CCBs) are the drugs of choice for this purpose. Digoxin is not recommended as a single agent, especially when the heart rate activity becomes uncontrolled during exercise. Oral or IV agents can lead to cardioversion in 70% to 90% of those cases with the onset of AF within the past 48 hours, but they are less effective in treating chronic AF cases appearing after 48 hours. **Amiodarone and dronedarone are useful medications when any structural heart disease is present; otherwise, propafenone or flecainide is used.** Most antiarrhythmic drugs are also proarrhythmic on their own. IV heparin should be started immediately in patients with newly diagnosed AF.

Risks of ECD in AF include thromboembolism, tachyarrhythmias, and bradyarrhythmias.

Surgical procedures. Catheter ablation is now frequently done to eliminate the aberrant conducting pathway. This is 99% effective with a mortality of only 1% to 3%. The Maze surgical procedure, in which a series of incisions are made in a maze-like pattern to reduce effective atrial size and prevent reformation of AF waves, is now used much less.

BRADYARRYHTHMIAS (<70 BEATS/MIN)

Atrioventricular Nodal Block

- **First-degree heart block:** The PR interval is >0.20 seconds on the ECG. All P waves are conducted and this condition requires no specific treatment. It is benign in most patients.

- **Second-degree heart block:** This heart block is characterized by intermittent nonconduction of P waves and "dropped" ventricular beats. Second-degree heart block consists of two types, Mobitz I and Mobitz II.

- **Mobitz type I second-degree heart block:** Mobitz type I second-degree heart block is characterized by a progressive prolongation of the PR interval until a dropped beat occurs (also called Wenckebach block) and does not progress to complete heart block. It is transient and usually requires no treatment. Type I may be associated with a bradycardia.

- **Mobitz type II:** Mobitz II second-degree heart block is characterized by non-conduction of P waves and subsequent "dropped" ventricular beats without the progressive prolongation of the PR interval (Figure 15–3). This is considered

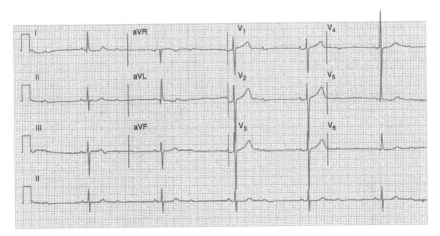

Figure 15–3. Second-degree heart block with bradycardia with ventricular HR of 30 beats/min. This is Mobitz II heart block with P waves of 60 beats/min. (Reproduced, with permission, from Longo DL, Fauci AS, Kasper DL, et al. *Harrison's Principles of Internal Medicine*. 18th ed. New York: McGraw-Hill Education, 2012. Figure e30–3).

malignant since it tends to proceed to complete heart block or third-degree heart block. Mobitz II heart block is associated with evidence of additional disease in the conduction system, such as bundle branch block (BBB) or bifascicular or trifascicular block. Mobitz type II heart block suddenly and unpredictably progresses to complete heart block and is usually treated with a pacemaker.

- **Third-degree heart block:** Third-degree heart block is also referred to as complete heart block or atrioventricular disassociation (AVD). In third-degree heart block, the P rate is higher than the QRS rate and marches at the same interval through the rhythm. Insertion of a pacemaker is usually required for relief of third-degree heart block.

Sinus Node Dysfunction

Sinus node dysfunction (SND) has also been called sick sinus syndrome (SSS) and refers to abnormalities in the formation of sinus node impulses. These conditions include sinus bradycardia, sinus pause/arrest, chronotropic incompetence, and sinoatrial exit block. SND is frequently associated with various SVTs, such as AF and atrial flutter. When associated with SVTs, SND is often termed tachy-brady syndrome or SSS, is seen frequently in the elderly, and is a common cause for the insertion of a pacemaker.

Treatment: The treatment of bradycardia begins with removing all drugs that are capable of causing a bradycardia. **Atropine** is used in an emergency or cases of symptomatic bradycardia. Atropine IV therapy and external or internal pacing are the main treatment options. Vagal maneuvers and constipation (straining) should be avoided since they can worsen bradycardia. Pacing is indicated for the treatment of symptomatic bradycardia, tachy-brady syndrome, complete heart block, and asymptomatic patients with asystolic pauses >3 seconds or ventricular escape rhythms of <40 beats/min. Permanent pacing improves survival in complete heart block, especially if syncope has occurred previously.

Drug therapy: One should consider a BB or CCB such as verapamil to treat AVNRT. CCBs slow calcium channel influx and decrease AVN conduction and increase AVN refractoriness. **Amiodarone has the least proarrhythmic effect and is the drug of choice for any patient with LV dysfunction or structural heart disease.** Dronedarone has a similar therapeutic effect as amiodarone without the iodine load of amiodarone. One should monitor the QT interval on patients on antiarrhythmic drugs and compare it to baseline ECGs. Watch patients closely for potential side effects of antiarrhythmic drugs. All patients on amiodarone need to be evaluated every 6 to 12 months with pulmonary function tests, to assess for problems of diffusion capacity for carbon monoxide (DLCO), chest x-ray, thyroid-stimulating hormone level, and liver function tests. This testing evaluates the most common side effects seen with the use of amiodarone. The iodine content of amiodarone is so high that CT scans may appear to have contrast even when done without contrast. When using **procainamide, one should follow CBC and WBC values since it has been associated with agranulocytosis.**

Procainamide can also cause a drug-induced lupus with positive antinuclear antibody (ANA, as in RNA not DNA) values.

VENTRICULAR ARRHYTHMIAS

To evaluate and diagnose an arrhythmia, one needs to obtain a 12-lead ECG as well as continuous ECG monitoring. Vital signs including O_2 saturation should be monitored. Ischemic heart disease (IHD) should be suspected, and old ECGs should be compared with the current ones. Reversible causes of ventricular arrhythmias such as drugs, electrolyte abnormalities, CAD, ischemia, IHD, hypoxia, or drug toxicity should be sought.

Ventricular Tachycardia

Ventricular tachycardia (VT) is defined as a wide- or narrow-complex tachycardia with continuous rapid depolarizing bursts in the ventricular His-Purkinje system. VT needs rapid attention and reversal with ECD, as **it is the main cause of sudden death.** VT is a reentrant pathway arrhythmia with abnormal impulse conduction. It is often comorbid with underlying structural heart disease, most commonly ischemic heart disease (IHD), electrolyte imbalances such as $\downarrow K^+$ and $\downarrow Mg^+$, drug toxicity with QT-prolonging drugs (psychiatric medications), prolonged QT syndrome, valvular heart disease, and nonischemic cardiomyopathy (viral, alcohol, etc.). VT is subdivided into sustained VT, lasting >30 seconds or requiring termination with ECD, and nonsustained VT, consisting of three straight PVCs with PVCs being <30 seconds. The morphology of the QRS can also be used to evaluate the origin and cause of VT. Concurrent treatment for IHD and CAD has begun because of their high correlation as underlying disorders in VT.

In families with a history of VT and death, one must consider a history of long QT syndrome. VT is also seen in arrhythmogenic right ventricular dysplasia and Brugada syndrome with RBBB. The symptoms and presentation that patients display depend upon the ventricular rate, duration of the arrhythmia, and presence of underlying heart disease.

Patients with nonsustained VT are usually asymptomatic but may complain of palpitations. Patients with sustained VT may present with syncope, near-syncope or sudden death. VT includes as a group VT, VF, and Torsade de pointes (TdP) or long QT syndrome arrhythmias. It is characterized by wide-complex QRS >0.12 seconds and ventricular rate >100 beats/min (Figure 15–4).

In VT, these rates are typically from 140 to 250 beats/min, in VF rates are >300 beats/min, and in TdP rates are 200 to 300 beats/min. When comparing SVT with aberrancy versus VT, **a history of structural or ischemic heart disease suggests that the arrhythmia is most likely VT.** The presence of AV dissociation or third-degree block also suggests VT. An RBBB morphology QRS >0.14 seconds or an LBBB morphology QRS >0.16 seconds is also more likely to be VT than SVT with aberrancy. A regular R-R interval in VT is more common than SVT with aberrancy. The presence of MI or CAD is almost diagnostic of VT. Profound depression in hemodynamics also point to a VT, but a BP near 100 mm Hg does not exclude it. Large "cannon" waves of atrial contraction against a closed tricuspid valve caused by the dissociation effect of the third-degree heart block are seen on

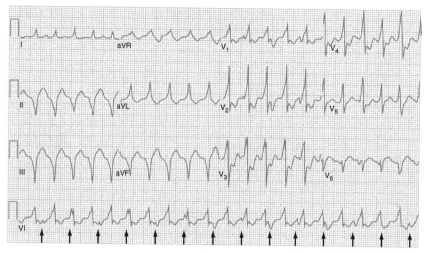

Figure 15–4. Ventricular tachycardia. ECG showing AV dissociation (arrows mark P waves), wide-complex QRS. (Reproduced, with permission, from Longo DL, Fauci AS, Kasper DL, et al. *Harrison's Principles of Internal Medicine.* 18th ed. New York: McGraw-Hill Education, 2012. Figure 233–10).

physical examination. **In unstable patients, VT should be assumed and treated with ECD, delivered in synchronized mode if a pulse is present and in nonsynchronized mode if a pulse is not present.** Definitive treatment of arrhythmias due to reentrant pathways is ablation of those pathways. In the absence of structural heart disease, ablation is the treatment of choice. If structural heart disease is present with an EF < 35%, an implanted cardiac defibrillator (ICD) is recommended. ICD use decreased mortality regardless of the etiology in all VT patients with EF < 35%.

Drug Therapy

Antiarrhythmic IV drug therapy for VT/VF serves to terminate arrhythmias, to prevent recurrence of arrhythmia, and to prevent life-threatening arrhythmias such as VF (along with insertion of an ICD). **For acute treatment of sustained monomorphic VT, IV lidocaine, procainamide, or amiodarone may be used.** Patients with recurrent VT need chronic therapy. Drug treatment of patients with VT and structural heart disease is inferior to implantation of an ICD. Drugs are used as adjuncts when ICD implantation is contraindicated. Pharmacological treatment for nonsustained VT can be avoided unless there is a history of structural heart disease or long QT syndrome. Here procainamide is the drug of choice. IV magnesium sulfate can be used to suppress polymorphic VT in patients with prolonged QT intervals. Treatment for CHF with BBs, ACE inhibitors (ACEI), and spironolactone will reduce the incidence of sudden death in patients with systolic dysfunction.

Ventricular Fibrillation

Ventricular fibrillation (VF) is an arrhythmia in which there is an uncoordinated and ineffective contraction of the ventricles in the heart, which stops pumping of blood. Although there is electrical activity in the heart, the mechanical activity is missing in this condition. VF is a medical emergency that requires prompt ECD and ACLS. VF will likely degenerate into asystole ("flatline"). The condition results in cardiogenic shock (CS), cessation of effective blood circulation, and sudden cardiac death (SCD) in minutes. If the patient is revived after an insufficient period (roughly 5 minutes) of cerebral hypoxia, the patient sustains irreversible brain damage. Brain death often occurs if NSR, return of spontaneous circulation (ROSC) or blood flow to the brain is not restored within 90 seconds of the onset of VF. This is especially the case if the VF has degenerated further into asystole with complete lack of cerebral and systemic blood flow.

Premature Pre-Ventricular Contractions

Premature pre-ventricular contractions (PVCs) originate from the ventricle (wide QRS) and are always followed by a compensatory pause as the electrical system resets. A premature atrial contraction (PAC) with aberrancy can mimic a PVC, but there is no compensatory pause. PVCs and arrhythmia rates increase as we age. PVCs appear to be benign unless an underlying left ventricular dysfunction is present. In patients with increased left ventricular dysfunction, PVCs are associated with an increased mortality, while reducing PVC frequency does not reduce mortality. SVT with wide QRS due to a BBB or preexcitation syndrome such as WPW can mimic VT.

Arrhythmias Associated With Long QT

Many common drugs cause TdP. The QT period is rate-dependent. Risk factors for TdP are female sex, hypokalemia, hypomagnesemia, structural heart disease, and a history of long QT or drug-induced arrhythmias (macrolides, quinolones, psychiatric drugs).

Torsade De Pointes

Torsade de pointes (TdP) is a form of polymorphic VT associated with a prolonged QT syndrome. For those patients who receive QT-prolonging drugs in the hospital, ECG monitoring of prolonged QT intervals is indicated. TdP should be avoidable if there is an awareness of individual risk factors and ECG signs of drug-induced long QT syndrome (LQTS) are seen. ECG risk factors for TdP include marked QT prolongation to >500 ms (with the exception of amiodarone- or verapamil-induced QT prolongation). Recognition of these ECG harbingers of TdP allows for treatment with IV magnesium, removal of the offending agent, and correction of electrolyte abnormalities. Other exacerbating factors include the prevention of bradycardia and long pauses where temporary pacing will be necessary.

CLINICAL CASE CORRELATION

- See also Case 4 (Hemodynamic Monitoring), Case 5 (Vasoactive Drugs and Pharmacology), and Case 16 (Acute Cardiac Failure).

COMPREHENSION QUESTIONS

15.1 A 76-year-old woman is evaluated in the ICU for dizziness, shortness of breath, and palpitations that began acutely 1 hour ago. She has a history of hypertension and heart failure with preserved ejection fraction. Medications are hydrochlorothiazide, lisinopril, and aspirin. On physical examination, she is afebrile, blood pressure is 80/60 mm Hg, pulse rate is 155 beats/min, and respiration rate is 30 breaths/min. Oxygen saturation is 80% with 40% oxygen by face mask. Cardiac auscultation reveals an irregularly irregular rhythm, tachycardia, and some variability in S1 intensity. Crackles are heard bilaterally in the lower third of the lung fields. Electrocardiogram demonstrates atrial fibrillation with a rapid ventricular rate. Which of the following is the most appropriate acute treatment?

A. Adenosine

B. Amiodarone

C. Cardioversion

D. Diltiazem

E. Metoprolol

15.2 A 54-year-old man is evaluated in the ICU for a 2-hour history of palpitations. He reports no syncope, presyncope, chest pain, or shortness of breath, and he has had no previous episodes of palpitations. Medical history is significant for nonischemic cardiomyopathy; ejection fraction was most recently measured at 38%. Medications are carvedilol and candesartan. On physical examination, he is afebrile, blood pressure is 125/86 mm Hg, and pulse rate is 110 beats/min. Cardiac evaluation reveals tachycardia and a regular rhythm, although the intensity of the S1 is variable. Cannon a waves are seen in the jugular venous pulsation. Which of the following is the most appropriate treatment?

A. Immediate cardioversion

B. Intravenous adenosine

C. Intravenous amiodarone

D. Intravenous verapamil

ANSWERS

15.1 **C.** This patient with atrial fibrillation is hemodynamically unstable and should undergo immediate cardioversion. She has hypotension and pulmonary edema in the setting of rapid atrial fibrillation. In patients with heart failure with preserved systolic function, usually due to hypertension, the loss of the atrial "kick" with atrial fibrillation can sometimes lead to severe symptoms. The best treatment in this situation is immediate cardioversion to convert the patient to normal sinus rhythm. Although there is a risk of a thromboembolic event since she is not anticoagulated, she is currently in extremis and is at risk of imminent demise if not aggressively treated. In addition, she acutely became symptomatic 1 hour ago, and while this is not proof that she developed atrial fibrillation very recently, her risk of thromboembolism is low if the atrial fibrillation developed within the previous 48 hours. Amiodarone can convert atrial fibrillation to normal sinus rhythm as well as provide rate control, but immediate treatment is needed and amiodarone may take several hours to work. In addition, she is in active heart failure, and metoprolol or diltiazem could worsen the pulmonary edema.

15.2 **C.** This patient likely has ventricular tachycardia based on the variable S1 heart sound, and the canon of waves illustrating AV dissociation. This should be confirmed on ECG. This patient appears to be stable. Amiodarone is the drug of choice for treating ventricular tachycardia in patients with heart failure. In unstable patients, DC cardioversion is the therapy of choice.

CLINICAL PEARLS

▶ The younger the patient with an arrhythmia, the more likely a congenital accessory pathway is present.

▶ Patients with atrial fibrillation or any arrhythmia who are hemodynamically unstable should undergo immediate cardioversion.

▶ Regularization of AF (at heart rates of 60 beats/min) can be a sign of digoxin toxicity.

▶ In nonvalvular AF, warfarin with a target INR of 2.0 to 3.0 decreases stroke risk by 62%.

▶ A pacemaker improves survival for patients with asymptomatic complete heart block.

▶ Patients with VT and structural heart disease are ideally treated with an ICD.

▶ Mobitz type II heart block progresses to complete heart block and is treated by a pacemaker.

▶ The longer the QT interval, the more the likelihood of an arrhythmia.

▶ Antiarrhythmic medications are proarrhythmic themselves.

▶ The location where the pulmonary veins enter the left atrium is a major site for the origin of AF.

▶ Procainamide is a classic medication causing drug-induced lupus and a positive ANA.

▶ In a patient with a wide-complex tachycardia and a history of coronary artery disease or cardiomyopathy, ventricular tachycardia is the most likely diagnosis.

REFERENCES

Colucci RA, Silver MJ, Shubrook J. Common types of supraventricular tachycardia: diagnosis and management. *Am Fam Physician.* 2010;82(8):942-952.

Dubin D. *Rapid Interpretation of EKGs.* 6th ed. Tampa, FL: Cover Publication Company; October 15, 2000.

Neumar RW, Otto CW, Link MS, et al. Part 8: adult advanced cardiovascular life support: 2010 American Heart Association guidelines for cardiopulmonary resuscitation and emergency cardiovascular care. *Circulation.* 2010;122(18 suppl 3):S729-S767. PMID: 20956224.

A 60-year-old Caucasian woman whose status is post myocardial infarction (MI) is admitted to the ICU for acute worsening dyspnea and chest pain that started this morning. On physical examination, her temperature is 98°F, heart rate is 108 beats/min, blood pressure 97/73 mm Hg, and respiratory rate 24 breaths/min. She speaks in short phrases. Her neck veins are prominent and distended to the mandible while sitting at 45 degrees upright. The heart rhythm is regular with normal S1 and S2 heart sounds, and an S3 heart sound is noted. A 4/6 holosystolic murmur that radiates to the axilla is heard. Lung rales are auscultated at the lung bases, bilaterally. There is 2+ pitting edema up to the knees, and her legs are cool to touch. Her laboratory report showed the following:

Serum Laboratory Studies		
Sodium (Na$^+$)	133 mEq/L (136-144) mEq/L	Hemoglobin 13 g/dL (12.0-15.5 g/dL)
Potassium (K$^+$)	4.0 mEq/L (3.7-5.2 mEq/L)	WBC 8.3×10^9 cells/L (4.3-10.10^9 cells/L)
Chloride (Cl$^-$)	95 mEq/L (101–111 mEq/L)	
Bicarbonate (HCO$_3^-$)	18 mEq/L (22-26 mEq/L)	
Arterial Blood Gas Studies		
pH	7.32 (7.35-7.45)	Central venous pressure (CVP) is 20 mm Hg (normal, 0-5 mm Hg)
Pa$_{CO_2}$	32 mm Hg (36-44 mm Hg)	Venous O$_2$ saturation 52%
Pa$_{O_2}$ (on room air)	40 mm Hg (75-100 mm Hg)	Arterial O$_2$ saturation 91%

▸ What is the most likely diagnosis?
▸ What complications should be anticipated in this patient?
▸ What treatment modalities should be initiated?

ANSWER TO CASE 16:

Acute Cardiac Failure/Cardiogenic Shock

Summary: This is a 60-year-old woman with acute decompensating heart failure (ADHF) with cardiogenic shock (CS). The central venous line pressure (CVP) is markedly increased and the cardiac output (CO) is decreased, as evidenced by the cool extremities and low SVO$_2$ saturation. Distention of the jugular vein is the most sensitive clinical sign for ADHF. Myocardial function deteriorated when she suffered a myocardial infarction (MI), which led to papillary muscle dysfunction and acute mitral insufficiency. The markedly decreased CO led to acute CS, as evidence by the decreased CO with hypotension and organ hypoperfusion (cool extremities, low serum sodium, and metabolic acidosis).

- **Most likely diagnosis:** Severe congestive heart failure (CHF) with acute cardiogenic shock.

- **Likely complications:** Acute mitral insufficiency, papillary muscle dysfunction or rupture.

- **Treatment modalities to initiate:** Endotracheal intubation (ETI) and mechanical ventilation (MV), ACE inhibitors, IV nitroglycerin, β-blockers, furosemide, and anticoagulation are all indicated. Although β blockers are a cornerstone of the treatment of acute MI, they should be carefully titrated in this case due to the acute CS. An aortic balloon pump (IABP) or ventricular assist device (VAD) should be considered to support the hemodynamic condition to bridge the patient to a PCI, CABG or open heart surgery to correct the papillary muscle dysfunction. IV nitroprusside and dobutamine can be added for improvement of CO by afterload reduction and positive inotropic effect.

ANALYSIS

Objectives

1. To understand how to diagnose acute cardiac failure.

2. To understand which drugs are effective in treating cardiac failure.

3. To understand the underlying causes for acute and chronic cardiac failure.

Considerations

This 60-year-old woman with an MI and heart disease was admitted with new-onset chest pain and cardiogenic shock from acute mitral regurgitation resulting from papillary muscle rupture. Inferior MIs are the most common cause of papillary muscle damage. She requires an intra-aortic balloon pump (IABP) to improve CO, BP, and flow to the coronary arteries. Vasopressors are also needed to improve the hemodynamic status. The new holosystolic murmur indicates mitral valve papillary muscle rupture or dysfunction, leading to severe mitral regurgitation. Mechanical ventilation is required to decrease the work of breathing and respiratory failure.

This patient's condition is an emergency and requires urgent intervention. Acute reversal of the mitral regurgitation (MR) is an important priority in this case.

APPROACH TO:
Acute Heart Failure

DEFINITIONS

CONGESTIVE HEART FAILURE (CHF): The inability of the heart to supply sufficient substrate to meet the needs of the body.

CARDIOGENIC SHOCK (CS): End-stage CHF and a largely irreversible condition; as such, it is more often fatal than not. It may be acute or end-stage occurrence.

PULMONARY EDEMA: Accumulation of fluid in the pulmonary air spaces and the interstitial spaces of the lungs, which inhibits oxygen and carbon dioxide diffusion, leading to impaired gas exchange and cardiogenic respiratory failure.

CLINICAL APPROACH

Acute heart failure is the leading cause of hospitalization in adults older than age 65. Ischemic heart disease is the leading cause of heart failure, followed by dilated cardiomyopathy, valvular heart disease, and hypertension. MI and CAD is the most common cause of CHF and may necessitate emergent revascularization with thrombolytic therapy (rTpa), percutaneous coronary intervention (PCI), or coronary artery bypass graft surgery (CABG). Other causes of CHF include anemia, hyperthyroidism, arrhythmia, NSAIDs, and renal failure. **Worsening CHF is a side effect of oral hypoglycemic drugs in the thiazolidinedione class (also known as glitazones), making these drugs contraindicated in patients with CHF** (Table 16–1). ADHD, pulmonary edema, and CHF are all multifactorial syndromes that result from CO impairment. In systolic heart failure, the heart cannot contract adequately, leading to fluid retention. Both the kidneys and the vascular baroreceptors sense the decrease in CO, inducing an increase in the renin-angiotensin-aldosterone system and the sympathetic system, as well as a contraction metabolic alkalosis. This increase ultimately leads to **irreversible cardiac dilatation and vascular remodeling,** as well as further fluid overload by a decreasing CO.

DIAGNOSIS

Symptoms of **ADHF** include dyspnea, fatigue, orthopnea, dyspnea on exertion, and paroxysmal nocturnal dyspnea. CHF can present atypically in patients with nonspecific complaints such as insomnia, nocturia, irritability, anorexia, fatigue, and depression. β-Type natriuretic peptide (BNP) is released by the atria when it becomes acutely dilated, a reflection of increased preload. **An elevated BNP level in the absence of renal failure is suggestive of CHF and can be used to diagnose CHF and to follow the effectiveness of treatment.** An increase in BNP induces diuresis and helps decrease fluid levels. A BNP value of <100 pg/mL is useful in ruling out CHF. However,

Table 16–1 • DIFFERENTIAL CAUSES OF CHF	
Disease	Clinical Findings
Ischemic heart disease (CAD)	History of myocardial infarction, presence of infarction pattern on (ECG), risk factors for coronary artery disease
Idiopathic dilated cardiomyopathy	HF in patients without risk factors or known coronary artery disease
Hypertension	History of poorly controlled hypertension, presence of an S4, left ventricular hypertrophy on electrocardiogram or ECG
Valvular heart disease	Mitral regurgitation, aortic stenosis; midsystolic murmur at base that radiates to carotid arteries
Infective endocarditis	Fever, positive blood cultures for typical organisms, risk factors for bacteremia (intravenous drug use, invasive intravenous lines)
Familial dilated cardiomyopathy	Family history of HF or sudden cardiac death
Toxic cardiomyopathies	History of exposure to the toxic agent (ETOH, anthracycline, radiation, cocaine, catecholamines, vitamin deficiencies)
Collagen vascular disease	History of systemic lupus erythematosus, polyarteritisnodosa, scleroderma, dermatomyositis; positive serology results
Endocrinologic disorders	Hyperthyroidism, hypothyroidism, acromegaly, pheochromocytoma, diabetes mellitus
Peripartum cardiomyopathy	HF symptoms with left ventricular dysfunction within 6 months of pregnancy
Hypertrophic cardiomyopathies	Family history of hypertrophic cardiomyopathy, ECG findings of ventricular hypertrophy. Outflow tract gradient by physical examination or echocardiography. Only murmurs that increase with a Valsalva maneuver (decreased venous return to heart)

there are some limitations of BNP, including insufficient specificity, limited correlation with Pulmonary Capillary Wedge Pressure (PCWP), and biologic variability (ie, BNP is decreased in obesity; BNP is increased with increasing age, female gender, chronic kidney disease). It is important to distinguish between the two types of CHF, **diastolic versus systolic,** since the treatment differs. This can be done via transesophageal echocardiogram (TEE) or transthoracic echocardiogram (TE).

The functional capacity in CHF can serve as a guideline for a stepwise strategy of treatment. A common classification scheme for CHF is that of the New York Heart Association (NYHA) (Table 16–2). CHF often presents with signs of both left and right heart failure. **The most common cause of right heart failure is left heart failure.** Right heart failure presents with elevated Jugular venous distention (JVD), dependent edema, and ascites, but with an absence of pulmonary congestion typical of left heart failure. When evaluating ADHF, one should first obtain a resting 12-lead ECG in all patients. An old ECG is extremely helpful for comparison with the current findings to determine progression of the disease and its time of onset.

A chest x-ray (CXR) often reveals signs of fluid overload and pump failure in the form of pulmonary edema accompanied by cardiomegaly, vascular congestion,

Table 16–2 • NEW YORK HEART ASSOCIATION CHF CLASSIFICATION; EFFORT NEEDED TO CAUSE SYMPTOMS	
NYHA CHF Class	Description
Class I Stage A	Asymptomatic, left ventricular dysfunction
Class II Stage B	Dyspnea with significant exertion
Class III Stage C	Dyspnea with minimal activity, including usual activities of daily living
Class IV Stage D	Dyspnea at rest

Kerley B lines (dilated lymphatics at bases of lungs), blunting of costophrenic angles, cephalization of the pulmonary vasculatures, and pleural effusions are common in ADHF/CHF. TE is used to determine the etiology of ADHF. TE evaluations assist in determining whether systolic dysfunction (ejection fraction [EF] <40%) or diastolic dysfunction (normal EF) exists. Significant valvular disease can also be revealed by TE determinations. Left ventricular remodeling with increased left ventricular end-diastolic volume and decreased contractility accompanies systolic dysfunction. Coronary artery disease (CAD), the main underlying cause of ADHF in two-thirds of all patients, must be aggressively treated. Patients who are post-MI often show evidence of ventricular remodeling.

Pulmonary artery catheterization can detect heart failure and monitor therapy. Routine PAC is not recommended, but it should be considered in selective cases when fluid status, perfusion, systemic or pulmonary vascular resistance is uncertain. Furthermore, if significant hypotension is present, renal function is worsening despite therapy, or cardiogenic shock is presumed, then PAC may be used.

Diastolic Dysfunction

Patients with diastolic dysfunction have EF values >40% and have normal left ventricular end-diastolic volumes. **Left ventricular hypertrophy (LVH) is frequently present with an increased stiffness in the ventricles** and a decreased compliance of the ventricular wall. Diastolic heart failure is common, especially in **elderly patients** with the previously described findings, which can be documented by TE/TEE and ECG studies.

TREATMENT

Nonpharmacological Therapy of CHF

When the CHF is compensated, limiting dietary sodium to <2 g/d and limiting fluids to 2 qt/d have decreased hospital readmissions for CHF. Mild exercise, specifically aerobic exercise, is known to improve hemodynamic values in patients with CHF. Exercise also eases the activities of daily living (ADL) and the quality of life (QOL). Identifying sleep disturbances and nighttime hypoxia is also an important step in the management of CHF. Accurately diagnosing and treating obstructive sleep apnea (OSA) can be lifesaving for these patients. Treatment of OSA will decrease BP, increase the capacity of exercise, decrease hospital admissions and improve QOL. The delivery of positive pressure decreases preload by delivering PEEP.

Patients with NYHA class III or class IV (Table 16–2) with a QRS >120 ms should be considered for biventricular pacing. If the EF is <35%, an implantable cardioversion device (ICD) is indicated. Cardiac resynchronization therapy via the pacer and ICD improves QOL and decreases mortality. Cardiac transplantation improves survival, functional status, and QOL in patients with NYHA of class III or class IV. Patients on maximal therapy but still displaying ADHF should be considered as subjects for transplantation if they are <65 years old. Contraindications for transplantation include end-organ damage from diabetes, vascular disease, cancer, cerebrovascular accident (CVA), lack of psychological support, and active psychiatric illness.

Drug therapy: CHF patients with systolic dysfunction have improved survival on angiotensin-converting enzyme inhibitors, β-blockers and for some patient groups, aldosterone antagonists. Recent studies also demonstrate combined neprilysin and renin-angiotensin system inhibition may be used for the treatment of heart failure. Digitalis used cautiously will decrease hospital readmission for CHF. In **African American with hypertension and CHF**, adding the combination of **hydralazine and nitrates** to standard therapy **increases survival rates**. Table 16–3 outlines the various pharmacological interventions that should be considered in patients with CHF. In patients with rare forms of CHF, efforts to treat diastolic dysfunction are designed to increase the cardiac output; these interventions include treating hypertension, maintaining NSR, and treating any form of ischemia. In treatment for acute heart failure, there is no significant benefit over placebo with vasopressin receptor antagonists, endothelin antagonists, novel inotropic medications, adenosine receptor antagonists, and nesiritide. These include inotropes, tolvaptan, tezosentan, levosimendan, and rolofylline. For acute heart failure patients with congestion and hypoperfusion, vasodilators are preferred to inotropes.

Management of right ventricular failure: Definitive therapy for an acutely decompensated right ventricular failure (RVF) requires primary treatment of the underlying condition in addition to hemodynamic support. Patients with right ventricular failure can be very resilient and can recover substantially if the underlying causes are successfully treated. Treatment options include percutaneous coronary intervention for RV infarction. Thrombolytic therapy should be applied if catheterization is not available. Open surgical embolectomy may be required for massive pulmonary emboli (PE) with heart failure due to acute pump failure.

Oxygen: Oxygen should be administered to all CHF patients whether the patient is hypoxic or not. This decreases the anxiety which usually accompanies CHF. The minimal FIO$_2$ is one that achieves an O$_2$ sat of 92% or greater. NIV and MV may be needed to assist the ventilatory and oxygenation requirements. The application of PEEP should also be considered.

Noninvasive ventilation (NIV): NIV is a perfect treatment modality for ADHF. It decreases the work in breathing, improves oxygenation and ventilation, and decreases preload. NIV may be helpful in pre-oxygenating patients with hypoxemic respiratory failure before ETI. NIV is increasing in ICUs throughout Europe and the United States. Closely monitor for mask tolerance and leaks, alterations

Table 16–3 • DRUG TREATMENT FOR HEART FAILURE DUE TO SYSTOLIC DYSFUNCTION

Drug Treatment	Drug Actions
Angiotensin-converting enzyme inhibitors (ACE), enalaprilat (IV only), captopril, lisinopril	ACE inhibitors are used for all classes of heart failure. They inhibit angiotensin-converting enzyme, resulting in decreased conversion of angiotensin I to angiotensin II and decreased metabolism of bradykinin. They improve exercise tolerance, hemodynamic status, and survival, and they may halt progression and cause regression of HF. Avoid in patients with history of ACE inhibitor–induced angioedema.
Valsartan/sacubitril and ivabradine	Recommended for heart failure in updated guidelines from the American Heart Association, the American College of Cardiology, and the Heart Failure Society of America. Valsartan/sacubitril is an angiotensin receptor-neprilysin inhibitor (ARNI). By blocking that receptor, it inhibits the break-down of bradykinin and in turn reduces blood volume. For heart failure with reduced ejection fraction, an ARNI, angiotensin II receptor blocker (ARB), or ACE inhibitor is recommended, together with a beta blocker and aldosterone antagonist. An ARNI should not be coadministered with an ACE inhibitor or in patients with an angioedema history. Since both drug classes affect bradykinin, they significantly increase angioedema risk.
Ivabradine	Ivabradine, a sinoatrial node modulator, may help reduce hospitalizations in patients with symptomatic stable chronic heart failure with reduced ejection fraction who are taking a maximum tolerated dose of a beta blocker and whose resting heart rate is $\geq$70 beats/min.
β-Blockers (carvedilol, metoprolol, bisoprolol)	Used for all classes of CHF. Inhibit adrenergic nervous system and improve survival. Reduce sudden death risk and may halt progression and cause regression of heart failure. Use with caution in patients with NYHA class IV heart failure. Avoid in patients with significant asthma and high-grade conduction system disease.
Aldosterone antagonists (spironolactone, eplerenone)	Improve survival in patients with NYHA II-IV heart failure. Improve survival after MI with left ventricular dysfunction. Follow potassium level closely, especially in patients taking ACE inhibitors and NSAIDs.
Angiotensin-receptor antagonists (losartan, valsartan)	Use in patients who cannot take ACE inhibitors. Inhibit renin-angiotensin system at angiotensin receptor level. Lead to improvement in hemodynamics, symptoms; patients have less incidence of cough.
Hydralazine and nitrates (isosorbide dinitrate, isosorbide mononitrate)	Reserved for patients intolerant to ACE inhibitors and angiotensin receptor blockers (ARB). Reduce afterload and preload. Improve survival in patients with heart failure but not so well as ACE inhibitors. Indicated to reduce mortality in African American when added to ACE inhibitors and β-blockers.
Digitalis glycoside (digoxin)	Positive inotropic agent. Slows heart rate through vagal effects, improves exercise tolerance, and reduces hospitalizations. No survival benefit. Aim for level < 2.0 mg/mL. Use lower dose in elderly and in patients with renal insufficiency. Avoid hypokalemia.
Loop diuretics	Palliative in patients with congestive symptoms. No survival benefit.
Positive inotropic agents (dobutamine, milrinone)	Used to improve hemodynamics in patients with severe CHF and maintain patients until cardiac transplant; can be used continuously at home in nontransplant candidates for palliation. Arrhythmogenic; no survival benefit.

in the respiratory rate, the use of accessory muscles, and their synchrony with the ventilator. Within 1 to 2 hours of admission, determine the success or failure of NIV use see NIV Case 12.

Surgical treatment: Coronary artery bypass graft (CABG) surgery is the removal of an autologous vein and using it to replace the blocked coronary artery in the heart. When the valve responsible for CHF requires modification due to excess valve tissue, valve repair is considered. In some cases, annuloplasty is required to replace the ring around the valve. If repair of the valve is not possible, it should be replaced with an artificial heart valve. The last level in the treatment of CHF is replacement of the heart. When severe heart failure is present and medication or other procedures are not effective, the diseased heart needs to be replaced or augmented. Unfortunately, the number of patients who qualify for heart replacement outnumber the supply of available donors.

Pacemaker: Pacemakers function by sending electric pulses to the heart, forcing it to beat at a rate that is considered normal or required by the patient. Pacemakers with sensory capacity can adjust their output rate depending on the cardiac demand of the patient. These devices are used to treat patients with arrhythmias or rhythm problems such as symptomatic bradycardia and tachycardia.

CARDIOGENIC SHOCK

Management of CS should focus on the augmentation of oxygen delivery and BP to maximize tissue perfusion. Delay in the diagnosis or therapy of CS increases mortality. The management of CS can be accomplished by pharmacological and mechanical means, or by revascularization.

Pharmacologic therapy: The initial treatment for patients with CS focuses on the restoration of normal hemodynamics, oxygenation, and reestablishment of a normal heart rhythm. In patients without significant pulmonary edema, a fluid challenge before vasopressor therapy is advised to improve splanchnic blood flow. If pulmonary edema is present or there is a lack of response to the fluid challenge, pharmacologic therapy should be initiated. The initial therapy should include medications that have both a **positive inotropic and vasopressor effect.** Cardiogenic shock requires both rapid diagnosis and appropriate therapy. ICU patients often have multiple-organ failure, and differentiating CS from other forms of shock can be difficult. Drugs considered for use as first-line treatments include norepinephrine, dopamine, dobutamine, epinephrine, and phenylephrine. In patients with heart failure, an increased mortality has been described in those given adrenergic inotropic agents. The improved hemodynamics resulting from the use of these agents comes at the cost of increased myocardial consumption of oxygen.

Using vasopressin instead of epinephrine resulted in similar hemodynamic effects via a direct effect on vasopressin receptors. **Vasopressin has been recommended as the drug of choice to be given during cardiac arrest, supplanting epinephrine.** Therapy with phosphodiesterase inhibitors (eg, milrinone) may be considered, particularly in cases with right ventricular dysfunction, although the hemodynamically unstable patient often poorly tolerates the resultant decrease in SVR. Levosimendan, an investigational calcium sensitizer that also promotes coronary vasodilation, continues to show promise as a novel treatment for CS. The maintenance of normal physiologic parameters (eg, MAP, cardiac index) should be the goal of therapy with any drug intended to correct CS, although high-dose vasopressor treatment has been associated with poorer patient survival.

Mechanical therapy: In patients who are unresponsive to pharmacologic therapy, mechanical augmentation of blood flow may be of benefit. **The placement of an IABP in patients with CS decreases the 6-month mortality.** IABP counterpulsation devices can be put in place at the bedside to improve diastolic pressure, simultaneously reducing left ventricular afterload without increasing myocardial oxygen demand. The incidence of major complications (eg, arterial injury and perforation, limb ischemia, visceral ischemia) associated with IABP insertion is 3%. IABP is contraindicated in patients with severe aortic insufficiency, severe peripheral vascular disease, and aortic aneurysm or dissection. In these conditions the placement of a ventricular assist device (VAD) may be considered.

Other potentially useful procedures include extracorporeal membrane oxygenation (ECMO) and placement of a ventricular assist device or a new heart. These have varying degrees of success. Newer percutaneous VADs are a more feasible choice in smaller medical-surgical centers. Patients with LVAD demonstrated significant improvement in hemodynamics, in renal function, and in the clearance of serum lactate compared to the use of IABP. There are a limited number of centers that have access to such technology. Experience in the placement of LVAD devices and in hemodynamic management is necessary to achieve an optimal benefit for patients. The use of IABP was independently associated with survival in the centers most experienced in its use. These devices are intended to serve as a bridge to cardiac transplantation, and resources must be available to continue this often-lengthy workup.

Revascularization therapy: Because AMI is frequently the cause of CS, reestablishing blood flow to the affected myocardial area is critically important and decreases mortality. Reestablishing coronary arterial flow by the administration of **thrombolytic** agents works, but the preferred modality of revascularization remains **either PCI or CABG.** Thrombolytic therapy for CS after STEMI is only for patients in whom definitive therapy is contraindicated or unavailable. **Fibrinolytic agents may still be considered in those situations in which PCI is not attainable for >90 minutes or if patients are within 3 hours of their MI and free of contraindications.** Early revascularization reduces mortality by 22% in patients with CS and by 16% in those who developed CS subsequent to admission. Early revascularization therapy is recommended for patients <75 years with complications of ACS. Revascularization in NSTEMI did result in a significant decrease in mortality. Therefore, it is just as important to revascularize NSTEMI patients. Both acute hemodialysis and ultrafiltration are used to remove the overload of fluid, especially in renally compromised patients.

Prevention

Long-standing hypertension is associated with both systolic and diastolic ventricular dysfunction leading to CHF. Hypertension is an independent risk factor for CAD.

Controlling hypertension markedly lowers the mortality and the risk for developing CHF. **Diabetics** suffer from increased cardiac events, independent of CAD and hypertension. Diabetes is also associated with LVH and arterial vessel wall stiffening. Aggressive BP control and lipid control with statins have beneficial effects in diabetic patients beyond those seen in the general population. Patients with CHF should avoid exposure to cardiotoxins such as alcohol, smoking, and illicit drugs. Smoking markedly increases the risk of CAD. Cocaine use has both direct and indirect cardiac effects that increase the risk for CHF and sudden cardiac death.

Other common occurrences that lead to ADHF include myocardial ischemia, arrhythmias, AF, severe hypertension, renal dysfunction, an unbalanced diet, and noncompliance with treatment. An elevated heart rate can lead to ADHF; thus, causes of tachycardia such as fever, anemia, hyperthyroidism, and infection should be addressed. In CHF the use of BB is indicated in almost all patients. Tachycardia in CHF decreases LV filling time, leading to a drop in CO. Patients with CHF frequently use concomitant medications such as NSAIDs and thiazolidinediones. Thiazolidinedione use for the control of diabetes is contraindicated in patients with CHF.

Daily weight determination at home is still the best evaluator of overall fluid volume. The actual weight is not important; rather, the difference from the last measurements and an increased trend in weight is important. The patient or the doctor may increase or decrease the diuretic therapy. Electrolyte imbalances in CHF are mostly related to its treatment. A blood Na^+ level ≤ 134 mEq/L is an independent risk for mortality, and Na^+ levels must be monitored in patients with CHF.

CLINICAL CASE CORRELATION

- See also Case 4 (Hemodynamic Monitoring), Case 5 (Vasoactive Drugs and Pharmacology), Case 12 (NIV), Case 14 (Acute Coronary Syndromes), and Case 15 (Cardiac Arrhythmias).

COMPREHENSION QUESTIONS

16.1 A 60-year-old man is evaluated in the ICU for acute chest discomfort after being pain-free for 72 hours post STEMI and PCI. The patient was treated with ASA, a β-blocker, and nitroglycerin. The ECG revealed an inferior wall STEMI. Troponins were elevated. On physical examination, the heart rate was irregular and feeble with a BP of 78/60 mm Hg. The JVD was elevated to the angle of the jaw. Pulseless cardiac activity is observed. Which of the following is the most likely cause for this patient's findings?

A. Acute cardiac tamponade

B. Aortic dissection

C. Left ventricular free-wall rupture

D. Right ventricular myocardial infarction

16.2 A 65-year-old African-American man presents to the clinic with dyspnea on exertion. He also complains of fatigue and difficulty completing his usual half hour workout on the treadmill. He denies a history of smoking but admits to drinking two six-packs of beer every weekend. Physical examination shows elevated Jugular venous pulse (JVP) crackles in both lower lung fields, and 2+ pitting edema to the knees. Which test would provide the most information to assess his condition?

A. Pulmonary function tests

B. Chest x-ray

C. Arterial blood gas

D. Echocardiograph

E. Electrocardiogram

16.3 An 80-year-old Hispanic woman with a past medical history of chronic obstructive pulmonary disease, congestive heart failure, and diabetes mellitus type II was admitted to the hospital because she could not catch her breath. Her heart rate is 105 beats/min, her respiratory rate is 30 breaths/min, her blood pressure is 178/112 mm Hg and her oxygen saturation is 90% on her home oxygen at 2 L/min. On physical examination, she is using accessory muscles. Rales are appreciated bilaterally. What is the goal of CHF treatment?

A. Decrease preload, increase afterload

B. Decrease force of contraction, increase afterload

C. Decrease preload, decrease afterload

D. Increase force of contraction, increase preload

ANSWERS

16.1 **C.** The most common cause of myocardial rupture is a recent myocardial infarction (MI). Myocardial rupture after acute MI may occur from 1 day to 3 weeks after infarction, with most ruptures occurring 3 to 5 days after infarction. Ischemic myocardial rupture after acute MI may involve the left ventricular and right ventricular free walls, the ventricular septum and the left ventricular papillary muscle. Myocardial rupture after infarction is more common in patients aged 60 years or older. Acute chest pain, shortness of breath, shock, diaphoresis, cool and clammy skin, and syncope may indicate a ventricular septal rupture after acute MI. Cardiac tamponade is caused by the accumulation of fluid in the pericardial space, causing reduced ventricular filling and hemodynamic compromise. Electrical alternates can be seen on ECG. Aortic dissection is a separation of the layers within the aortic wall and can be commonly described as a tearing or ripping pain that radiates to the back between the scapula. A right ventricular infarction is an atherosclerotic occlusion of the right coronary artery. ECG findings can show ST-segment elevation in leads V3 through V6.

16.2 **D.** Echocardiograph would provide the most information because not only can assessment of size and function of the heart chambers can be carried out, the heart valve function and diastolic function can also be assessed. Right atrial pressure, left atrial pressure, stroke volume and pulmonary artery pressure can also be estimated by echocardiography.

16.3 **C.** The heart cannot produce a normal stroke volume in CHF. Goals of CHF therapy include the following: (1) decreasing the preload to decrease the stroke volume pumped out by the left atrium and ventricle. This can be done with diuretics. (2) decreasing the afterload to decrease the resistance the heart is pumping against. This can be done with vasodilators. (3) increasing the force of contraction. This can be done with positive inotropes. Vasodilators and inotropes should only be used as a bridge to definitive therapy, or for palliation in medically refractory patients.

CLINICAL PEARLS

▶ Jugular venous distention is the most sensitive clinical sign of acute cardiac decompensation.

▶ Echocardiography confirms the diagnosis of ADHF and aids in directing its management.

▶ In patients with right ventricular MI, echocardiography demonstrates right ventricular enlargement with reduced systolic function.

▶ The use of IABP in severe ADHF serves as a bridge to surgery or angioplasty.

▶ Medications have not lowered morbidity or mortality in CHF secondary to diastolic dysfunction.

▶ In CHF, reversible factors that can cause exacerbations should be identified and treated. A sodium concentration <134 mEq/L is an independent risk factor for greater mortality in CHF.

▶ When ECG changes suggest myocardial ischemia, early revascularization is needed.

▶ Vasopressin can be added to dobutamine and norepinephrine for improvement in MAP.

REFERENCES

Chinnaiyan KM, Alexander D, Maddens M, McCullough PA. Curriculum in cardiology: integrated diagnosis and management of diastolic heart failure. *Am Heart J.* 2007;153:189-200.

Yancy CW, Jessup M, Bozkurt B, et al. 2013 ACCF/AHA guideline for the management of heart failure. *J Am Coll Cardiol* 2013;62(16):1495-1536.

Loscalzo J. *Harrison's Pulmonary and Critical Care Medicine.* New York, NY: McGraw-Hill; 2013.

CASE 17

A 45-year-old man was brought to the emergency department (ED) in January because of fever, confusion, and "inability to talk." His wife reported that he had generalized malaise, headache, and low-grade fever for 3 days with no other specific symptoms. Several hours before coming to the ED, he was noted to have progressive lethargy and confusion and lost his ability to speak. He did not have nausea, vomiting, diarrhea, focal weakness or seizures. He was previously in good health, took no medications, and denied recent travel outside of the United States. There were no recent insect bites or pet exposures. On physical examination, his temperature was 38.3°C (101°F) and other vital signs were normal. Expressive aphasia was noted, but there were no focal findings and the pupils were equal and reactive to light. There was some nuchal rigidity noted. There were no petechiae, splinter hemorrhages, subconjunctival hemorrhages, or heart murmurs. The fundi were normal without papilledema. A lumbar puncture was performed, and the findings from the cerebrospinal fluid (CSF) were as follows: leukocyte count 150 cells/µL with 90% lymphocytes, erythrocytes 500/µL, protein 125 mg/dL, glucose 50 mg/dL, and no organisms were seen on a Gram stain. After the lumbar puncture he developed progressive weakness of the right upper extremity.

▶ What is the most likely diagnosis?
▶ What is the best treatment for this patient?
▶ What other diagnostic tests may be performed to support the diagnosis?

ANSWERS TO CASE 17:
Meningitis/Encephalitis

Summary: A previously healthy 45-year-old man developed a sudden onset of fever, headache, expressive aphasia, and focal weakness in January. A lumbar puncture (LP) reveals no organisms, elevated protein and leukocytes with lymphocyte predominance. He has progressive weakness of his right upper extremity.

- **Most likely diagnosis:** Herpes simplex virus type 1 (HSV-1) encephalitis.

- **Best treatment:** Admit to the ICU and immediately start intravenous acyclovir. Until definitive confirmation of etiology, also initiate antibacterial therapy.

- **Confirmatory tests:** A brain biopsy is definitive (usually not done if the HSV PCR test is positive and/or empiric acyclovir results in clinical improvement). A PCR on the CSF for HSV-1 should be performed and is often positive. MRI of the brain and EEG add support to the diagnosis.

ANALYSIS

Objectives

1. To describe the most common causes of meningitis and encephalitis.

2. To find the differences in the CSF examination in meningitis and encephalitis etiologic agents.

3. To discuss the options for treating meningitis and encephalitis.

Considerations

This patient has a typical presentation of sporadic HSV-1 encephalitis. His acute onset of low-grade fever, generalized malaise, and headache which progressed to lethargy, aphasia, and then focal weakness of the right upper extremity is strongly suggestive of HSV-1 encephalitis. Seizure is often present. Encephalitis viruses include Eastern equine encephalitis, St. Louis encephalitis, La Crosse encephalitis, California encephalitis, Powassan fever, and all others, which are less common than West Nile virus (WNV) and HSV-1 encephalitis. In the absence of a known outbreak of WNV, the presentation suggests that the most likely diagnosis is viral encephalitis due to HSV-1. Herpes encephalitis is the most common cause of fatal sporadic encephalitis in the United States and should always be considered in the differential diagnosis "treatable" with antiviral medication. The CSF findings of a lymphocytic pleocytosis with a significant number of RBCs and an elevated protein on LP are suggestive of HSV encephalitis. Decreased CSF glucose levels may also be present in HSV encephalitis but are rarely present in other kinds of viral encephalitis. A positive polymerase chain reaction (PCR) for HSV-1 in the CSF would confirm the diagnosis. Supporting information for HSV-1 encephalitis may include CT or MRI of the brain, EEG, brain biopsy, and culture of the CSF for HSV. Other considerations would include rickettsia (RMSF); nonspirochetal treponemes (lyme); fungal (cryptococcosis); protozoal (acanthoamoeba, Nagleria); and bacterial etiologies. Therapies should consider geographic exposures, vector exposure (ticks, mosquitoes), occupation, hobbies and immune defects.

APPROACH TO:
Meningitis/Encephalitis

CNS infections are medical emergencies. These include meningitis due to a bacterial or viral infection of tissues surrounding the cerebral cortex (meninges) and encephalitis, which is a viral infection of the cerebral cortex. There may be a combination of meningitis and encephalitis (meningoencephalitis), which is most often viral in etiology.

BACTERIAL MENINGITIS

Early diagnosis and appropriate therapy (within 2 hours of presentation) of suspected bacterial meningitis is crucial. More than 75% of all cases of bacterial meningitis in the United States are due to *Streptococcus pneumoniae* or *Neisseria meningitidis*. Meningitis due to *Haemophilus influenzae* has markedly decreased due to widespread immunization with the Haemophilus B influenza conjugate vaccine. *Listeria monocytogenes* remains an infection of at-risk patients, and infections by this bacterium are sporadic. Less commonly, meningitis due to *Streptococcus agalactiae* (Group B Streptococcus) and *Escherichia coli* may be seen in at-risk patients (neonates, infants, and immunocompromised patients).

Streptococcus pneumoniae is the most common etiologic agent of community-acquired bacterial meningitis and is often seen in patients with other foci of infection: pneumonia, otitis media, mastoiditis, sinusitis, or endocarditis. It may also be one of the causes of meningitis following **CSF leaks** due to trauma, iatrogenesis, or congenital defects of the meninges. The pneumococcal 13-valent for children and 23-valent vaccine for adults are effective in preventing invasive disease.

Neisseria meningitidis is the **second most common sporadic agent of bacterial meningitis** and the most common cause of outbreaks and epidemics of bacterial meningitis in the United States. It occurs **primarily in children and young adults.** Patients with persistent deficiencies in the terminal complement components (C5-C9) are predisposed to infection with *N. meningitidis*. A quadravalent (A, C, Y, or W-135) conjugate vaccine is available but does not protect against serogroup B, the agent of one-third of cases in the United States. The Advisory Committee on Immunization Practices (ACIP) has recommended vaccination be used for the prevention of meningococcal disease in the following individuals:

1. Routine vaccination of adolescents at age 11 to 12 years with a booster at age 16

2. A two-dose primary series administered 2 months apart for persons aged 2 to 54 years with persistent complement deficiency (C5-C9), or functional or anatomic asplenia, or HIV infection

Other less common causes of bacterial meningitis include *L. monocytogenes*, Group B streptococci (*S. agalactiae*), aerobic gram-negative bacilli, and staphylococcus species. **Listeria monocytogenes meningitis** is associated with **extremes of age**, namely neonates and persons >50 years of age. Alcoholism, malignancy, immunosuppression, diabetes mellitus, hepatic failure, renal failure, iron overload, collagen vascular disorders, and HIV infection are also predisposing factors.

Group B streptococcal meningitis, an important cause of infection in **neonates**, can be seen in adults with the same underlying conditions that predispose to listerial meningitis. **Aerobic gram-negative bacilli** (*Klebsiella* species, *E. coli*, *Serratia marcescens*, and *Pseudomonas aeruginosa*), *Staphylococcus aureus*, and *S. epidermidis* may cause meningitis in patients with **head trauma** (subsequent to neurosurgical procedures and placement of CSF shunts) or following bacteremia due to catheters, indwelling devices, and urinary tract infection. **Community-acquired Methicillin-resistant S. aureus** (CA-MRSA) is an emerging cause of community-acquired meningitis. The differential diagnosis of bacterial meningitis is broad and includes organisms that may be mycobacterial, fungal, protozoal, and viral.

Diagnosis of Meningitis

Meningitis should be considered if a patient has **fever, headache, neck stiffness, and altered mental status.** On examination "jolt accentuation" of the headache elicited with rapid horizontal movement of the head is considered to be more sensitive for the diagnosis of meningitis than the traditional Kernig or Brudzinski signs of meningeal irritation. **Nuchal rigidity** is the inability to flex the head forward due to rigidity of the neck muscles. **Kernig sign** is positive when the leg is bent at the hip and knee at an angle of 90 degrees, and subsequent extension of the knee is painful. **Brudzinski sign** is the appearance of involuntary lifting of the legs when the patient's head is lifted from the examining couch when the patient is lying supine. These findings are not specific and may indicate subarachnoid hemorrhage as well as meningitis. Nuchal rigidity, altered mental status, and Kernig and Brudzinski signs may be absent, but this should not deter an evaluation for meningitis.

The diagnosis of meningitis is established by the analysis of a CSF specimen (Table 17–1). At times CT imaging may be necessary prior to performing a lumbar

Table 17–1 • CEREBROSPINAL FLUID FINDINGS IN PATIENTS WITH MENINGITIS					
CSF Parameter	Normal	Bacterial	Viral	TB	Cryptococcal
Opening pressure (mm H$_2$O)	80-200	200-500	≤ 250	180-300	> 200
Leukocyte count (cells/μL)	0-5	1000-5000	50-1000	50-300	20-500
Leukocyte count differential	Lymphs[a]	PMN[b] > 80%	Lymphs[a] predominate	Lymphs[a] monocytes	Lymphs[a]
Glucose (mg/dL)	50-70	< 40	> 45	≤ 45	< 40
Protein (mg/dL)	15-40	100-500	< 200	50-100	> 45

[a]Lymphocytes.
[b]Polymorphonuclear neutrophils.

puncture to reduce the risk of brain herniation; however, this imaging should not delay empiric antibiotic therapy. **Specific indications for a CT imaging prior to an LP include: focal neurological findings (including seizure), increased intracranial pressure or papilledema, age >65 years, underlying immune deficiency, and coma.** A CSF white cell count $\geq 500/\mu L$, a CSF lactate acid ≥ 3.5 mmol/L, or a CSF-to-serum glucose ratio ≤ 0.4 are highly predictive of bacterial meningitis. Latex agglutination testing is available for the evaluation of bacterial meningitis (*H. influenzae* type B; *S. pneumoniae*; *N. meningitidis* groups A, B, C, Y, or W135; *S. agalactiae* and *E. coli* K1; **BD Directigen Meningitis Combo Test**). A polymerase chain reaction (PCR) should be considered as a diagnostic aid, especially for meningitis due to enteroviruses, which cause about 85% of the viral meningitis seen in the United States (echovirus, coxsackievirus A and B, and the nonpolio enteroviruses).

Tuberculous meningitis can mimic enteroviral and herpes simplex virus infections. IgM antibody captures enzyme-linked immunosorbent assay (ELISA) testing which is useful in identifying arbovirus infections, especially those due to WNV, St. Louis encephalitis, California encephalitis, Eastern equine encephalitis, La Crosse encephalitis, and Powassan viruses. This is especially important in patients whose CSF evaluation is consistent with aseptic meningitis. Aseptic meningitis is meningeal inflammation without identification of a causative bacterial agent and accompanied by a monocytic pleocytosis of the CSF. Seasonality, geography, exposure to ticks or mosquitoes, and concomitant symptoms and signs are usually helpful in determining the etiology.

The natural history of aseptic meningitis is usually benign and often subclinical or underappreciated due to its low-grade presentation (eg, mumps, enteroviral infections). However, at times, especially WNV can cause devastating effects with severe morbidity and mortality. Testing for fungal, mycobacterial, HIV, and nontreponemal spirochetal agents (Lyme disease) should be performed when clinically indicated (eg, immunosuppression, exposure history) in nonbacterial meningitis. A Venereal Disease Research Laboratory (VDRL) test should be considered on all abnormal CSF samples to exclude syphilis. Noninfectious causes of meningitis should be considered, including drug-induced causes (nonsteroidal anti-inflammatory drug [NSAID] use and collagen vascular diseases, especially systemic lupus erythematosus).

Treatment of Meningitis

If the examination of CSF reveals the presence of purulent meningitis and a positive Gram stain suggests a specific etiology, targeted antimicrobial therapy must be initiated as quickly as possible (optimally within 30 minutes of arrival in the ED). If the Gram stain is negative, empiric antibiotic therapy is determined by the patient's age and underlying conditions (Table 17–2). The administration of dexamethasone concomitant with or just prior to the first dose of antimicrobial therapy will attenuate the inflammatory response created by the lysis of certain meningeal pathogens (*H. influenzae*, *Mycobacterium tuberculosis*, *S. pneumoniae*, and *Cryptococcus neoformans*) by antimicrobial agents. If *L. monocytogenes* is proven or suspected, ampicillin should be included in the antibacterial regimen, to which gentamicin may be added for synergy.

Table 17–2 • EMPIRIC ANTIMICROBIAL THERAPY FOR PURULENT MENINGITIS		
Predisposing Factors	Common Bacterial Pathogens	Recommended Antimicrobial Agents
Age 2-50 years	S. pneumoniae, N. meningitidis	Vancomycin + a third-generation cephalosporin
Age > 50 years	S. pneumonia, N. meningitidis, L. monocytogenes,[a] aerobic gram-negative bacilli	Vancomycin + ampicillin + a third-genaration cephalosporin
Basilar skull fracture	S. pneumonia, H. influenzae, Group A β-hemolytic streptococci	Vancomycin + a third-generation cephalosporin
Postneuro surgery or head trauma	S. aureus, S. epidermidis, aerobic gram-negative bacilli (including P. aeruginosa)	Vancomycin + either ceftazidine or cefepime
Cerebrospinal fluid shunt	S. aureus, S. epidermidis, aerobic gram-negative bacilli (including P. aeruginosa), diphtheroids (including P. acnes)	Vancomycin + either ceftazidime or cefepime

[a]Gentamicin may be added for synergy in Listeria, S. aureus, and gram-negative meningitis.

In the treatment of bacterial meningitis, time is of the essence. Antimicrobial treatment should not be delayed while awaiting the results of a CT scan or an MRI. If a CT scan is indicated prior to an LP, **antibiotics should be started empirically** after an appropriate examination and septic workup.

VIRAL ENCEPHALITIS

Viruses are by far the most common cause of encephalitis. Approximately 20,000 cases of encephalitis occur in the United States each year, with the predominant endemic sporadic cause being the HSV-1. **The most common epidemic cause of viral meningitis is WNV,** followed by other sporadic and epidemic viral etiologies. Rabies encephalitis is now rare in North America. Viral encephalitis presents as an acute-onset, febrile illness associated with headache, altered level of consciousness, and occasionally focal neurologic signs. The clinical presentation of encephalitis can be similar to meningitis, but the two differ in that meningitis is not always characterized by focal neurologic signs and change in mental status. While fever and headache are the principal manifestations of both syndromes, nuchal rigidity is characteristic only of meningitis.

Arboviral diseases such as Eastern equine encephalitis and St. Louis encephalitis have affected humans in the United States for years. These viral infections may be fatal or have significant morbidity; the prevalence in humans has been low and effective treatments and human vaccines have not been developed. This situation changed in 1999 when the first cases of WNV occurred in the United States. The virus spread throughout the United States and has now been diagnosed in thousands of patients annually with significant morbidity and mortality.

WNV encephalitis is most severe in the older age groups, with the highest mortality and morbidity rates occurring in those ≥65 years of age. While most cases of WNV infection are subclinical or mild, the disease can be severe and most often occurs during seasonal outbreaks or epidemic conditions. These severe clinical presentations of WNV include encephalitis, meningitis, flaccid paralysis, and fever. Vaccines have been developed for veterinary use in preventing WNV as early as 2001; however, there are currently no approved vaccines for human use for WNV.

In the United States nonepidemic, sporadic, or focal encephalitis is most frequently due to HSV-1, with one-third of the cases occurring in patients <20 years of age and one-half occurring in those over 50 years old. **HSV-1 encephalitis results from a reactivation of the latent virus in the trigeminal ganglion, resulting in inflammatory necrotic lesions in the temporal cortex and limbic system.** Most HSV-1 cases occur in the absence of an antecedent illness.

Diagnosis of Encephalitis

After a history and physical examination is completed, CSF analysis should be performed including cell count, glucose, protein, and cultures (both viral and bacterial). PCR should be performed for specific viral diagnoses including HSV-1, and IgM antibody capture ELISA tests should be based upon suspected viral etiologies. CSF cultures for HSV-1 and arboviruses are usually negative, but the sensitivity of the PCR for HSV and the arboviral IgM antibody capture ELISA exceeds 90%. **In HSV encephalitis, MRI typically demonstrates unilateral or bilateral abnormalities in the medial and inferior temporal lobes,** which may extend into the frontal lobe. The EEG findings include focal delta activity over the temporal lobes and periodic lateralizing epileptiform discharges (PLEDs). Brain biopsy with fluorescent antibody and histopathology is reserved for patients who do not respond to empiric acyclovir or have negative PCRs of the CSF. CT imaging is not as sensitive as MRI with gadolinium.

The **CSF typically shows a lymphocytic pleocytosis,** an increased number of erythrocytes and an increased concentration of protein; glucose levels are usually normal but may be low early in the infection. With early HSV-1 encephalitis, the CSF may initially show a Polymorphonucleocytes (PMN) predominance which then shifts to a lymphocytosis. Acyclovir should be started immediately when HSV-1 infection is suspected. PCR for HSV-1 DNA in CSF should be obtained, but treatment should not be delayed waiting for results. A temporal lobe abnormality on MRI (eg, a hemorrhagic lesion) is considered to be a poor prognostic sign for neurologic recovery, although CMV, EBV, and echoviruses can cause the same syndrome of encephalitis infection.

WNV infection is more frequently associated with a poliomyelitis, Parkinson-like syndrome, or a Guillain-Barre type of presentation. Vector-borne diseases such as WNV infection are unlikely events during a Minnesota winter, especially when there is no evidence of an outbreak or epidemic. **The diagnosis of HSV-1 encephalitis is critical because it is the only viral infection of the CNS for which antiviral therapy with acyclovir has been proven effective.** In HSV encephalitis, prompt acyclovir treatment reduces mortality to approximately 25% in adults and older children. Unfortunately, over 50% of the patients who survive will have neurologic sequelae.

HIV-RELATED CENTRAL NERVOUS SYSTEM DISEASES

HIV-infected individuals are susceptible to CNS toxoplasmosis infection when their CD4 lymphocyte counts are below 200/µL and are at high risk with CD4 counts below 50/µL. Localized or focal encephalitis is the most common presentation of toxoplasmosis. **Toxoplasmosis is the most common cause of a CNS mass lesion in AIDS**, followed by CNS lymphoma (B cell or non-Hodgkin), which occurs in approximately 2% to 12% of HIV-infected individuals. Unlike the situation in immunocompetent hosts, HIV-associated lymphoma is strongly associated with **Epstein–Barr virus infection.** In patients with AIDS, lymphoma was second only to toxoplasmosis as the most common source of central nervous system mass lesions. A negative PCR for Epstein–Barr virus and the diffuse nature of an MRI abnormality exclude central nervous system lymphoma.

Cryptococcal meningitis (CM) is a subacute infection of the central nervous system associated with a CSF pleocytosis of 40 to 400 cells/µL with lymphocyte predominance and slightly low glucose levels. Diagnosis of cryptococcal CNS infection can be made in >98% of patients by combining the use of rapid antigen detection tests for **cryptococcal antigen, India ink preparation, and CSF cultures for fungi.**

Progressive multifocal leukoencephalopathy (PML) is an opportunistic infection caused by polyomavirus JC, which is associated with gradual demyelination of the central nervous system and thereby expressed as a progressive neurologic deficit. The lesions of PML are generally bilateral, asymmetric, nonenhancing or with delayed peripheral enhancement, and are periventricular or subcortical in distribution. Radiographic studies reveal no unusual tissue mass effects. This is in contrast to primary central nervous system lymphoma and toxoplasmosis in which mass effect may occur.

Risk factors for AIDS-related opportunistic infections include late-stage HIV infection (CD4 cell count <100/µL), no prior treatment, and the presence of thrush. Patients with PML usually display focal neurologic signs, and an MRI will reveal multiple white matter lesions without mass effect, involving the right lateral frontal, right frontoparietal, and left frontal lobes, right pons, bilateral brachium pontis, and right cerebellum. In addition, the PCR is positive for polyomavirus JC in PML. While the gold standard for the diagnosis of PML is brain biopsy, the CNS lesions are usually quite deep and relatively inaccessible. When the preponderance of clinical evidence supports a diagnosis of PML, biopsy can usually be deferred. Approximately 50% of patients with AIDS and PML will survive the PML if highly active antiretroviral therapy is administered, presumably because of the effects of immune reconstitution in arresting the disease process. Neurologic deficits typically persist in survivors proportionate to the disease severity at the time of presentation.

PROTOZOAL MENINGOENCEPHALITIS

Primary amoebic meningoencephalitis may be due to any of the four free-living amoebae, for example, *Naegleria fowleri, Balamuthia mandrillaris, Sappinia diploidea,* and *Acanthoemba castelanii.* Other parasitic infections such as those caused by

Trypanosoma brucei, Trypanosoma cruzi, and *Toxoplasma gondii* are among those with a protozoan etiology. These pathogens are uncommon causes of CNS infections in North America. *Naegleria fowleri* produces primary amebic meningoencephalitis (PAM), and its symptoms are indistinguishable from acute bacterial meningitis. Other amoebae cause granulomatous amoebic encephalitis (GAE), which is more apt to be subacute and can present as an indolent or asymptomatic chronic infection. Amoebic meningoencephalitis can mimic a brain abscess, aseptic or chronic meningitis, or even a CNS malignancy. Infection with *Strongyloides stercoralis* can lead to a devastating systemic infection often involving the CNS with polymicrobial bacterial meningitis. Termed "hyperinfection syndrome," it is seen in severely immune-compromised patients, such as those with HIV or HTLV 1 and 2, and those receiving anti-TNF therapies.

CLINICAL CASE CORRELATION

- See also Case 18 (Antimicrobial Use in ICU), Case 19 (Sepsis), and Case 20 (Immune-Compromised Patient With Sepsis).

COMPREHENSION QUESTIONS

17.1 A 44-year-old man who is HIV infected is hospitalized because of a 1-week history of progressive weakness of the left lower extremity and an inability to walk. He has also had a rapid loss of weight, night sweats, and frequent low-grade fever. His CD4 cell count at the time of diagnosis was 88/μL. On physical examination he appears cachectic and chronically ill. His temperature is 38.1°C (100.6°F). Other significant findings included the presence of oral thrush, splenomegaly, bilateral lower extremity weakness, and hyperreflexia. An LP is performed, and examination of his CSF shows the following: opening pressure normal; leukocyte count 21/μL with 98% lymphocytes and 2% neutrophils; erythrocyte count 1/μL; protein 85 mg/dL, and glucose 55 mg/dL. The India ink stain, cryptococcal antigen test, and culture for fungi were negative. The PCR was positive for polyomavirus JC and negative for EBV virus. Which of the following is the most likely diagnosis?

A. Cerebral lymphoma

B. Cerebral toxoplasmosis

C. Cryptococcal meningitis

D. Progressive multifocal leukoencephalopathy

E. Tuberculosis

17.2 A 25-year-old man is evaluated in the ED for fever, headache, and mental status changes of 4 hours' duration. He underwent a cadaveric kidney transplantation 10 months ago, and his immunosuppressive regimen includes prednisone and azathioprine. He has no allergies. On physical examination, his temperature is 38.7°C (101.6°F), heart rate is 115 beats/min, respiratory rate is 25 breaths/min, and blood pressure is 100/60 mm Hg. He is oriented to the year and his name but cannot recall the month. His neck is supple, and Kernig and Brudzinski signs are absent. The neurologic examination is normal. His peripheral leukocyte count is 20,000/μL. A CT scan of the head shows no sign of hemorrhage, hydrocephalus, mass effect, or midline shift. An LP is performed, and examination of the CSF shows leukocyte count 2000/μL (60% neutrophils, 40% lymphocytes), erythrocyte count 20/μL, glucose 25 mg/dL, protein 150 mg/dL, and a negative Gram stain. The opening spinal pressure is normal. Results of blood, urine, and CSF cultures are pending. Which of the following is the most appropriate empiric antibiotic therapy?

A. Ampicillin and ceftriaxone

B. Ampicillin, ceftriaxone, and vancomycin

C. Ceftriaxone and moxifloxacin

D. Ceftriaxone and vancomycin

E. Moxifloxacin

17.3 A 5-day-old newborn is brought into the ED with fever, poor feeding, and a seizure. On examination the infant appears lethargic, and temperature is 101.4°F rectally. Lumbar puncture shows numerous white blood cells and an elevated protein level. Which of the following is the most likely organism?

A. *Streptococcus pneumoniae*

B. *Neisseria meningiditis*

C. *Toxoplamosis gondii*

D. *Listeria monocytogenes*

ANSWERS

17.1 **D.** The most likely diagnosis is PML. PML is an opportunistic infection caused by polyomavirus JC, leading to demyelination of the CNS that causes gradually progressive neurologic deficits. Radiographically, there is no mass effect. The lesions are generally bilateral, asymmetric, nonenhancing, and peri-ventricular or subcortical in distribution. This late-stage HIV infection is based on a CD4 cell count <100/μL. The presence of thrush in this patient represents or reveals a high-risk status for AIDS-related opportunistic infections. He also has focal neurologic signs and an MRI that shows multiple white matter lesions without mass effect involving the right lateral frontal, right frontoparietal, and left frontal lobes and cerebellum. A PCR analysis is positive for polyomavirus JC. The gold standard for diagnosis of PML is a brain biopsy, but with the preponderance of evidence supporting a diagnosis of PML, a biopsy can be deferred. If HAART is administered, 50% of AIDS patients will survive PML. Neurologic deficits typically persist in survivors. In patients with HIV infection and CD4 cell counts <200/μL, localized or focal encephalitis is the most common presentation of toxoplasmosis and is the most common CNS system mass lesion. A negative serologic test for toxoplasma-specific IgM would add additional support to the exclusion of toxoplasmic encephalitis. CNS lymphoma occurs in approximately 2% to 12% of HIV-infected individuals. It is strongly associated with Epstein–Barr virus infection. In patients with AIDS, lymphoma was second only to toxoplasmosis as the most common CNS mass lesion.

17.2 **B.** Risk factors for listerial meningitis include immunosuppression, neonatal status or age >50 years, alcoholism, malignancy, diabetes mellitus, hepatic failure, renal failure, iron overload, CVDs, and HIV infection. The most appropriate empiric therapy is ampicillin (the drug of choice for *Listeria*), with ceftriaxone and/or vancomycin. The CSF fluid supports a diagnosis of meningitis. Empiric vancomycin and ceftriaxone are recommended for the treatment of meningitis in patients 2 to 50 years of age. This covers *S. pneumoniae* and *N. meningitidis*, the most common organisms responsible for meningitis in this age group. The analysis of CSF in patients with listerial meningitis often fails to reveal typical gram-positive rods with characteristic "tumbling motility" in wet mount preparations, but often shows pleocytosis and may demonstrate a significant number of lymphocytes in addition to neutrophils. Patients usually have ↑ CSF protein levels; ↓ CSF glucose levels are found less commonly and less profoundly with listerial meningitis. The fluoroquinolones may be effective but do not penetrate the CNS well. Gentamicin is synergistic with ampicillin despite poor CNS penetration.

17.3 **D.** *Listeria monocytogenes*, Group B Streptococcus, and *E. coli* are the most common bacteria encountered in newborn meningitis. Pneumococcus is the most common community acquired organism in adults, and *N. meningiditis* is the second most common organism. Toxoplasmosis is common in HIV infected and other immunocompromised patients.

CLINICAL PEARLS

▶ Meningitis has a high morbidity and mortality rate, especially in high-risk patients.

▶ LP and CNS imaging are central to the diagnosis of meningitis and encephalitis.

▶ Each year 20,000 cases of encephalitis occur in the United States, with the predominant sporadic cause being HSV and the most common epidemic cause being West Nile Virus WNV.

▶ PML is caused by polyomavirus JC, with demyelination of the CNS and neurologic deficits.

▶ If HAART is administered, 50% of patients with AIDS and PML will survive the latter disease.

▶ HSV is the most common cause of fatal sporadic encephalitis in the United States.

▶ HSV encephalitis involves fever, headache, seizures, focal neurologic signs, and impaired multiple sclerosis (MS).

REFERENCES

Attia J, Hatala R, Cook DJ, Wong JG. The rational clinical examination. Does this adult patient have acute meningitis? *JAMA*. 1999;282:175-181. [PMID:10411200.]

Fitch MT, Van de Beek D. Emergency diagnosis and treatment of adult meningitis. *Lancet Infect Dis.* 2007;7:191-200.

Kennedy PG. Viral encephalitis. *J Neurol*. 2005;252:268-272. Epub 2005 Mar 11. [PMID: 15761675.]

A 74-year-old woman with a history of cerebral vascular accident and residual neurological deficits has been hospitalized for the past 3 weeks and has been in the ICU for 8 days for management of recurrent urinary tract and blood-borne infections. You are notified by her nurse of a temperature of 39.4°C. On examination, her pulse rate is 100 beats/min, respiratory rate is 22 breaths/min, and blood pressure is 110/84 mm Hg. The patient is currently on the third day of ciprofloxacin for empiric treatment of her recurrent urinary tract infection. Her serum creatinine is 2.02 mg/dL. Her urine culture reveals multidrug-resistant *Acinetobacter baumannii*, and the blood culture reveals the same organism in addition to fungus.

▶ What is the most appropriate next step in the management of this patient?
▶ What are the underlying processes that predispose to this condition?
▶ What are appropriate strategies in the prevention of this problem?

ANSWERS TO CASE 18:
Antimicrobial Use in ICU

Summary: A 74-year-old woman with a prolonged hospitalization and renal dysfunction now has a recurrent urinary tract infection and bacteremia with a multidrug resistant (MDR) bacteria species. She has elevated temperature despite antibiotic treatment, and she has fungus identified in her blood culture.

- **Next Step:** Administer appropriate therapy to cover the multi-resistant bacterial infection and fungal infection. The antimicrobial therapy selection needs to take into account the patient's renal dysfunction (serum creatinine of 2.02 mg/dL).

- **The underlying processes predisposing this condition:** Prolonged hospitalization, comorbid conditions, recurrent or persistent infections in a relatively immunecompromised host, and previous antibiotic exposures are likely the causes contributing to the current infection by MDR bacterial species and fungus.

- **Prevention of resistance:** Provide prompt broad-spectrum antibiotics for empiric therapy followed by deescalation after culture sensitivities become available and when the patient shows good clinical responses to the initial therapy.

ANALYSIS

Objectives

1. Learn the principles of antimicrobial selection and treatment endpoints in ICU patients.

2. Learn antimicrobial treatment strategies that may reduce the occurrence of antimicrobial resistance.

3. Learn the supportive care that may improve responsiveness to antimicrobial treatment in the ICU population.

Considerations

This is a 74-year-old woman with significant residual neurologic deficits and renal insufficiency after suffering a cerebral vascular accident. She has had a prolonged hospital course and is now in the ICU with a nosocomial infection and sepsis. She is currently on antibiotics but does not appear to be improving. When a patient does not respond to antimicrobial therapy, it is generally important to determine if another source of infection is present and/or if the antibiotic treatment regimen is inappropriate or insufficient against the microorganisms responsible for the infection.

The culture results at this point are helpful in directing her management. As the same bacteria are isolated from her urine and her blood stream, it appears that the infection is severe, systemic, and inadequately controlled with the current antimicrobial regimen. In addition, fungal species identification in the blood suggests that fungal sepsis may be also contributing to the worsening clinical picture. Infection with drug-resistant organisms contributes to increased hospitalization and hospital costs and a poorer prognosis. Unfortunately, this patient represents a common clinical scenario in many modern ICUs.

Selection of the correct antimicrobial agents and dosages and appreciation of the patient's renal dysfunction are the most important considerations in this patient's current management, which begins with determination of the sensitivity spectrum of the cultured MDR *A. baumannii* and fungal species. Assistance from the institution's microbiology laboratory and infectious disease specialists should be sought out to coordinate the management of her complicated infections. The emergence of antibiotic-resistant bacteria is a significant problem in intensive care units. This resistance makes antimicrobial therapy more difficult as the patient's disease process and illness severity continue to increase. The administration of the wrong broad-spectrum antibiotics can lead to even more difficult to treat infections.

APPROACH TO:
Antimicrobial Use in ICU

DEFINITIONS

NOSOCOMIAL INFECTIONS: Infections acquired in a healthcare facility. Generally, the infectious organism is first cultured for >48 hours after hospital admission.

HEALTHCARE-ASSOCIATED INFECTIONS: Infections in patients with prior hospitalization for >3 days within the past 90 days, patients transferred from nursing home, or patients with a history of exposure to transfusion/dialysis centers.

EMPIRIC ANTIBIOTIC THERAPY: Antibiotic therapy started without culture evidence of infection. The therapy is started based on clinical suspicion of infection based on clinical and physiologic parameters.

ANTIMICROBIAL DE-ESCALATION: The goal of the deescalating strategy is to strike a balance between providing prompt, appropriate initial antimicrobial therapy and minimizing the emergence of antimicrobial resistance. Patients with suspected infections are treated with broad-spectrum antibiotics aimed at the most probable organisms causing the infections, and antibiotic coverage is narrowed (or discontinued altogether) as soon as culture results become available, or if no infections are documented. Similarly, duration of treatment may be shortened or terminated when patients with uncomplicated infections show clinical improvement/resolution.

ANTIBIOTIC RESISTANCE: The ability of microorganisms to grow in the presence of antibiotic levels that would normally suppress growth or kill susceptible bacteria.

CLINICAL APPROACH

Healthcare-related infections affect ICU patients with far greater frequency than patients residing elsewhere in the hospital. Consequently, antibiotics are one of the most common therapies utilized in the intensive care unit. Additionally, **up to 70% of all nosocomial infections isolated in the ICU are due to multidrug resistant bacteria.** The reason for this elevated level of drug resistant infections is multifactorial. ICU patients have more severe underlying disease processes, are crowded into small areas of the hospital, and are often malnourished and immunecompromised. They are more likely to be subjected to multiple invasive procedures including endotracheal tubes, indwelling urinary catheters, and central venous lines. In addition to the patient-specific risk-factors, there are other general factors such as excessive antimicrobial use, poor aseptic technique, and inadequate hand hygiene of healthcare providers that contribute to the increased risk of infection. The inappropriate choice and duration of antibiotics can also contribute to the overgrowth and infection of drug-resistant bacteria.

Microbial resistance is increasing in both gram-negative and gram-positive bacteria. These bacteria strains are increasingly resistant to broad-spectrum antibiotics. The inadequate empiric coverage of these resistant bacteria can lead to an increase in morbidity and mortality. At the same time, the inappropriate use of broad-spectrum antibiotics can contribute to the increase in emergence of resistant bacteria. Thus, the challenge for the physician is to utilize antibiotics that will cover the resistant bacteria without overtreatment that can lead to resistance.

When a patient is septic, antibiotics must be initiated promptly. **Preferably, antibiotics should be administered within 1 hour of diagnosis, as each hour of delay over the next 6 hours has been shown to contribute to a decrease in survival of 7.6%.** For most septic patients, the culture results are not known at the time of the initial presentation; therefore, antibiotic choices are made based on clinicians' suspicions of the infected source. The initial choices of the preemptive antimicrobial therapy need to adequately address the potential infective organisms in order to minimize the mortality associated with the infection. Inadequate initial therapy usually involves either the failure to cover a specific microbe or the selection of antibiotics to which the organism is resistant. Therefore, high-risk patients admitted to the ICU with serious infections should be treated aggressively with broad-spectrum antibiotics until the bacteria cultures are isolated. Cultures should be obtained before antibiotics are started. Once the culture isolates with their associated antibiotic sensitivities are identified, the antimicrobial therapy should be immediately adjusted to more narrow coverage antibiotics that have bactericidal activity against the bacteria. This deescalation therapy allows for treatment of the infection while reducing the risk of antimicrobial resistance. It is also crucial to consider the basic pharmacokinetics (necessary dosage to achieve adequate levels, tissue penetrance, etc.) of the drug so that underdosing does not occur, as underdosing can lead to an increase in the emergence of resistant organisms. This is particularly important in patients with renal insufficiency; adjustments of drug dosing and frequency are often needed when patients are receiving hemodialysis.

Table 18–1 • INITIAL EMPIRIC ANTIBIOTIC COMBINATIONS FOR HOSPITAL ACQUIRED PNEUMONIA	
Common Pathogens	Antibiotic Choices
• Methicillin-sensitive *S. aureus* • *Streptococcus pneumoniae* • *Haemophilus influenza* **Antibiotic-sensitive enteric Gram-negative bacilli:** • *Escherichia coli* • *Enterobacter spp.* • Klebsiella • *Proteus spp.* • Serratia	Ceftriaxone *or* Levofloxacin, moxifloxacin, or ciprofloxacin *or* Ampicillin/sulbactam *or* Ertapenem
Possible MDR bacteria: • *P. aeruginosa* • Klebsiella • Acinetobacter • Methicillin-resistant *S. aureus*	Antipseudomonal cephalosporin (cefepime, ceftazidime) *or* Antipseudomonal carbepenem (imipenem or meropenem) *or* β-lactam/β-lactamase inhibitor (piperacillin–tazobactam) *plus* Antipseudomonal fluoroquinolone (ciprofloxacin or levofloxacin) *or* Aminoglycoside (amikacin, gentamicin, or tobramycin) *plus* Linezolid or vancomycin

Recognizing when patients are at high risk for developing infections associated with MDR organisms is important in selecting appropriate initial broad-spectrum antibiotics. These high-risk patients include those who have had prior antibiotics treatments during their hospitalization, those with prolonged hospitalization, and patients with indwelling devices (such as endotracheal tubes, central venous catheters, and urinary catheters). Infected high-risk patients should be started on combination broad-spectrum antibiotics based on presumed infectious sources and local antibiograms (Table 18–1).

Knowledge of the source of infection should also be sought after in order to select the most appropriate initial antibiotic regimens. Antibiotics have different tissue penetrations that should be taken into account when treating infections. Source control of the infection, such as abscess drainage, should be performed immediately. The choice of antibiotics is somewhat dependent on the local hospital flora. Different resistant rates are found at different hospitals, so antibiograms showing local antibiotic susceptibility should be used as a guide for initiating therapy that will cover local resistance. Once the cultures return with susceptibility, antibiotic therapy should be deescalated.

Along with appropriate antibiotic selection and deescalation, the duration of antibiotic therapy is important in reducing antimicrobial resistance. Once empiric broad-spectrum antibiotics have been started, if there is no organism isolated after 72 hours, serious consideration should be given to stopping the antibiotic administration. In a study evaluating the duration of therapy in treating patients with ventilator-associated pneumonia (VAP), it was determined that treating patients for 8 days instead of the standard 15 days had no difference in mortality;

however, there was significant decrease in the incidence of MDR bacterial infections among patients treated for only 8 days. Patients with spontaneous bacterial peritonitis receive no additional benefits from being treated for more than 5 days of cefotaxime. Antibiotics should be stopped after a predetermined time course for other infections. This allows for shorter therapy with decreased risk for resistance organisms. It is also more economical not to provide prolonged, unnecessary antibiotic therapy. However, these maneuvers must all be taken into consideration with the patient's clinical status. If the patient remains septic or is clinically deteriorating, antibiotic administration can be prolonged. Likewise, patients who are immune-compromised or elderly may benefit from longer durations of antibiotics therapy.

There are other strategies used in the ICU to decrease infection rates. Specific strategies that have been shown to decrease the rate of central line-associated bloodstream infections (CLABSI) when used in combination include **hand hygiene, the use of full sterile barriers during central-line insertion, skin antisepsis with 2% chlorhexidine solution, subclavian vein insertion site, chorhexidine-impregnated sponge dressings at the line sites, centralizing equipment in central line carts during catheter insertion, and daily assessment of central line necessity.** Strategies that may reduce ventilator-associated pneumonia include elevation of the head of bed and protocols for sedation medications and ventilation, which are associated with reduced ventilation days. The early administration of enteral nutritional support also seems to decrease infection rates, allowing for decreased use of antibiotics. As compared to parenteral feeding, enteral feeding is associated with a decrease in overall infections. Additionally, the use of enteral feeding allows for maintenance of nonspecific mechanisms of immune protection by maintaining gut epithelium. Normal gut epithelium provides for absorption of nutrients, exclusion of pathogenic organisms, mucus production, and maintenance of normal gap junctions. These mechanisms all protect against potentially harmful bacteria. Not only does enteral feeding aid in nonspecific immune protection, but it also helps provide continued function of gut-associated lymphoid tissue (GALT), which is home to lymphocytes that can produce cytokines and immunoglobulins. All of these factors help to provide improved immune function, thus decreasing the need for antibiotics.

CLINICAL CASE CORRELATION

- See also Case 9 (Ventilator managment), Case 19 (Sepsis), and Case 20 (Immunosuppressed patients).

COMPREHENSION QUESTIONS

18.1 An 82-year-old woman is admitted to the ICU for presumed urosepsis. Her initial blood pressure is 80/50 mm Hg, heart rate is 110 beats/min, and oxygen saturation is 100% on 2 L O_2 nasal cannula. Urine, blood, and sputum cultures were collected in the emergency department. Her hemodynamics improve to blood pressure of 120/80 mm Hg and heart rate of 80 beats/min after 2 L of normal saline, and remain stable. She is started on IV vancomycin. Three days later, all of her cultures return with no growth to date. The next step in management should be:

A. Continue IV vancomycin for 8 more days

B. Continue IV vancomycin for 3 more days

C. Switch to ciprofloxacin PO for 3 days

D. Discontinue antibiotics completely

E. Reculture the patient

18.2 A 34-year-old man is seen in the emergency department with fever, chills, nausea, and vomiting 2 days after injecting heroin intravenously. Which of the following is the correct order of antibiotic management?

A. Obtain cultures, start specific monotherapy antibiotic, change to broad-spectrum antibiotics if resistant bacteria are found.

B. Start broad-spectrum antibiotics, pan culture (blood, urine, sputum), narrow coverage after 72 hours.

C. Start broad-spectrum antibiotics, culture in 3 days if no improvement, deescalate antibiotics based on culture results.

D. Obtain blood cultures and obtain a CT scan of the abdomen. If the CT is normal, observe the patient until cultures become available.

E. Pan culture, start broad-spectrum antibiotics, deescalate after culture results return.

18.3 Which of the following measures decreases the risk of developing antibiotic resistance in the ICU?

A. Central-line skin preparation using betadine

B. Antibiotic deescalation

C. Restricting broad-spectrum antibiotics usage

D. Continued antibiotic administration for 2 weeks

E. Use of peripherally inserted central venous catheters (PICC) rather than standard central venous catheters

18.4 A 32-year-old woman with a history of poorly controlled Type 1 diabetes had a below the knee amputation 2 months ago for gangrene of her foot. Her postoperative course was complicated by a UTI and pneumonia. Her amputation wound spontaneously opened 2 days ago, and she was pancultured. Her wound was satisfactorily debrided in the operating room, and she was started on IV vancomycin and IV Zosyn. She is now being transferred to the ICU for worsening hyperglycemia and dehydration. Her wound culture has grown methicillin-resistant *Staphylococcus aureus* (MRSA) that is sensitive to vancomycin. All other cultures were negative. What is the next step in management?

A. Glucose control and narrow her current coverage to vancomycin

B. Glucose control, continue her current antibiotics, and add cefepime

C. Glucose control and continue her current regimen

D. Stop her current antibiotics and perform above knee amputation for source control

E. Continue current antibiotics and obtain additional cultures

18.5 An 89-year-old woman who is significantly malnourished is in the ICU with *Pseudomonas aeruginosa* pneumonia. She has received 5 days of antibiotics, but she still has copious amounts of sputum and is continuing to require a significant amount of ventilatory support. The most appropriate course of action is:

A. Continue her current regimen, but reculture for any spikes in temperature.

B. Discontinue her antibiotics on day 8 of therapy.

C. Broaden her antibiotics for the next 24 hours and then stop antibiotics.

D. Stop antibiotics, reculture and await culture results before re-starting antibiotic therapy.

E. Emperically add an antifungal agent.

ANSWERS

18.1 **D.** This patient presented to the emergency department hypotensive and tachycardic, and although it was initially thought that she might be septic, none of her cultures returned with any bacteria. Additionally, she improved with simple rehydration, indicating that she was possibly just dehydrated. Thus, there is no need to continue her antibiotics. Furthermore, continuation of her antibiotics could lead to the formation of resistant bacteria.

18.2 **E.** It is essential to obtain cultures prior to starting antibiotic therapy for presumed sepsis. Although the unnecessary use of broad-spectrum antibiotics can lead to increased antimicrobial resistance, it is important that all bacteria are initially covered when starting empiric antibiotic therapy. Once the bacterial cultures return, then the antibiotics can be deescalated to the appropriate monotherapy.

18.3 **B.** The use of broad-spectrum antibiotics for prolonged duration contributes to the increase in antimicrobial resistance. However, their use is necessary in the initial empiric therapy in order to cover the majority of probable pathogens. Once the cultures have returned, the therapy can be deescalated so that the patient's infection can be appropriately treated and broad-spectrum antibiotic use can be limited. Using aseptic technique and limiting the duration of antibiotic administration also helps reduce antimicrobial proliferation and resistance. Chlorhexadine skin preparations have been shown to cause fewer central-line associated infections in comparison to betadine skin preparations. The use of PICCs in hospitalized patients has not been shown to be associated with reduced catheter-associated infections in comparison to standard central venous catheters.

18.4 **A.** The hyperglycemia can contribute to poor response to antimicrobial therapy in this patient and needs to be better managed. This patient has multiple risk factors for infection with resistant bacteria. Her wound has grown MRSA that is sensitive to vancomycin. This is the most likely source of her sepsis. The addition of Zosyn does not provide additional benefits. Her wound has been recently inspected and debrided to satisfaction; therefore, there is no indication at this time to perform an above the knee amputation. Fungal infections are reasonably common in relatively immunocompromised patients; however, there is no indication of this process at this time.

18.5 **A.** This is an elderly patient who is being treated for pneumonia. Although she is nearing the end of a standard 8-day course of antibiotics for ventilator-associated pneumonia, she is malnourished and still requiring a significant amount of ventilatory support. Because of her age and relative immune-compromised status, it is reasonable to extend her antibiotics past the standard 8 days, with reculturing if she spikes temperatures through her current antibiotic coverage and continued vigilance for other causes of her fever.

CLINICAL PEARLS

▶ Broad-spectrum antibiotics should be started on septic patients based on presumed location of infection and local antibiograms.

▶ Once culture sensitivities have returned, antibiotics should be de-escalated to minimize the use of broad-spectrum antibiotics.

▶ The duration of antibiotic administration should be limited to specific time courses. If there is no growth of initial cultures after 72 hours, serious consideration should be given to discontinuing the antibiotics.

▶ Prolonged administration of antibiotics may be necessary in the elderly, immunecompromised, and clinically deteriorating patient.

▶ Nonpharmacologic strategies for decreasing the need for antibiotics in the ICU include aseptic technique, handwashing, and early enteral nutrition.

REFERENCES

ATS/IDSA. Guidelines for the management of adults with hospital-acquired, ventilator-associated, and healthcare-associated pneumonia. *Am J Resp Crit Care Med.* 2005;171:388-416.

Bhalodi AA, Nicolau DP. Principles of antimicrobial therapy and the clinical pharmacology of antimicrobial drugs. In: Hall JB, Schmidt GA, Kress JP, eds. *Principles of Critical Care.* 4th ed. New York, NY: McGraw-Hill Education; 2015:544-551.

Cioffi Jr WG, Connolly MD. The septic response. In: Cameron JL, Cameron AM, eds. *Current Surgical Therapy.* 11th ed. Philadelphia, PA: Elsevier Saunders; 2014:1262-1267.

File TM, Jr. Recommendations for the treatment of hospital-acquired and ventilator-associated pneumonia: review of recent international guidelines. *Clin Infect Dis.* 2010;51(Suppl1): S42-S47.

Ho VP, Barrie PS. Antibiotics for critically ill patients. In: Cameron JL, Cameron AM, eds. *Current Surgical Therapy.* 11th ed. Philadelphia, PA: Elsevier Saunders; 2014:1271-1278.

Leone M, Martin C. How to break the vicious circle of antibiotic resistances? *Current Opinion in Critical Care.* 2008;14:587-592.

Masterton RG. Antibiotic de-escalation. *Crit Care Clin.* 2011;27:149-162.

A 59-year-old woman with a history of Type II diabetes mellitus was found unconscious at home by her family members. In the emergency center, she was noted to have a temperature of 38.6°C, pulse rate of 112 beats/min, blood pressure of 96/50 mm Hg, and respiratory rate of 26 breaths/min. After 2L of normal saline, the patient became more alert and began to answer questions appropriately. Laboratory values reveal WBC 26,000 cells/mcL, hemoglobin 12 g/dL, normal platelet count, and a serum glucose level of 280 g/dL. An indwelling urinary catheter was placed and showed return of concentrated and cloudy urine. The urinalysis revealed 50 WBC per high power field. A CT scan of the abdomen without contrast revealed no free fluid in the abdomen and an inflamed right kidney with perinephric fat stranding. Shortly after the patient was transferred to the ICU, her nurse notifies you that her blood pressure is 78/50 mm Hg and heart rate is 120 beats/min.

▶ What is the most likely diagnosis?
▶ What are the priorities in this patient's management?
▶ How would you monitor and support this patient's status?

ANSWERS TO CASE 19:
Sepsis

Summary: A 59-year-old diabetic woman is unconscious with fever, tachycardia, and hypotension. Laboratory analysis reveals a leukocytosis with likely urinary tract infection, and imaging shows inflammation of the upper urinary system. Her presentation is consistent with septic shock.

- **Most likely diagnosis:** Urinary Tract Infection and septic shock.

- **Priorities in management:** Resuscitation and antimicrobial therapy.

- **Monitoring and support of organ perfusion:** Intravascular fluid status can be assessed and monitored with CVP catheters or echocardiography. Mean arterial pressure and mixed-venous O_2 measurements are helpful to determine the patient's responses to therapy. The patient's mental status, urine outputs, and serum lactate levels during the course of resuscitation are useful indicators of response to the resuscitation efforts. Specific monitoring and support guidelines were initially outlined by the Surviving Sepsis Campaign publications from over 10 years ago, and these recommendations have been further refined with emerging evidence-based practices.

ANALYSIS

Objectives

1. Learn the guidelines and principles for the management of septic patients.
2. Learn the monitoring and strategies for managing patients with septic shock.
3. Learn the pharmacologic support for patients with septic shock.
4. Learn the role of glucocorticoid therapy for septic shock.

Considerations

This patient is suffering from shock. Shock is defined as inadequate oxygen delivery to meet the patient's tissue metabolic demands. Her initial altered mental status and concentrated urine are overt signs of inadequate end-organ perfusion. There are many ways to classify shock. One useful way to think about the etiologies of shock is to divide them into hypovolemic, cardiac, or distributive processes. Hypovolemic shock is caused by hemorrhage or dehydration. Cardiac processes include intrinsic cardiac dysfunction as well as extrinsic causes, such as tamponade or tension pneumothorax. In contrast, sepsis is a distributive process caused by acute vasodilation without an accompanying increase in fluid volume. The acute vasodilation leads to the increase in the capacitance of the circulatory system without an increase in volume, causing a relative hypovolemia. Other distributive causes of shock include anaphylaxis, neurogenic shock and third spacing seen with systemic inflammation. Sepsis is related to the systemic inflammatory response syndrome

(SIRS), which is characterized by hypo or hyperthermia (T <36°C or >38°C), tachycardia, tachypnea, leukocytosis or leukocytopenia. Sepsis can be diagnosed when the features of SIRS are present and an infection is the suspected cause. The diagnosis of sepsis does not necessarily mean that shock is present. Septic shock is the diagnosis when there is ongoing hypotension despite fluid resuscitation.

Antimicrobial therapy should be initiated early to address the infectious process, and delays in the initiation of appropriate antimicrobial therapy has been clearly demonstrated to lead to worse outcomes associated with sepsis. The initial approach toward the correction of hypotension is to restore intravascular volume with crystalloid administration, and once this is accomplished, persistent hypotension is further addressed with the addition of vasoactive pharmacologic agents and possibly corticosteroids as indicated.

APPROACH TO:
Sepsis

DEFINITIONS

SHOCK: Inadequate oxygen delivery to meet the needs of the body's tissues.

CENTRAL VENOUS PRESSURE (CVP): The pressure measured in the superior vena cava reflecting right ventricle end-diastolic pressure. It is measured with a centrally inserted venous catheter usually inserted in the internal jugular or subclavian vein. CVP is used clinically to assess volume status in critically ill patients. The CVP is not reliable for intravascular volume estimation in patients with tricuspid valve disease.

SIRS: The systemic inflammatory response syndrome (SIRS) is a clinical syndrome describing the derangement of the body's inflammatory response. A patient with two or more of the findings below meets criteria for the diagnosis of SIRS:

- Temperature <36°C or >38°C
- Heart Rate >90 beats/min
- Respiratory Rate >20 breaths/min
- White Blood Cell Count >12,000 or <4,000 cells/mcL

SEPSIS: When the etiology of SIRS is presumed to be infectious in origin, the diagnosis of sepsis is made.

SEVERE SEPSIS: Sepsis with at least one organ system dysfunction.

SEPTIC SHOCK: Septic shock is present when there is ongoing hypotension despite fluid resuscitation.

EARLY GOAL-DIRECTED THERAPY: A treatment strategy for sepsis with the goal of rapid restoration of tissue perfusion by manipulation of cardiac preload, afterload, contractility, and oxygen carrying capacity.

CLINICAL APPROACH

Guidelines and Principles for the Management of Septic Patients

There is a spectrum of severity in sepsis. Uncomplicated sepsis may be caused by gastroenteritis or the flu and may only require supportive care with or without antibiotic therapy. Severe sepsis is generally associated with mortality rates of 25% to 30%. Septic shock is the most severe form of sepsis, where mortality can be as high as 50%.

When confronted with a patient in septic shock, there are two main early treatment goals: (1) address the source of the infection, and (2) restore perfusion to the tissues to prevent reversible and irreversible organ injuries. Addressing both goals should occur simultaneously and as soon as the patient is encountered. Randomized trials have shown that patient survival is improved with early intervention, so patients who meet criteria for the diagnosis of septic shock should be treated as rapidly as possible, even if that means starting treatment in the emergency department rather than in the ICU.

Ideally, resuscitative efforts should be guided by information gained from continuous monitoring. Since the vasodilation associated with sepsis may produce relative hypovolemia and distributive shock, aggressive initial fluid resuscitation is frequently needed to restore intravascular volume and blood pressure. The first goal is to achieve a CVP of 8 to 12 mm Hg, mean arterial pressure (MAP) of >65 mm Hg, and urine output of >0.5 mL/kg/h. Sometimes this can be achieved with fluids alone. However, if fluids alone do not achieve these goals, a vasopressor should be initiated. One of the targets of resuscitation is to improve central venous oxygen content (CVO_2) to >70%; if this target is not accomplished with fluids in individuals with anemia, blood transfusions can be given to maintain an appropriate hematocrit. In some patients with severe primary cardiac dysfunction, dobutamine infusion may be initiated to improve cardiac output, CVO_2 and tissue oxygen delivery.

While the patient is being resuscitated, the source of their infection needs to be rapidly identified. Antibiotics should not be withheld during the investigative period. **Empiric, broad-spectrum antibiotics should be started within 1 hour of recognition of septic shock.** The work up includes obtaining blood, urine, and sputum cultures as well as any other appropriate cultures. Imaging may be required to identify other etiologies, such as pneumonia or intra-abdominal infectious sources. Once the source of the infection is identified, antibiotic therapy can be tailored based on cultures and antibiotic-resistance profiles.

Monitoring and Strategies for Patients With Septic Shock

The treatment of shock requires continuous monitoring of hemodynamic status. A central venous catheter is helpful to monitor central venous pressure (CVP) as well as CVO_2. CVO_2 reflects overall oxygen demand and consumption. A low CVO_2 suggests inadequate oxygen delivery to the tissue beds. An arterial catheter is placed to monitor blood pressure and more specifically, mean arterial pressure. Finally, a Foley (urinary) catheter is used to ensure adequate urine output (>0.5 mL/kg/h), which generally suggests sufficient end-organ perfusion. It is important to recognize that the placement of vascular and urinary monitoring devices are adjuncts to the resuscitation and should not be prioritized over the resuscitation process.

In some instances a Swan-Ganz catheter, also known as a pulmonary artery catheter (PAC) may be used to obtain more information about cardiac status. For instance, the PAC can be used to determine the cardiac filling pressures, cardiac output, and systemic vascular resistance. The utility of PAC in critically ill patients is controversial; specifically, there is no good clinical evidence to support that its use improves survival, and the decision to place a PA catheter is a highly individualized process. The PA catheter is being used less frequently in the ICU setting, as much of the information gained through PAC monitoring can also be determined by echocardiography.

Laboratory analysis can also help determine the adequacy of resuscitation. For instance, serial blood lactate levels can be used to monitor the response to treatment. Decreasing trend (normalization) in lactate levels may indicate that tissue oxygenation is being restored. Similarly, base excess measurements on the arterial blood gases should begin to normalize when oxygen delivery to the tissues improves.

Pharmacologic Support for Patients With Septic Shock

A primary therapeutic goal in the treatment of septic shock is to restore tissue oxygenation. This is achieved through optimization of preload, cardiac contractility, afterload and oxygen carrying capacity. While fluid resuscitation and blood transfusions can improve preload and oxygen carrying capacity, in severe cases additional pharmacologic support may be required to improve cardiac contractility and increase afterload.

In patients with hypotension unresponsive to fluids, vasopressor therapy should be initiated. When the MAP is low, autoregulation of blood pressure to the tissue beds is impaired such that perfusion is entirely dependent on the blood pressure. A vasopressor can improve perfusion pressure and improve blood flow to the tissues. The Surviving Sepsis Campaign has recommended norepinephrine (levophed) or dopamine at the lowest dose necessary to maintain tissue perfusion as the initial pharmacologic support. Epinephrine may be given if an additional agent is needed. The assessment of the adequacy of tissue perfusion can be determined using blood pressure, CVO_2, urine output, normalization of blood lactate concentrations, and normalization of base excess on arterial blood gas. Some patients with septic shock do not respond appropriately to vasopressors due to relative vasopressin deficiency and would benefit from the addition of vasopressin at a constant infusion rate of 0.03 units/min.

Dobutamine is a β agonist that increases cardiac contractility and therefore increases cardiac output. Dobutamine is given when the CVO_2 is low or when myocardial dysfunction is suspected based on elevated filling pressures or low cardiac output. By increasing cardiac output, oxygen delivery to the tissues may be improved in these individuals. One of the drawbacks of dopamine administration in septic patients is the severe tachycardia and arrhythmias that dopamine can produce.

The Role of Glucocorticoid Therapy in Septic Shock

Some critically ill patients may experience relative adrenal insufficiency and may benefit from glucocorticoid supplementation. In a randomized controlled French multicenter trial involving septic patients with persistent hypotension after appropriate fluid and vasopressor therapy, improvements in shock reversal and a reduction in mortality when patients received corticosteroids were demonstrated, and they determined it was not necessary to prove that a patient has adrenal insufficiency with cortisol stimulation testing prior to giving supplementation. Subsequently, another large European randomized controlled trial (CORTICUS) showed that septic patients who did not require vasopressors failed to benefit from corticosteroids treatments. Taken together, it appears that septic patients with refractory hypotension after appropriate fluid and vasopressor administration are the most appropriate patients for corticosteroid replacement therapy.

CASE CORRELATION

- See also Case 18 (Antibiotic use in ICU) and Case 20 (Immunosuppressed patients).

COMPREHENSION QUESTIONS

19.1 A 52-year-old man presents with right upper quadrant pain and jaundice. In the emergency department he is found to have a fever of 39.2°C, a heart rate of 112 beats/min and a blood pressure of 92/40 mm Hg. He has not urinated for 12 hours. He is tender in the right upper quadrant and has a leukocytosis of 19,000. What is the next step in his treatment?

   A. Admission to the ICU

   B. Right upper quadrant ultrasound

   C. Intravenous fluid administration

   D. Placement of a pulmonary artery catheter

   E. Place a Foley catheter for urine output monitoring

19.2 Which of the following is not a therapeutic endpoint in the treatment of sepsis?

   A. Central venous oxygen >70%

   B. Urine output >0.5 mL/kg/h

   C. Mean arterial pressure >65

   D. Central venous pressure of 8 to 12 mm Hg

   E. Temperature <38.5°C

19.3 A 62-year-old woman is diagnosed with sepsis due to an intra-abdominal abscess from perforated diverticulitis. While awaiting CT-guided drainage of the abscess, what is the best way to treat her infection?

A. Start broad-spectrum antibiotics now.

B. Start antibiotics based on gram stain from the abscess fluid.

C. Wait to start antibiotics until blood culture results return.

D. Only give antibiotics if she does not improve after drainage of the abscess.

E. Once CT-guided drainage is performed, there would be no need for antibiotic therapy.

ANSWERS

19.1 **C.** This patient meets criteria for the diagnosis of SIRS given his fever, tachycardia, hypotension, and leukocytosis. Additionally, his clinical presentation is consistent with infectious cholangitis. Since he meets the criteria for SIRS and an infection is suspected, the diagnosis of sepsis should be made; furthermore, his ongoing hypotension and low urine output indicate that he is in septic shock. Early goal-directed therapy with the goal of restoring tissue oxygen delivery improves survival from sepsis. So the first step in the treatment of this patient should be fluid resuscitation. Antibiotics should be initiated within 1 hour of presentation. After fluids have been started, monitors for CVP and blood pressure can be placed. Diagnosing the source of his infection should be done as well, but a right upper quadrant ultrasound is not the initial step in his treatment. While he may ultimately require admission to the ICU, therapy should not be delayed while awaiting transfer to the ICU.

19.2 **E.** The goals of therapy for early goal-directed treatment of sepsis reflect the need to restore oxygen delivery to the tissues. Temperature is not an endpoint used to measure the adequacy of tissue oxygenation. Central venous pressure allows for an assessment of overall fluid status; a CVP <8 is consistent with hypovolemia. Adequate urine output (>0.5 mL/kg/h) indicates good end-organ perfusion. Normal central venous oxygen saturation similarly implies adequate oxygen delivery to the end organs.

19.3 **A.** In septic patients, institution of early antibiotic therapy is very important. While cultures should be obtained, it is not necessary to prove that infection exists or to identify the infecting organism before starting therapy. It is better to start broad-spectrum antimicrobials initially and then tailor them when culture data are available or stop them entirely if no source is identified.

CLINICAL PEARLS

▶ Sepsis is diagnosed when there are two or more criteria for SIRS and an infection is suspected.

▶ Rapid reversal of hypoperfusion improves survival in sepsis.

▶ The goal of treating sepsis is to improve oxygenation of tissue. This involves fluid administration, vasopressor therapy, blood transfusions as needed, antibiotics, and infectious source control.

▶ The definition of septic shock is hypotension refractory to resuscitation.

REFERENCES

Cioffi Jr WG, Connolly MD. The septic response. In: Cameron JL, Cameron AM, eds. *Current Surgical Therapy.* 11th ed. Philadelphia, PA: Elsevier Saunders; 2014:1262-1267.

Dellinger RP, Levy MM, Carlet JM, et al. Surviving Sepsis Campaign: International guidelines for management of severe sepsis and septic shock: 2008. *Crit Care Med.* 2008;36:296-327.

Han J, Cribbs SK, Martin GS. Sepsis, severe sepsis, and septic shock. In: Hall JB, Schmidt GA, Kress JP, eds. *Principles of Critical Care.* 4th ed. New York, NY: McGraw-Hill Education; 2015:562-576.

Rivers E, Nguyen B, Haystad S, et al. Early goal-directed therapy in the treatment of severe sepsis and septic shock. *N Engl J Med.* 2001;345:1368-1377.

Surviving Sepsis Campaign; available from http://www.survivingsepsis.org. Accessed January 15, 2017.

A 65-year-old man is admitted to the ICU after becoming hypoxic, tachypneic and febrile (temperature of 103.2°F). The patient complains of pleuritic chest pain and shortness of breath, and his sputum is blood tinged. He is status post-allogenic bone marrow transplant (BMT) 24 days ago for acute myelogenous leukemia (AML) following a long period of treatment for myelodysplastic syndrome (MDS). Posttransplant he noted soreness of the mouth and rectal area but had no prior pulmonary symptoms and was continued on immunosuppressive therapy to prevent graft versus host disease (GVHD). On examination he appears acutely ill, toxic, and tachypneic. Examination of his oropharynx reveals mucositis with thrush. His chest is clear to auscultation, though he is tachypneic and tachycardic. A port-a-cath is present in the right subclavian position without signs of inflammation. The abdomen is benign without tenderness or mass. Extremities are without lesions. Neurologically, he is alert and without focal deficits. His WBC is 540/mm^3 with 10% neutrophils (absolute neutrophil count ~54/mm^3). He is anemic and thrombocytopenic. A chest CT scan is below (Figure 20–1). Empirical antimicrobial therapy was started.

▶ How should this patient be diagnosed and treated?
▶ What are some specific causes of the patient's immunosuppresion?

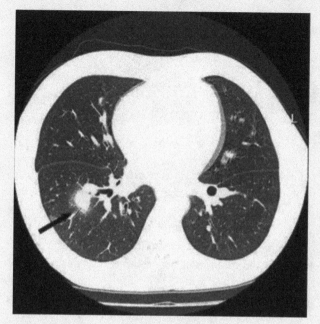

Figure 20–1. Chest CT scan shows a contrast enhanced lesion with a "halo sign" (arrow).

ANSWERS TO CASE 20:
Sepsis in the Immune-Compromised Patient

Summary: This 65-year-old man who is status post-allogenic BMT for AML on immunosuppressive therapy is admitted to the ICU for shortness of breath and fever, which have progressed over the past 48 hours. He has profound and prolonged neutropenia with an absolute neutrophil count (ANC) of 54/mm^3. There is a cavitary lesion on chest CT that shows the "halo sign." Broad-spectrum antimicrobial therapy (covering bacterial and fungal pathogens) and supportive care are instituted.

- **Diagnosis and treatment:** After a septic work up, start IV antibiotics (eg, vancomycin and piperacillin-tazobactam) and empirical antifungal therapy (in this case voriconazole), and institute neutropenic precautions.

- **Cause(s) for immunosuppression:** Long-term stay in the hospital, disruption of mucous membranes and skin (mucositis, proctitis, IV access with a port-a-cath), immunosuppressive therapy of GVHD, prior prophylactic antimicrobials post chemotherapy and BMT, and most importantly, profound and prolonged neutropenia.

ANALYSIS

Objectives

1. Discuss immunosuppression and its causes in the intensive care setting.

2. Know the likely pathogens based on the specific types of immunosuppression that might be encountered in the ICU.

3. Understand the immune dysfunction seen in infected patients who become septic with resultant immune and coagulation dissonance (sepsis and sepsis associated coagulopathy).

4. Discuss the modalities for monitoring the immune status of critically ill patients with infection.

Considerations

The patient is a 65-year-old man with multiple defects of immunity following an allogenic BMT for AML, which was subsequent to his history of MDS. During the pre-engraftment phase of his transplant and while on preventive therapy (prophylaxis) for GVHD, he became critically ill with pulmonary infiltrates and a cavitary lesion demonstrated in one of the infiltrates. Pulmonary infections can occur at any stage of transplant, but about one-third of these infections occurs during pre-engraftment. The common problem of recovering a causative organism in a patient with pneumonia is compounded in the severely compromised patient due to issues of hypoxia and coagulopathy (especially thrombocytopenia). Thus, invasive diagnostic procedures are often avoided or contraindicated. Prophylactic antimicrobials (eg, ciprofloxacin, trimethoprim-sulfamethoxazole, and fluconazole) are routinely adopted in BMT patients. This has resulted in a reduction of bacterial and *Candida albicans* infections in this population. However, about 10% of these patients will develop opportunistic fungal infection (especially *Aspergillus* and other non-albicans *Candida* species) following immunosuppression and *prolonged and profound neutropenia*. Other fungal infections that may be identified in this population include *Fusarium, Cryptococcus,* non-albicans *Candida,* and *Mucor.* The early diagnosis and treatment of invasive fungal infections (IFI) of the lung is critical for the patient's survival while in this tenuous immunological state. Fortunately, newer methods of microbial diagnosis and more effective antifungal therapies have seen improved survivability.

Monitoring of BMT patients with serial Aspergillus galactomanan assays coupled with clinical findings such as the "halo sign" on CT scan in the setting of profound/prolonged neutropenia allows for the presumptive diagnosis of invasive Aspergillus infection (IAI). The halo sign shows a "ground glass" surrounding an enhanced mass indicating early inflammation. Serum galactomannan increases can be detected before other diagnostic features appear, on average between 7 and 14 days prior (Mayo Clinic, 2016). Currently, two azole drugs are approved for the treatment of invasive pulmonary aspergillosis: voriconzole and as of 2015, isavuconazole. These drugs are more effective and safer than amphotericin B, including its lipid formulations. An echinocandin (eg, caspofungin) may be added to the azole drug (eg, voriconazole or isavuconazole) in some circumstances. The diagnosis of IAI may be further supported by the demonstration of angioinvasive fungi on tissue specimens, as seen on special stains (eg, PAS or silver stain), demonstrating **septate hyphae with acute angle branching (highly suggestive but not diagnostic of *Aspergillus*)**. Subsequent fungal culture of tissue specimens is conclusive when *Aspergillus* is grown.

APPROACH TO:

Pneumonia and Sepsis in an Immunocompromised ICU Patient

DEFINITIONS

ABSOLUTE NEUTROPHIL COUNT (ANC): The absolute number of neutrophils per microliter (mm^3) is the percentage of neutrophils in the WBC. ANCs of $<100/mm^3$ is neutropenia and creates a high risk for certain pathogens/opportunistic organisms such as *Aspergillus* sp., especially if neutropenia lasts >7 days. For example, WBC = $1000/mm^3$ with 10% neutrophils = 10% = $1,000 \times 0.1$ = ANC of $100/mm^3$.

IMMUNNOSUPPRESSION: A dissonance or lack of the host's immune response to fight infection.

OPPORTUNISTIC PATHOGEN or OPPORTUNISTIC INFECTION (OI): Organisms (bacterial, viral, fungal, parasitic) which are usually not pathogens in immunocompetent hosts.

MRSA: *Staphylococcus aureus* resistant to methicillin due to the presence of β-lactamases.

VISA: *Staphylococcus aureus* that is partially resistant to vancomycin based on decreased penetration of vancomycin across the cell wall.

MDRO: Gram-negative rod-shaped bacteria that are resistant to multiple antimicrobials. This resistance is usually plasmid mediated (eg, *Klebsiella pneumoniae, Pseudomonas aeruginosa, Escherichia coli, Enterobacter* sp., *Acinetobacter* sp.).

ESBL: Extended spectrum β-lactamase.

CRE: Carbapenem-resistant Enterobacteriaceae.

SEPSIS: Sepsis is a clinical term used to describe a dysregulated systemic inflammatory response to infection, with or without organ dysfunction. Sepsis is a complex syndrome that is difficult to define, diagnose, and treat. It is a range of clinical conditions that extends from bacteremia to multisystem failure and death in severe instances. It is a major cause of mortality, killing approximately 1400 people worldwide every day. The term *severe sepsis* has been abandoned as all sepsis is severe, with high mortality.

GRAFT VERSUS HOST DISEASE (GVHD): Occurs when the patient's immune system is dominated by the donor's tissue immune system. This results in the donor immune system considering the host's tissue as foreign. Symptoms may include severe rash, pruritus, mucositis, GI disturbances, and liver dysfunction. This may be a life-threatening condition.

CLINICAL APPROACH

Immunosuppression may be subdivided into congenital, acquired, and iatrogenic or due to drug/therapy origins (Table 20–1). **The most common inherited cause in adults is described as common variable immunodeficiency (CVI), where there is**

Table 20–1 • MAJOR TYPES OF IMMUNE DEFECTS: SPECIFIC DEFECTS, CONDITIONS, AND DISEASES

- Disruption or inflammation of mucosa and/or skin (including indwelling "lines")
- Phagocytic defects: neutropenia, chemotaxis, killing defects
- Humoral or antibody (B-cell) defects: hypogammaglobulinemia, IgA deficiency
- Complement system defects: low complement deficiencies, C3 and C5 (*S. pneumoniae, Haemophilus influenzae* infection); high complement deficiencies, C5b, C6, C7, C8, C9 (*Neisseria meningitidis, Neisseria gonorrhoeae* infection)
- Cell-mediated (T-cell) defects: e.g., HIV/AIDS and lymphoma

insufficient production of antibodies to infectious agents. CVI can be treated with pooled human immune globulin supplementation. Immunosuppression can result from infections such as HIV, measles, and cancers. HIV/AIDS and lymphomas can cause significant decreases in T—cell-mediated immunity. **AIDS has emerged as the most common cause of suppressed cell-mediated immunity (CMI).** Fortunately, ART (antiretroviral therapy, formerly HART) and the application of antimicrobial prophylaxis have made a deep impact on the survival of AIDS patients. Therapy-induced immunosuppression may be caused by a variety of drugs and treatments. These include corticosteroids, azathioprine, methotrexate, mycophenolate mofetil, cyclophosphamide, infliximab, rituximab, an increasing number of chemothera-peutic agents, and irradiation or radiation therapy, to list a few.

Infection Prevention

The immune system's primary function is to prevent infection. When the immune system is suppressed, dysfunctional, or absent, the patient's ability to combat infec-tions is reduced and the incidence of infections increases. These infections may arise from microorganisms called **opportunistic infections (OI)** that normally do not cause disease. Infections are usually more severe in immunosuppressed patients and have a greater likelihood of resulting in death. The best methods to protect these patients are to avoid unnecessary or overly aggressive immunosuppressive therapy when possible, avoid exposure to infectious agents, and reconstitute the immune system when possible. Other preventive strategies include appro-priate immunizations, prophylactic antimicrobials, and following isolation and hand washing policies.

For neutropenic patients, reverse isolation is important, and raw vegetables should be avoided unless they are irradiated** to prevent the transfer of bacteria to the patient's gastrointestinal system via food. Indwelling catheters should be avoided and monitored closely when used. Attention to hand washing and the proper use of gloves, facial masks, and protective clothing are essential. While hand hygiene is critical in the prevention of infections, compliance with proven guidelines among healthcare workers is below 40%. In some cases, **granulocyte colony-stimulating factor (G-CSF)** is needed to hasten bone marrow recovery. Healthcare associated infections are the most common adverse events resulting from hospitalization, with approximately 5% to 10% of hospitalized patients in the developed world acquiring such infections.

ICU Care

Improvements in patient survival with comorbid disease and advances in critical care management have resulted in an increase in the number of patients in the ICU who are immunocompromised. An immunocompromised host with altera-tions in phagocytic, cellular, or humoral immunity has an increased risk of infec-tious complication(s) and provides a breeding ground for an opportunistic process to occur.

Patients may also become immunocompromised if they have an alteration in or a breach of their skin or mucosal defense barriers that permits microorganisms to initiate a local or a systemic infection (eg, indwelling vascular catheters, Foley

Table 20–2 • IMMUNE DEFECTS AND COMMONLY ASSOCIATED PATHOGENS	
Immune Defect	Commonly-Associated Pathogens
Skin and mucosal disruption	Burns: *P. aeruginosa, S. aureus*, MRSA, VRE, VISA; traTuma: *Streptococcus pyogenes, Streptococcus epidermidis*
Phagocytic defects: Neutropenia Chemotaxis Killing defects	Gram-positive cocci > GNR ("enteric"), *P. aeruginosa, Aspergillus* and *Candida* sp., *S. aureus*, GNR ("enterics") *S. aureus, Burkholderia cepacia*, GNR, *Aspergillus*
Humoral immunity, hypogamma-globulinemia, IgA deficiency, asplenia, hyposplenism	*S. pneumoniae, H. influenzae*, pyogenic bacteria, *Giardia lamblia*
Cell-mediated immunity	Intracellular bacteria (*Listeria monocytogenes*), viruses (HSV, VZV, CMV), fungi (*Candida* sp., *Cryptococcus neoformans*), parasites (*Toxoplasma gondii*)
Complement defects: C3 or C5, C5b, C6, C7, C8, C9	*S. pneumoniae, H. influenzae, N. meningitidis, N. gonorrhoeae*

catheters, endotracheal tubes, and erosions of the mucosa or skin). Specific organisms must be considered in the setting of immunosuppression based on the type of defect(s) present.

Specific Organisms

Although the causes of fever in immunocompromised hosts are numerous and often never elucidated, some guidance to therapy is given by knowing the specific immunological defect or defects present in the patient (Table 20–2). The **duration of immune defense alteration has an extremely important effect on the types of infectious complications** that are likely to occur. This includes ICU patients who are immunocompromised because of cancer or its treatment, those undergoing bone marrow or solid organ transplantation, patients who have had a splenectomy, and patients with human immunodeficiency virus (HIV) infection or the acquired immunodeficiency syndrome (AIDS). Recognizing specific issues and challenges in the management of immunocompromised patients and focusing on infectious complications is vital to patient survival and well-being in the ICU setting. See Table 20–3 for guidance on immunosuppression and site of infection.

Sepsis

Sepsis is a major cause of morbidity and mortality in ICUs and affects more than a million Americans annually with a mortality of over 28%. Despite advances in the management of sepsis, the mortality remains high worldwide at 18% to 50%. Early fluid resuscitation, early antibiotics, and early goal-directed therapy (EGDT), along with newer modalities of respiratory therapy, have all contributed to decreasing the mortality from sepsis. The immune compromised patient with sepsis remains at

Table 20–3 • CAUSES OF FEVER BY IMMUNOSUPPRESSION AND SITE

Site	Bone Marrow Transplant	Kidney Transplant	Liver Transplant	Lung Transplant	Heart Transplant	Adult HIV/AIDS Infection
Blood	Bacteremia, fungemia	Bacteremia	Uncommon	Uncommon	Uncommon	S. pneumoniae
Lung	Sinusitis, fungal Bacterial/fungal pneumonia with neutropenia Cytomegalovirus 30-60 days after allogenic transplant	Uncommon	Uncommon	Common pneumonia, local or diffuse; many are fungal	Common, local or diffuse	Bacterial sinusitis, otitis Pneumonia: Pneumocystis jirovecii, S. pneumoniae, Cryptococcus, Pseudomonas
Liver	Hepatosplenic candidiasis while recovering from neutropenia	Uncommon	Hepatitis, cholangitis, abscess	Uncommon	Uncommon	Hepatitis A, B, and C Perianal herpes simplex
CNS	Toxoplasma, Nocardia, Cryptococcus (uncommon), Aspergillus sp.	Listeria (uncommon)	Listeria (uncommon)	Listeria (uncommon)	Listeria (uncommon)	Toxoplasma, cryptococcal meningitis, neurosyphilis, Cytomegalovirus
Skin	Bone marrow same as high risk	CMV	Uncommon	Uncommon	Uncommon	Herpes simplex virus, Cytomegalovirus, Varicella zoster virus

even greater risk of death than the immune competent patient. Understanding the dysregulation or dissonance of the immune system in sepsis and septic shock is key to intervening in this multifactorial syndrome. Currently, the mainstay of therapy in these critically ill patients remains early administration of appropriate antimicrobials, aggressive fluid resuscitation/deresuscitation, and EGDT coupled with excellent management of respiratory embarrassment and host homeostasis. At present there are no specific medications targeting sepsis/septic shock and sepsis associated coagulopathy ("SAC") available in the USA. However, several molecules and interventions are under investigation following the withdrawal of activated protein C from the market.

The period of immune dysregulation in the compromised host limits and disorganizes host defenses against primary and latent infections, thereby predisposing the patient to sepsis, septic shock, multiorgan dysfunction, and in many patients, death. The pathophysiology of these events is still not completely understood but can be viewed as a basic deterioration or dysregulation of homeostasis controls by intercellular communications systems when faced with systemic injury due to microbial invasion. The importance of the endothelial system's role in this event cannot be overemphasized.

Host Response

The host response to infection is complex and varies depending on the type of infection/organism, the infective dose (bacterial load), and host genetic factors (genomics). Microbial invasion of a healthy patient may activate both the acquired and innate immune systems. During an infectious process, the host's leukocytes respond to exogenous danger signals via *pathogens-associated molecular patterns* (PAMP's). Endogenous mediators are released by the host cells and modify the immune response to infection. The resultant pro-inflammatory state helps to localize infections by recruiting phagocytes and immune surveillance cells to the area(s) of infection. When the response is exaggerated, sepsis, septic shock and multiorgan dysfunction (MODS) can result.

When antigen(s) are presented to naïve T-cells, they are primed to differentiate into either Type 1 (Th1) or Type 2 (Th2) helper cells (and other more recently described Th17 and Treg cells). This polarity of determination of CD4 T-cells is complex and intimately involved in the evolution of the sepsis syndrome and its outcome. Th1 cells are involved in cell-mediated immunity and secrete interferon-gamma (IFN-γ) and IL-2, whereas Th-2 cells participate in humoral-antibody-mediated immunity and secrete IL-10, IL-4, IL-5, and transforming growth factor-β (TGF-β). The shift from Th1 cells to Th2 cells is a hallmark of how the inflammatory response is down-regulated and is referred to as the *compensatory anti-inflammatory response syndrome* (CARS). CARS may occur in patients who survive the initial sepsis syndrome and then enter a state of immune suppression and dysfunction. The ratio of pro-inflammatory/anti-inflammatory cytokines has been associated with the time of death in sepsis. These ratios (especially IL-10/TNF-α ratio) may be of use in not only predicting severity and mortality in sepsis, but also assisting in the precise management of the patient. Most deaths in sepsis occur late in the course of the syndrome, during the later phase

Table 20–4 • THE PRO-INFLAMMATORY AND ANTI-INFLAMMATORY CYTOKINES AND STATES	
Pro-Inflammatory Cytokines: Early Sepsis	Anti-Inflammatory Cytokines: Compensatory Anti-Inflammatory Response (CARS)
TNF-α	Th-2 cells, IFN-γ
IL-6	IL-10
IL-1	IL-4
Release of acute phase reactants (APRs): C-RP, ESR, PCT	IL-13, TGF-β

APRs: acute phase reactants released due to pro-inflammatory cytokine activity; C-RP: C-reactive protein; ESR: erythrocyte sedimentation rate; PCT: procalcitonin.

of immune suppression. It is also important to note that immune reconstitution, such as that seen in some AIDS patients when started on anti-retroviral therapy (ART), can result in a severe inflammatory syndrome, which occurs especially when the CD4 count is less than 50. The **immune reconstitution inflammatory syndrome** (IRIS) is seen when a previously existing OI such as tuberculosis or cryptococcosis (either undiagnosed or previously treated) is responded to by the recovering immune system with an abrupt onset of fever and organ damage. This is based in part on the "reconstitution" of antigen-specific Th1 immunity following ART therapy. See Table 20–4 for summary of proinflammatory and inflammatory cytokines and states.

Posttransplant Immunosuppression

Advances in immunosuppression have resulted in a significant reduction in the incidence of acute graft rejection. Fortunately, there has not been a commensurate increase in infection and resultant malignancy with the use of these newer, more effective agents. There are four basic groups of immunosuppressive agents used in transplantation:

- Calcineurin inhibitors: Cyclosporin, Tacrolimus (Prograf)

- Rapamycin (mTOR) inhibitors: Sirolimus (Rapamune), Everolimus (Zortress)

- Antimetabolites: Mycophenolate (Cellcept), Azathioprine (Imuran)

- Corticosteroids

The introduction of the newer immunosuppressants such as tacrolimus, mycophenolate mofetil (MMF), leflunomide, and sirolimus have actually shown a significant reduction in the incidence of acute rejection free of increases in infection and malignancy. Treatment of immunocompromised patients with new fever is based on the type and degree of immune dysfunction contingent to each setting (Table 20–5).

Table 20–5 • TREATMENT OF IMMUNOCOMPROMISED PATIENTS WITH NEW FEVER

Condition	Treatment Plan
Low-risk cancer patient	Broad-spectrum antibiotics with a single parenteral agent (levofloxacin and amoxicillin plus clavulanate potassium)
High-risk cancer patient	Same as low risk or use a combination regimen; consider additional treatment or modification if the patient has a persistent fever or neutropenia
Bone marrow transplantation	**Immediately postoperative:** same as high-risk cancer after receiving transplant; patients are at risk for CMV, varicella zoster virus, other viral syndromes, as well as parasitic and fungal infections **Greater than 100 days posttransplant (late infection):** likely from encapsulated bacteria, which are managed with antibiotic therapy
Kidney transplantation	Postoperatively, treatment should be directed empirically with broad-spectrum antibiotics for septicemia, pyelonephritis, or pneumonia (consider CMV, viral, or parasitic infections)
Liver transplantation	Immediately postoperatively, treatment should be directed empirically for bacteremia, enteric organisms, and ascending cholangitis
Lung transplantation	**Immediately postoperative:** treat for a gram-negative bacteria from pneumonitis. Patients with cystic fibrosis and pseudomonas have a significant risk for this infection. **Late infection:** consider *Aspergillus*
Heart transplantation	**Immediately postoperative:** treat for gram-positive or gram-negative bacteria with a consideration for pneumonia or mediastinitus Common postoperative viral infections are CMV, EBV Common postoperative fungal infections are *P. jirovecii* and *Toxoplasma*
Splenectomy	Give antibiotic regimen for encapsulated organisms
HIV/AIDS in children	Focus therapy for specific-site of infection (ie, URI vs UTI, etc). Treatment depends on the age-corrected CD4 count for low CD4 counts. Opportunistic infections: *P. jirovecii*, *Mycobacterium avium*, and Cytomegalovirus should be considered and treatment should be directed empirically
HIV in adults	Treatment similar to children; with the exception of *S. pneumonia*, bacterial infections are less common. When the CD4 count is < 200 mm^3, treatment directed toward PCP or Toxoplasmosis With CD4 count <50 mm^3, treatment should be directed toward *Mycobacterium tuberculosis*, *M. avium*, and *Cryptococcus*
Anti-TNF therapies	**On therapy:** Tuberculosis; Histoplasmosis; Pneumocystis; Nocardiosis; Listeria; Legionella; Cryptococcosis; PML; Varicella **Pre-Treatment:** Patients should be screened for latent TB and endemic mycoses prior to starting therapy. Vaccinations should be up to date prior to treatment with Anti-TNFs. No live vaccines during therapy.

Table 20-6 • POSSIBLE DIAGNOSTIC MARKERS OF IMMUNE DYSFUNCTION
Increased initial and sustained IL-10 levels
High IL-10/ TNF-α ratios
Decreased mHLA-DR expression
Interleukin-10 (IL-10); monocyte human leukocyte antigen type (mHLA-DR), tumor necrosis factor-α (TNF-α)

Identifying Immune Dysfunction in the Septic Patient

The host response in sepsis is complex and involves the endothelial cell/organ responses and generation/regulation of circulating mediators. Some cytokines have been demonstrated to correlate with sepsis and sepsis mortality. Markedly elevated levels of circulating IL-6 and soluble TNF receptors have been correlated with severity of disease and 28-day mortality. This type of information may be useful in determining when anti-inflammatory therapy may be effectively instituted in sepsis. Measuring blood levels of circulating cytokines can help determine presence and degree of immunosuppression and the presence or absence of infection. **Elevated and sustained levels of IL-10 and high IL-10/TNF-α ratios have been demonstrated to be predictive of poor outcome in sepsis.** IL-10 and TGF-β are anti-inflammatory cytokines associated with the down-regulation of the immune system during sepsis. Currently, several assays are being used routinely in ICUs and emergency rooms to predict presence and severity of infection and sepsis. These include C-RP, PCT, and D-dimer. PCT has been used to assist in modifying antibiotic therapy (early termination of treatment with low levels of PCT suggesting viral infection). Some of these biomarkers may be of greater use in the early diagnosis of sepsis and sepsis-associated coagulopathy (Table 20–6).

Potential Therapies Aimed at Immune Dysfunction in Sepsis

Anti-inflammatory therapies have not clearly decreased overall mortality in patients with sepsis. Trials with TNF-α antagonists, IL-1 receptor antagonists, anti-endotoxin antibodies, corticosteroids, granulocyte colony-stimulating factor (G-CSF), activated protein-C and other molecules have not been clearly successful. Current studies are evaluating molecules and devices that may be used in sepsis. Intravenous Immunoglobulin (IVIG) can supply specific antibodies in immune deficiency states, infection, or sepsis-induced pathological settings such as *Clostridium difficile* infection, endotoxemias, depressed immunoglobulin states, meningococcemia, severe streptococcal infections, and respiratory tract infections. IVIG has been used as adjunctive therapy in septic shock with variable results.

CLINICAL CASE CORRELATION

- See also Case 17 (Meningitis/Encephalitis), Case 18 (Antibiotics), Case 19 (Sepsis), and Case 33 (Multiorgan Dysfunction).

COMPREHENSION QUESTIONS

20.1 A previously healthy 27-year-old man was admitted to the ICU after a motor vehicle accident (MVA). He was intubated and given fluid resuscitation and blood transfusions prior to transfer to the operating room (OR) for laparotomy due to a ruptured viscus (stomach). After surgery he was managed in the ICU with TPN, Foley catheterization, and a completed four-day course of preventive antibiotic therapy for the ruptured viscus. He was extubated on the third day in ICU but was maintained on TPN following the laparotomy. On the sixth day in the ICU, his temperature spiked to > 102°F. Upon examination he was noted to be toxic but had no identifiable focus of infection. A chest x-ray showed no lung infiltrates. What empiric therapy would you initiate pending the result of cultures for common pathogens?

A. Gram-negative bacterial sepsis from ruptured viscus. Start broad-spectrum antibiotics.

B. Candidemia. Start fluconazole or echinocandin (eg, caspofungin).

C. Influenza. Start rimantadine.

D. Invasive aspergillosis. Start voriconazole.

E. Hospital-acquired pneumonia (HAP). Start vancomycin and ceftazidime.

20.2 A 55-year-old man is transferred to the ICU for evaluation of a fever of 103°F, pleuritic chest pain, shortness of breath, and hemoptysis. He is 21 days status post-allogenic bone marrow transplant (BMT) for acute myelogenous leukemia (AML). Chest x-ray reveals the presence of an infiltrate and a CT of the chest reveals a cavitary lesion with a "halo" sign. He remains profoundly neutropenic (<100 neutrophils/mm^3) and thrombocytopenic (10,000/mm^3). Examination reveals that he is tachypneic and tachycardic. Bronchoscopy shows hyphae budding at 45 degrees. What empiric therapy should be instituted?

A. Amphotericin B given IV and open lung biopsy or transthoracic biopsy

B. Voriconazole and Gram stain of sputum; determine galactomannan level

C. Fluconazole IV and bronchoscopy with transbronchial biopsy

D. Echinocandin IV and VATS with directed biopsy for culture and sensitivity, and silver stain

E. Treat empirically for tuberculosis

ANSWERS

20.1 **B.** The patient is at high risk for candidemia due to the ruptured viscus and upper GI surgery, indwelling lines with total parenteral nutrition (TPN), prior use of broad-spectrum antibiotics for the ruptured viscus, and blood transfusion. Other risk factors for candidemia in the ICU include neutropenia, hematological malignancies, hemodialysis, burns, prior enteric bacteremia, and recent fluconazole use (<30 days). Unstable patients should be started preemptively (empirically) on an echinocandin (eg, caspofungin): patient outcomes are related to both the early intervention and the choice of an effective therapy. Stable patients may be started on fluconazole pending the result of fungal cultures. Over 50% of patients in the ICU who develop candidemia are colonized with non-albicans species of *Candida* (eg, *Candida glabrata*, *Candida parapsilosis*, *Candida tropicalis*, and *Candida lusitaniae*). In ICU patients with invasive candidiasis/candidemia, the removal or replacement of indwelling venous catheters and any other catheters and an evaluation of TPN need should be routine and considered in all patients unless absolutely not feasible.

20.2 **B.** The patient has had an allogenic bone marrow transplantation (BMT) with prolonged and severe neutropenia. The finding of a "halo" sign and hyphae budding at 45 degrees is highly consistent with an *Aspergillus* lung infection (seen in 10%-20% of patients with BMT). *Aspergillus* is most prominent due to effective prophylaxis against *Candida* with current protocols. Therapy of suspected *Aspergillus* lung infections must be instituted as early as possible to improve outcomes. Voriconazole is now the drug of choice for this infection. The diagnosis of pulmonary *Aspergillus* infection is confirmed by demonstrating the branching hyphae at an acute angle on tissue biopsy silver stains, as it is a vaso-invasive hyphae and has subsequent positive cultures. Finding *Aspergillus* in his sputum and seeing a rise in his baseline galactomannan level (done weekly posttransplant) would be consistent with the diagnosis of IAI.

CLINICAL PEARLS

▶ Common variable immunodeficiency is the most common inherited immunodeficiency of adults.

▶ Profound and prolonged neutropenia is a high risk for invasive Aspergillosis, especially in the lungs.

▶ When fever persists ≥ 4 days despite appropriate empiric antibiotic therapy, attention/therapy should be directed at *Candida*/yeast and *Aspergillus*/mold.

▶ Patients with both suppressed (chemotherapy/immunosuppression) and reconstituted (ART in AIDS) immune systems are at high risk for predictable infections of cell-mediated immunity.

▶ Hand washing is the most important preventive strategy to reduce hospital-acquired infection.

REFERENCES

Loscalzo J. *Harrison's Pulmonary and Critical Care Medicine*. New York, NY: McGraw-Hill; 2013.

Mayo Clinic (2016) *Mayo Medical Laboratories* [Online]. Available at http://www.mayomedicallaboratories.com/test-catalog/Clinical+and+Interpretive/84356. Accessed May 6, 2016.

Pizzo PA. Fever in immunocompromised patients. *N Engl J Med*. Sep 16 1999;341:893-900.

A 63-year-old man is hospitalized and is recovering from an acute myocardial infarction that occurred 6 days ago. He began to complain of vague epigastric pain for the past day, and an myocardial infarction (MI) was ruled out by ECG and cardiac enzymes. Several hours later, he began to feel dizzy and passed a large amount of dark bloody stool per rectum. Shortly thereafter, he vomited approximately 100 mL of blood. At this point, his blood pressure is 90/60 mm Hg and pulse rate is 85 beats/min. He is transferred to the ICU for further monitoring.

► What are the priorities in this patient's management?
► What are the risk factors for this patient's condition?
► What are the factors that may adversely affect the outcome?

ANSWERS TO CASE 21:

Gastrointestinal Bleeding

Summary: A 63-year-old man who is hospitalized for a recent myocardial infarction develops signs and symptoms of acute upper gastrointestinal (GI) hemorrhage. His vital signs are concerning for hemorrhagic shock.

- **Priorities in management:** Priorities in this particular patient include establishing a secure airway and maintaining adequate circulating blood volume and definitive hemorrhage control. The patient should be resuscitated with a combination of crystalloids and blood products to optimize cardiac function and maintain a normal coagulation process. This includes potential transfusions of packed red cells, platelets, and fresh-frozen plasma to correct for any coagulation defects. Once the patient's physiologic status is stabilized, he should be prepared for upper GI endoscopy to diagnose and potentially treat his gastrointestinal bleeding.

- **Risk factors for this patient's condition:** This patient is recovering from a recent myocardial infarction. The stress related to his current illness is a risk factor. In addition, patients with unstable cardiac conditions often receive antiplatelet therapy, which can increase the risk for bleeding complications.

- **Factors that adversely affect the outcome:** There are many reported clinical and endoscopic factors that influence outcomes.

  - Clinical contributors to adverse outcomes:

    1. Shock on admission

    2. Comorbid illnesses

    3. Prior history of bleeding requiring transfusion

    4. Admission Hgb <8g/dL

    5. Transfusion requirement of >5 units of PRBCs

    6. Blood in the nasogastric (NG) aspirate that does not clear with lavage

    7. Age >65 years

  - Endoscopic contributors of adverse outcome in acute upper gastrointestinal hemorrhage:

    1. Visible vessel in ulcer base (~50% rebleeding risk)

    2. Active bleeding from ulcer base

    3. Adherent clot at ulcer base

    4. Location of ulcer (worse prognosis when located on posterior lesser curvature of stomach or posterior duodenal bulb)

    5. Ulcer diameter >2 cm

ANALYSIS

Objectives

1. Learn the initial management and diagnostic strategy for patients with upper gastrointestinal bleeding.
2. Learn the management of patients with nonvariceal- and variceal-related upper gastrointestinal bleeding.
3. Learn the differences in the management approaches to patients with upper GI bleeding and lower GI bleeding.

Considerations

This patient has an acute upper gastrointestinal hemorrhage. He is in his sixties with underlying cardiovascular disease; therefore, he is at increased risk for a low-flow state due to diminished cardiac output (from his recent myocardial infarction). Additionally, he has been in the hospital for 6 days and is at risk for stress-related ulcer formation and hemorrhage. Antiplatelet therapy has most likely been prescribed for his cardiac condition, which further increases his risk for bleeding complications. A major goal at this time is to optimize the support of his hemodynamic status without creating increased physiological stress to his heart. Normalization of his vital signs would avoid additional ischemic injury to his heart. The packed red blood cell replacement for his blood loss must not be given excessively, as restoration of hemoglobin to a target hemoglobin of >9 g/dL has been demonstrated to be associated with worse outcome in comparison to replacement with a target hemoglobin of 7 g/dL. In addition to volume and blood product resuscitation, pharmacological therapy needs to be initiated as we determine whether his bleeding is most likely nonvariceal or variceal in origin. Appropriate resuscitation followed by timely diagnostic studies, including endoscopy, would be important.

APPROACH TO:
GI Bleeding

DEFINITIONS

UPPER GI BLEEDING: Bleeding source proximal to the ligament of Treitz (esophagus, stomach, and duodenum).

LOWER GI BLEEDING: Bleeding source distal to the ligament of Treitz (jenunum, ileum, colon, and rectum).

OCCULT GI BLEEDING: Slow bleeding originating anywhere along the GI tract. Patients do not complain of bleeding symptoms and commonly present with anemia, fatigue, and hemoccult positive stool.

GASTRODUODENAL ULCERATION: Ulcers of the stomach or duodenum. These comprise the majority of upper GI bleeding episodes (50%), and the condition is very often due to *Helicobacter pylori* infections (80%-90%).

PORTAL HYPERTENSION-ASSOCIATED BLEEDING: Esophagogastric varices are present in 30% to 60% of patients with cirrhosis. Significant mortality is attributable to the first bleeding episode (30%-50%).

STRESS GASTRITIS: Inflammation of the lining of stomach. The physiologic stress from trauma, burns, major surgery, or severe medical illness is associated with the development of hemorrhagic gastritis, or stress erosions in the fundus or gastric body.

ESOPHAGITIS: Inflammation of the esophagus, often caused by gastroesophageal reflux disease (GERD), which can predispose patients to mucosal ulceration and upper GI bleeding. Bleeding can also occur from erosion by a nasogastric tube (NGT), typically in the chronic patient.

NSAID EROSIVE GASTROPATHY: Nonsteroidal anti-inflammatory drug (NSAID)-related ulcers. These can develop within 1 to 2 days of treatment and usually appear in the antrum of the stomach. Ulcers typically present asymptomatically and resolve after cessation of treatment.

GASTRIC ANTRAL VASCULAR ECTASIA (GAVE): GAVE is a rare cause of upper GI bleeding overall. It is commonly referred to as "watermelon stomach" because of the watermelon-like striped appearance of mucosal erythema stemming from the pylorus (usually limited to the antrum). GAVE is associated with bone marrow transplants, scleroderma, and cirrhosis. A direct cause is not identified.

DIEULAFOY'S LESION: Dieulafoy is a large ectatic submucosal arteriole that erodes through the mucosal layer of the stomach. Most appear in the proximal stomach (up to 95%), predominantly on the lesser curvature and within 6 cm of the gastroesophageal junction.

PERCUTANEOUS TRANSARTERIAL EMBOLIZATION: This interventional radiology approach is an alternative to surgery in patients for whom endoscopic therapy has failed. The rate of technical success has been reported to range from 52% to 98% with recurrent bleeding in 10% to 20% of patients.

CLINICAL APPROACH

The initial management and diagnostic strategy for patients with upper gastrointestinal bleeding is noted in Figure 21–1. All patients with upper GI bleeding should undergo the ABCs of resuscitation. Hemodynamically unstable patients (SBP ≤90, orthostatic hypotension), those with evidence of severe bleeding (HCT drop of >6%), or those with a transfusion requirement of greater than 2 units PRBCs should be admitted to the ICU for resuscitation and close monitoring. Central venous pressure monitoring should be considered, especially in patients with significant cardiopulmonary and renal comorbidities. The decision to initiate blood transfusions for patients should be based on individual patient's underlying conditions and hemodynamic and perfusion statuses rather than any predetermined hemoglobin values. Correction of coagulopathy (INR >1.5 and/or platelet count <50,000)

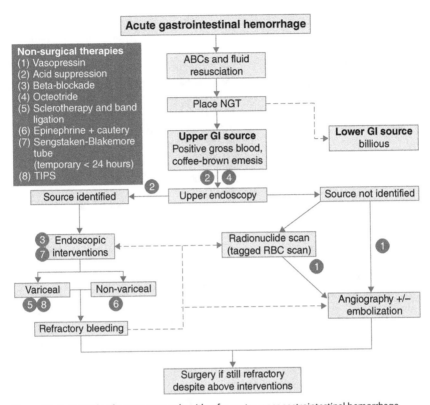

Acute gastrointestinal hemorrhage

Non-surgical therapies
(1) Vasopressin
(2) Acid suppression
(3) Beta-blockade
(4) Octeotride
(5) Sclerotherapy and band ligation
(6) Epinephrine + cautery
(7) Sengstaken-Blakemore tube (temporary < 24 hours)
(8) TIPS

ABCs and fluid resuciation

Place NGT

Upper GI source
Positive gross blood, coffee-brown emesis

Lower GI source
billious

Source identified ← ② Upper endoscopy → Source not identified

③ ⑦ Endoscopic interventions

Radionuclide scan (tagged RBC scan)

Variceal ⑤ ⑧   Non-variceal ⑥

Angiography +/− embolization

Refractory bleeding

Surgery if still refractory despite above interventions

Figure 21–1. Example of management algorithm for acute upper gastrointestinal hemorrhage.

with fresh-frozen plasma or platelet transfusion is important in patients with ongoing bleeding. Patients receiving antiplatelet therapy should have platelet transfusions to provide functioning platelets since platelet counts in these individuals do not necessarily indicate normal platelet functions. Decisions to reinitiate or terminate antiplatelet therapy should be based on the risks/benefits of individual patients' cardiovascular comorbidities versus bleeding risks.

After resuscitation, an initial attempt at determining whether the source is an upper or lower source should be made. In patients with massive upper GI tract bleeding, agitation, or impaired respiratory status, endotracheal intubation should be considered prior to the initiation of endoscopy. After the ABCs are stabilized and resuscitation is underway, an NGT should be considered, and NGT placement may be beneficial in preventing aspiration for patients with active hematemesis. If the NG-aspirate is coffee-ground or bloody in nature, an upper GI source is confirmed. Even if there is a clear aspirate, there still exists a small possibility that bleeding could be from the duodenum (closed pylorus). Absence of blood or coffee-ground emesis in the presence of an open pylorus (presence of bilious NG aspirate) localizes bleeding to the lower GI tract. In upper GI bleeding cases, the patient should proceed to upper endoscopy to definitively localize and potentially treat the lesion.

Upper GI endoscopy can identify the source and status of bleeding in 90% of cases. Early endoscopy (within 12 hours) is recommended for most patients with acute upper gastrointestinal hemorrhage, as it has been demonstrated to improve the diagnostic sensitivity of the procedure. Endoscopic findings are often helpful to risk stratify patients to low or high risk for recurrent or life-threatening hemorrhage. This may assist in selecting patients who may be suitable for early hospital or ICU discharges or, alternatively, further ICU monitoring.

Administration of intravenous erythromycin (3 mg/kg IV over 20-30 minutes) 30 to 90 minutes prior to endoscopy can often improve visibility, shorten endoscopy time, and reduce the need for second-look endoscopy. Erythromycin is a motilin agonist in the GI tract that promotes antegrade flow of gastric and duodenal contents.

Patients who are found to have mucosal ulcerations during EGD (esophogogas-troduodenoscopy, or upper endoscopy) should undergo biopsy of the gastric and antral mucosa to evaluate for *H. pylori*. Patients who are *H. pylori* positive should receive triple-therapy (clarithromycin 500 BID, amoxicillin 1 g BID, and a proton pump inhibitor) for at least 1 week. At 4 weeks, repeat *H. pylori* testing should be performed; proton pump inhibitor therapy should be stopped 1 week prior to this to prevent false negative results.

In situations where endoscopy fails to identify the site or control the bleeding, angiographic techniques can also be applied to diagnose and treat the upper GI bleeding. Although the role of angiography is better defined for lower GI bleeding, selective angiography is successful for localization and embolization of upper GI bleeding in up to 75% of patients with active bleeding.

MANAGEMENT OF UPPER GI BLEEDING

Medical Treatment for Both Variceal and Non-Variceal Related Acute GI Hemorrhage:

1. **Vasopressin:** Vasopressin can dramatically decrease the splanchnic blood flow and reduce upper GI bleeding. However, vasopressin and vasopressin analogues are now in disfavor due to the systemic vasoconstrictive effects, and for that reason octreotide is the preferred adjunctive therapy in conjunction with EGD for variceal upper gastrointestinal hemorrhage patients.

2. **Acid Suppression:** Acid suppression with high-dose proton pump inhibitors (pantoprazole 80 mg bolus followed by 8 mg/h infusion) given before or after endoscopy has been shown to significantly reduce the occurrence of rebleeding, decrease hospital stay, reduce the number of actively bleeding ulcers, and reduce transfusion requirements. In patients with NSAID-related ulcers, 4 weeks of outpatient PPI therapy is suggested.

3. **Endoscopic Intervention:** For nonvariceal bleeding, endoscopic hemostasis may be achieved with the use of epinephrine injections followed by thermal therapy. Permanent hemostasis occurs in roughly 80% to 90% of patients. Patients' physiologic statuses, clinical presentations, and endoscopic findings are all important determinants of the success of endoscopic interventions for these bleeding patients.

Medical Treatment for Variceal-Related Acute GI Hemorrhage:

1. **Octreotide:** Prior to endoscopy, octreotide (loading dose 50 µg, followed by 25-50 µg/h × 5 days) should be administered which may reduce the risk of bleeding. Octreotide can also be used as adjunctive therapy if endoscopy is unsuccessful, contraindicated, or unavailable. Although it has been best studied in the variceal bleeding population, octreotide is also loosely indicated for treatment of acute nonvariceal upper gastrointestinal bleeding.

2. **Beta-Blockers:** Used as maintenance therapy after acute upper GI bleeding from portal hypertension has been controlled. Oral beta blockade plus endoscopic therapy has been shown to reduce the rebleeding rate over endoscopic therapy alone. Endoscopic band ligation followed by beta-blockade is the recommended treatment strategy for variceal bleeding.

Interventions for Upper GI Hemorrhage from Variceal Sources:

1. **Sclerotherapy and Band Ligation:** Endoscopic sclerotherapy and/or band ligation for esophageal varices is the mainstay of emergent treatment. However, the risk of rebleeding after a single treatment is significant—up to 50% with sclerotherapy and 35% with band ligation. Some evidence a suggest that band ligation, when compared to sclerotherapy, is associated with fewer treatment-related complications. Lower rebleeding rates and improved survival have been reported with band ligation.

2. **Sengstaken-Blakemore Tube (SB Tube):** In rare circumstances where bleeding cannot be controlled endoscopically, the Sengstaken-Blakemore (Minnesota) tube can be used with the caveat that it must not be inflated for greater than 48 hours due to the high risk of tissue necrosis. The gastric balloon is inflated first, and if bleeding is not controlled, the esophageal balloon is inflated. SB tube placement is helpful for the temporary control of bleeding so that arrangements can be made for definitive care (eg, TIPS or endoscopic therapy).

3. **Transjugular Intrahepatic Portosystemic Shunt (TIPS):** Ideally applied in Child's B or C cirrhotic patients. TIPS can provide a bridge to liver transplantation. In comparison to sclerotherapy or band ligation, rebleeding rates are lower with TIPS. However, TIPS is associated with an increased occurrence of hepatic encephalopathy but no difference in overall survival. Rebleeding following TIPS can occur when shunt thrombosis occurs.

Surgical Treatment for Upper GI Hemorrhage:

The Child (or Child-Pugh) scores are used to assess severity of liver disease and prognosis. Serum bilirubin, albumin, INR, presence or absence of ascites, and presence or absence of encephalopathy are used. Class A has the best survival, and Class C has the worst.

1. **Surgical Shunts:** Patients who are Child's A are considered for surgical decompression (eg, distal splenorenal shunt) since the likelihood of occlusion for TIPS at 2 years outweighs the potential benefit of TIPS.

2. **Operative Exploration:** Operative exploration for upper gastrointestinal hemorrhage is generally reserved for individuals who fail endoscopic treatment. Depending on the source of the hemorrhage, procedures may include bleeding vessel ligation, lesion resection, and/or acid reduction procedures (eg, vagotomy) to prevent future ulcer formation. Transplantation is a rare last resort for Child's B and C patients in the emergent setting due to variceal-related bleeding.

MANAGEMENT OF LOWER GI BLEEDING

The initial management is to rule out an upper GI bleeding source. If available, urgent colonoscopy following mechanical bowel preparation is helpful for early identification of the bleeding source and endoscopic therapeutic options. Other initial diagnostic options for the localization of lower GI bleeding sources include CT angiography and tagged RBC scan. The advantage of the CT angiography over the tagged RBC study is better anatomic localization of bleeding sites (eg, localizing bleeding from the cecum rather than the right lower quadrant). Once the bleeding site is localized, the therapeutic options include microembolization by angiographic approach, endoscopic treatment, and surgical treatment. The decision for the selection of diagnostic and therapeutic management of lower GI bleeding patients is generally based on the availability of personnel, technology, and resources available at the individual institutions. The overall outcome of lower GI bleeding patients is much better than that of upper GI bleeding patients because of the inherently different natural histories of clinical conditions. In contrast to the upper GI bleeding patients in the ICU, the majority of the bleeding episodes do not produce hemodynamic instability, and the majority of bleeding cases are self-limiting.

> ### CASE CORRELATION
> - See also case 22 (Liver Failure) and case 41 (Hemorrhage and Coagulopathy).

COMPREHENSION QUESTIONS

21.1 A 55-year-old alcoholic with history of alcoholic cirrhosis arrives to the ED vomiting copious amounts of blood, hypotensive (BP 88/50 mm Hg), tachycardic (HR 115 beats/min), and with an O_2 saturation of 95% on the monitor. He is intubated, resuscitated, and taken to the endoscopy suite for further therapy. Which of the following therapeutic modalities has the highest bleeding recurrence rate for the variceal population after initial endoscopic treatment?

A. Sclerotherapy alone

B. Band ligation alone

C. Sclerotherapy and band ligation

D. TIPS

E. Operative portal-systemic shunt

21.2 A 60-year-old man with a history of *H. pylori* antral ulcer treated with triple therapy 5 weeks ago comes to clinic for follow up. He says his clinical condition has improved. He continues to take omeprazole for symptoms of GERD (last dose was this morning). What is the best laboratory measure for confirmation of eradication of *H. pylori* in this patient during this visit?

A. Repeat endoscopy with histologic examination

B. Anti-IgG against *H. pylori*

C. Urea breath test

D. Campylobacter-like organism (CLO) test

E. None of the above

21.3 A 65-year-old cirrhotic woman is brought to the emergency department with acute hematemesis and altered mental status. She is hypotensive, tachycardic, and vomiting blood. After intubation and fluid resuscitation, she is taken to the endoscopy suite, where multiple large varicosities are seen at the gastroesophageal (GE) junction. The gastroenterologist infuses octreotide and vasopressin, attempts band ligation, sclerotherapy and a Minnesota tube, all of which slow down but do not stop the bleeding. The patient's laboratory studies reveal the following: Hgb 5.8 g/dL, platelets 90,000/µL, INR 2.8, AST/ALT 86/90 IU/L, albumin 1.8 g/dL, total bilirubin 2.1 mg/dL, BUN/Cr 80/2.6 mg/dL. After 8 units of PRBCs, 6 units of FFP and 10 packs of platelets she remains borderline hypotensive (95/60 mm Hg) and has continued bleeding. What would be the next best intervention?

A. Try another Sengstaken-Blakemore tube

B. Continued fluid resuscitation and transfusion

C. TIPS

D. Hepatic transplantation

E. Distal Splenorenal (Warren) shunt

21.4 A 40-year-old man with a history of alcoholic cirrhosis presents with hematemesis. He is intubated and admitted to the ICU. Which of the following is proven beneficial for his management?

A. Resuscitation to keep his systolic blood pressure greater than 130 mm Hg

B. The initiation of vasopressin drip

C. Blood product replacement to keep the Hgb value above 9 g/dL

D. Early placement of TIPS

E. Blood product replacement to keep the Hgb value above 7 g/dL

ANSWERS

21.1 **A.** Multiple randomized trials have compared sclerotherapy versus sclerotherapy and band ligation versus band ligation alone. Meta-analyses suggest that rebleeding rates are highest in patients who undergo sclerotherapy alone (particularly patients with large varices). There is no additional benefit with regard to rebleeding if band ligation is accompanied by sclerotherapy in the same setting versus band ligation alone. For this reason, band ligation is the preferred first endoscopic modality, with a 35% chance of rebleeding. TIPS is superior to endoscopic therapy, with rebleeding rates far less than band ligation and sclerotherapy. Operative portal-systemic shunts are associated with low rebleeding rates but high procedural-associated mortality.

21.2 **E.** This patient is >4 weeks out of treatment for *H. pylori* but continues to take a PPI, which can cause false negative results. The patient should be instructed to stop taking his omeprazole for a week and then return to clinic to perform a urea breath test to confirm eradication of his infection.

21.3 **C.** TIPS is the best option for this patient who is classified as a Child's C cirrhotic. Of the other interventions, (A) is incorrect because it is a temporizing measure. (B) is incorrect because the patient is likely developing a consumptive coagulopathy and progressing into DIC. (D) is not a good choice because it is not likely she will receive a donor liver in an acute situation, and (E) is incorrect, as Warren shunts are indicated only in Child's A patients.

21.4 **E.** In a randomized trial examining resuscitation strategies for patients with acute upper GI hemorrhage, the patients who were randomized to hemoglobin endpoints of 7 g/dL had fewer transfusions, shorter ICU stays, and improved survival in comparison to patients who were randomized to Hgb endpoints of 9 g/dL. The subset analysis showed that patients with variceal hemorrhage were those who experienced the greatest benefits. Resuscitation of bleeding patients to excessively elevated blood pressures is not beneficial and in fact may contribute to excessive bleeding. Vasopressin is helpful for some patients, but vasopressin infusions can cause vasoconstrictive complications, and this treatment modality has been largely replaced by octreotide administration in patients with variceal bleeding. Early TIPS administration can be helpful to control bleeding for some patients; however, selection of the appropriate patients for this treatment remains less certain.

CLINICAL PEARLS

▶ Incidence of upper GI bleeding is approximately 170/100,000 patients a year, greater than lower GI bleeding.

▶ The mortality rate of upper GI bleeding is between 5% to 11%.

▶ Maintaining a CVP of <10 mm Hg for variceal bleeding patients is associated with lower rates of rebleeding.

▶ Resuscitation of upper GI bleeding patients with a target Hgb of 7 g/dL is associated with lower mortality, lower transfusion requirement, and shorter ICU stay than resuscitation to a target Hgb of >9 g/dL.

▶ Most upper GI bleeding cases are due to gastroduodenal ulceration, the majority of which can be managed endoscopically.

▶ Variceal hemorrhage is best managed by endoscopic techniques or with TIPS as an alternative. Surgical shunts have fallen out of favor in the acute setting, and TIPS is a viable bridge for some patients prior to hepatic transplantation.

▶ Priorities in management for acute upper GI bleeding include securing an airway, volume resuscitation, and early upper endoscopy.

REFERENCES

Jutabha R, Jensen D. Approach to upper gastrointestinal bleeding in adults. www.uptodate.com. Accessed on October 8, 2010.

Qayed E, Subramanian RM. Gastrointestinal hemorrhage. In: Hall JB, Schmidt GA, Kress JP, eds. *Principles of Critical Care*. 4th ed. New York, NY: McGraw-Hill Education; 2015:1008-1021.

Shanmugan S, Stein SL. Lower gastrointestinal bleeding. In: Cameron JL, Cameron AM, eds. *Current Surgical Therapy*. 11th ed. Philadelphia, PA: Elsevier Saunders; 2014:302-306.

Shuhart M, Kowldley K, Neighbor B. GI bleeding. http://www.uwgi.org/guidelines/ch_07/ch07txt .htm (Online Review). Accessed on April 5, 2011.

A 26-year-old woman was brought to the emergency center after being found by her roommate to be lethargic and vomiting at home. The patient's roommate had been on a business trip and had not seen the patient for one and a half days. On examination, the patient appears lethargic and mildly jaundiced. Her CBC is within normal limits. The serum transaminases are 2,500 IU/mL and 3,100 IU/mL. Serum glucose is 50 mg/dL, and total bilirubin is 2.8 mg/dL. Her prothrombin time is 45 seconds (INR 4), creatinine level is 2.6 mg/dL, and her arterial pH is 7.35. The serum acetaminophen concentration is 20 mg/L (NI < 10 mg/L). The patient had an nasogastric (NG) tube placed in the ED followed by gastric lavage and evacuation of gastric contents. In addition, she had activated charcoal treatment in the ED. She is now admitted to the ICU.

▶ What is the next step in treatment?
▶ What are the complications associated with this process?
▶ What are other treatment options in addition to medications and supportive measures?

ANSWERS TO CASE 22:
Acute Liver Failure

Summary: A 26-year-old woman is brought to the hospital with vomiting and lethargy. Her laboratory studies demonstrate marked elevation of the serum transaminases, serum bilirubin and creatinine. Her blood glucose and artery pH are low. Her elevated acetaminophen level is highly suggestive of acetaminophen toxicity. Initial treatment with gastric lavage and activated charcoal has already been given prior to arrival to the ICU.

- **Next step:** Administer *N*-acetylcysteine (NAC) therapy by mouth. This can be mixed with a carbonated beverage to improve tolerance. The initial loading dose is 140 mg/kg followed by 70 mg/kg every 4 hours for 17 doses or until the INR decreases to <1.5. If the patient is unable to tolerate oral intake, then intravenous *N*-acetylcysteine can be administered.

- **Complications:** Complications that may occur as the result of acute liver failure include cerebral edema, infections (including bacterial and fungal), acute kidney injury, high-output hyperdynamic process, and coagulopathy and bleeding complications.

- **Treatments other than medications and supportive measures:** Patients with severe acute liver failures may need liver transplantation. Alternatively, some limited experiences have shown that acellular liver support devices or bioartificial liver support devices may be temporarily implemented to provide support while liver recovery occurs. Alternatively, bioartificial liver devices can also be used as a bridge for the support of patients with fulminant hepatic failure prior to liver transplantation.

ANALYSIS

Objectives

1. Learn the initial evaluation and diagnosis of acute hepatic failure.

2. Learn the causes of acute hepatic failure.

3. Learn the management of acute hepatic failure.

4. Learn to identify patients with acute hepatic failure who may need referral for liver transplantation.

Considerations

This patient's presentation is highly suspicious for acute liver failure due to acetaminophen overdose. However, because the circumstances of this overdose are uncertain, the initial evaluation must also include a toxicology screen for other possible medications and illicit drug-related causes and a hepatitis screen for viral hepatitis. In addition, appropriate imaging and blood cultures should be done to rule out sepsis as the potential cause of this multiple organ dysfunction picture. Because there were no witnesses to the ingestion, it is difficult to determine the timing of the over-ingestion of acetaminophen; therefore, gastric lavage and activated charcoal therapy provided in the emergency department were appropriate early measures. NAC administration is vital to minimize the liver toxicity in this patient, and this should be initiated as early as possible in the emergency department and continued in the ICU. ICU admission for observation is very appropriate for this patient, given her altered mental status, acute kidney injury, and metabolic acidosis that suggest serious toxicity from ingestion. A detailed neurological examination needs to be completed in addition to a CT scan of the brain, given the patient's initial presentation of lethargy. Her neurological presentation suggests possible grade II encephalopathy, in which case the patient would be considered a potential candidate for referral to a liver transplant center. Even though acetaminophen-induced acute hepatic failure is the most common cause of acute liver failure in the United States, the survival is reported to be reasonably good at 78% to 80%, and >80% when NAC can be administered within 12 hours of ingestion.

APPROACH TO:
The Patient with Acute Hepatic Failure

DEFINITIONS

ACUTE HEPATIC FAILURE: Defined as the development of impaired liver synthetic function, coagulopathy, and hepatic encephalopathy in less than a 2 to 3 month period, in a patient without underlying liver disease.

GRADING OF HEPATIC ENCEPHALOPATHY: The West Haven grading system is based on level of impaired autonomy, level of consciousness, intellectual function, and behavior.

Grade 1 Trivial lack of awareness; shortened attentions span; euphoria or anxiety; impaired performance of simple addition or subtraction; minimal change in level of consciousness

Grade 2 Lethargy or apathy; disorientation for place or time; subtle personality change; inappropriate behavior; asterixis (liver flap)

Grade 3 Somnolence or semi-stupor but with response to verbal stimuli; marked confusion and disorientation

Grade 4 Comatose and unresponsive to verbal or noxious stimuli; decorticate or decerebrate posturing

N-ACETYLCYSTEINE (NAC): NAC helps to detoxify the acetaminophen toxic metabolite (*N*-acetyl-p-benzoquinone imine [NAPQI]). Ideally, when NAC is given within 8 to 10 hours after ingestion it protects against NAPQI-induced liver and renal injuries. NAC administration has been demonstrated to reduce the liver injury associated with acetaminophen overdose even when given within 16 hours after ingestion. The recommended dose is 140 mg/kg diluted in oral solution as a loading dose, followed by 70 mg/kg oral doses every 4 hours for 17 doses. Patients who are unable to tolerate oral intake can be given intravenous NAC with an initial loading dose of 150 mg/kg in D5W over 15 minutes, followed by a maintenance infusion dose of 50 mg/kg over 4 hours and then 100 mg/kg infusion over the next 16 hours.

LIVER SUPPORT SYSTEMS: Liver support devices are categorized as **acellular systems** that utilize albumin dialysis or **bioartificial liver (BAL) support systems.** The most common acellular system is the molecular reabsorbent and recirculating system (MARS). MARS has been shown to improve hemodynamic status, decrease encephalopathy, decrease intracranial pressure, and decrease serum bilirubin and creatinine. The bioartificial liver support systems are extracorporeal circulatory systems that utilize a veno-venal dialysis concept, where the patient's blood is circulated through a cell-based bioreactor. The bioreactors are loaded with either transformed human hepatocytes or porcine hepatocytes. Application of the BAL essentially provides patients with temporary liver filtering functions and biosynthetic functions. Clinical applications of BAL have been shown to improve the 30-day survival of patients with acute liver failure.

KING'S COLLEGE HOSPITAL (KCH) CRITERIA: This is the most widely applied criteria for the selection of patients with acute liver failure for liver transplantation.

The **KCH criteria for acetaminophen-induced failure** are:

1. pH <7.30 after resuscitation, irrespective of encephalopathy grade or

2. Prothrombin time >100 seconds and creatinine >300 µmol/L in patients with grade III or grade IV encephalopathy.

Modification to include lactate of >3.5 mmol/L after fluid resuscitation has been proposed by some. Patients with acetaminophen toxicity who meet the KCH criteria have a >90% mortality without liver transplantation. A recent meta-analysis showed that the KCH criteria are associated with sensitivity of 69% and specificity of 92% in predicting death without transplantation.

The **KCH criteria are different for patients with acute liver failure not induced by acetaminophen, and these** include: prothrombin time >100 seconds or three or more of the following criteria:

1. Age <10 or >40 years

2. Acute liver failure caused by non-A, non-B, non-C hepatitis, halothane hepatitis, or idiosyncratic drug reaction

3. Jaundice present for >1 week prior to onset of encephalopathy

4. Prothrombin time >50 seconds

5. Serum bilirubin >17.5 mg/dL

CLINICAL APPROACH

Acute liver failure can be produced by a variety of causes including toxins, viral infections, metabolic causes, vascular causes, and autoimmune causes. Acute liver injuries from these mechanisms can cause damages leading to hepatocyte apoptosis and/or necrosis. Injuries associated with mitochondrial permeability changes typically lead to apoptosis if the cells' ATP stores are preserved; examples of such include acute Wilson disease and Reye syndrome. When injuries producing mitochondrial permeability changes occur in the face of cellular ATP depletion, cell necrosis occurs. The site of injury within the liver architecture is important in determining the potential for cellular regeneration and recovery prognosis. Stem cells are located in the portal tract region, and preservation of these cells is important for regeneration; therefore, injury to the portal zone is associated with lower potential for regeneration and worse prognosis.

Toxin Induced Injuries

Acetaminophen is the most common type. Acetaminophen-induced liver injury can occur with ingestion of 4 g/d, but more often injuries are caused by the consumption of >10 g/d or 150 mg/kg/d. Acetaminophen is metabolized in the hepatocytes by cytochrome enzymes to the toxic metabolite N-acetyl p-benzoquinone imine (NAPQI), which is normally detoxified by conjugation with glutathione. Depletion of glutathione can increase the susceptibility of the individual to acetaminophen-induce liver injury. Acetaminophen-induced injuries are typically concentrated in the central zones, while the portal tracts are spared. Based on the architectural site of the injury, the potential for recovery is generally very good.

   Amanita (mushroom) poisoning is more commonly encountered in Western Europe than the United States. In the United States, Amanita species are most frequently encountered in coastal Pacific Northwest and to lesser extents in the Blue Ridge Mountains, Pennsylvania, New Jersey, and Ohio. Most Amanitas are encountered during late summer to early winter. Of the over 5000 species of mushrooms in existence, only approximately 50 species are poisonous to humans. Three of the Amanita species are responsible for >90% of all mushroom-related fatalities. Patients with mushroom poisoning typically present with vomiting, crampy abdominal pain, and diarrhea within 10 to 12 hours of ingestion. Clinical and laboratory findings associated with acute liver injury are often not manifested until 2 days after ingestion.

   Treatment measures include evacuation of duodenal contents by suction to interrupt the enterohepatic circulation of amatoxins. Sodium bicarbonate administration within 2 hours of ingestion may be helpful in elimination of urinary α-amanitin. Hemodialysis or hemoperfusion utilizing a charcoal filter may also be effective in removing amatoxins from the circulation. The overall prognosis of patients with Amanita poisoning is not good, as some patients who recover from the acute insult will go on to have chronic hepatitis and late liver failure.

Viral Hepatitis Induced Acute Liver Failure

Viral hepatitis caused by hepatitis A, B, and E viruses can produce acute liver injuries which generally result in spontaneous resolution; however, a small percentage of these patients may go on to develop acute hepatic failure. Antiviral treatments have not been demonstrated to reduce the occurrence of viral hepatitis-associated acute liver failure. The acute hepatitis associated with hepatitis B has been shown to be associated with a worse prognosis when co-infection with hepatitis D is present. Antiviral therapy may be indicated for patients with hepatitis B-induced acute liver failure when the patient is anticipated to require liver transplantation; the use of antiviral therapy in this setting reduces the risk of hepatitis B recurrences in the transplanted liver.

Metabolic Causes of Acute Liver Failure

Metabolic causes of acute liver failure include acute fatty liver of pregnancy. This is an unusual metabolic process where the metabolic abnormality in the fetus causes maternal liver injuries. These injuries typically occur during the third trimester of pregnancy, with some patients developing rapid progression of jaundice and liver failure. In approximately 50% of cases, this process occurs with preeclampsia. Delivery of the fetus is the treatment of choice for most patients. There have been limited reports suggesting plasma exchange therapy may also be of benefit in these patients.

Patients with Wilson disease may present with acute liver failure caused by copper toxicosis. Frequently, these patients have underlying chronic liver injuries prior to the onset of the acute injuries. The application of MARS has been shown to reverse some of the acute injuries associated with this process.

Vascular Causes of Acute Liver Failure

Acute obstruction of the hepatic veins (Budd-Chiari syndrome) may occur as the result of hypercoagulable states. Once identified, patients may benefit from portal venous decompression procedures, such as transjugular intrahepatic protosystemic shunt (TIPS) of operative portocaval shunts to reduce further liver parenchymal injuries.

Ischemia is a common cause of acute liver injury, and this is typically described as "shock liver." This type of injury is typically associated with a severe and/or prolonged hypotensive episode that causes injuries mostly in the central zone. Treatment is to address the underlying condition causing the global hemodynamic compromise.

Evaluation of Patients With Acute Hepatic Failure

Early recognition of this condition is important in improving prognosis, since early recognition permits the identification of the inciting events, initiation of cause-specific therapies, and early referral to specialty units for specialized support or transplantation. The history is useful to identify and determine possible substance ingestion and timing of ingestion. In addition, history of preexisting liver diseases or risk factors will help determine the chronicity of the liver injury.

During the physical examination, the focus is on liver and spleen sizes, and presence or absence of stigmatas of chronic liver disease. The neurological evaluation should be thorough, with noting of the papillary sizes and reactivity, deep tendon responses, mental status, and cognitive function. The West Haven

Criteria and the Glasgow coma score (GCS) are both helpful for quantification of neurological function. It is important to keep in mind that the neurological status may change as the patient's condition changes; therefore, neurological assessments should be repeated frequently to determine progress.

Laboratory evaluations should be performed to determine possible causes of injury, metabolic panels, coagulation panels, complete blood count, and blood and tissue typing if liver transplantation is anticipated. Imaging studies should be performed to assess liver characteristic and size, spleen size, and patency of hepatic vasculature. Management of acute liver failure patients is often optimized when a multidisciplinary team, including intensivists, transplant surgeons, transplant hepatologists, and nephrologists, is involved in the care of patients with the most severe injuries.

COMPLICATIONS ASSOCIATED WITH ACUTE HEPATIC FAILURE

Cerebral edema leading to intracranial hypertension is one of the most lethal complications associated with acute liver failure. Risk factors associated with this complication include grade III or IV encephalopathy, serum ammonia >150 to 200 μM, rapid progression of encephalopathy, super-infection, requirement for vasopressor support, and requirement for renal replacement therapy. Intracranial hypertension can be identified by CT imaging or intracranial pressure monitoring. Intracranial pressure monitoring is the most reliable way of identifying this complication; however, placement of monitors in these patients can be associated with 10% to 20% risk of bleeding complications. Moderate hypothermia (32°C-33°C) has been shown to be an effective treatment for patients with intracranial hypertension.

Hemodynamic failure is commonly seen in patients with acute liver failure. Typically, it is associated with high cardiac output and low systemic vascular resistance. Because this clinical picture closely resembles the septic response, it is important that all infectious causes are ruled out. Blood pressure support is important in these patients to maintain cerebral perfusion, and vasopressors are often needed.

Hematologic failure with coagulopathy occurs commonly in patients with acute liver failure. Empiric administration of 10 mg of vitamin K intravenously is recommended because subclinical vitamin K deficiency can contribute to coagulopathy. Prophylactic transfusion of blood products to correct coagulopathy has not been shown to improve outcome; however, for bleeding patients or prior to invasive procedures, transfusion to correct the INR to 1.5 and increase the platelet count to >50,000/mm^3 is generally recommended. Cryoprecipitate is recommended for bleeding patients with fibrinogen <100 mg/dL. Recombinant factor VIIa is sometimes helpful when bleeding patients do not respond to fresh frozen plasma (FFP) transfusions.

Acute kidney injury may accompany acute liver failure. Urinary sodium levels are low in patients who are volume depleted and in patients with hepatorenal syndrome. Volume assessment is important in these patients with either intravascular monitoring devices or echocardiography. Renal replacement therapy is often needed as the acute kidney injury progresses. For patients requiring renal replacement therapy, continuous veno-venal hemofiltration with dialysis is often better tolerated than intermittent dialysis.

Infections occur commonly in acute liver failure patients, and it is the most common cause of death in this patient population. It is believed that these patients have impaired Kuppfer cell function and abnormal clearance of gut bacteria and bacterial product, rendering the patients highly susceptible to bacterial and fungal infections. Although some groups believe that broad-spectrum prophylactic antibiotics should be administered in patients with acute liver failure, survival has not been shown to improve with prophylaxis. Clinicians should maintain high vigilance for possible infections in these patients and have low threshold for treatment.

Catabolism and nutritional failure occurs commonly in this patient population. Oral feeding is advisable until patients develop grade 2 to 3 encephalopathies. Caloric targets for patients should be 25 to 30 kcal/kg. Enteral tube feeding or parenteral nutrition should be initiated when oral intake is not feasible. Protein intake should be limited to 1 g/kg/d to minimize excess ammonia production. Supplemental glutamine should be avoided, as it appears to contribute to excess ammonia production and worsening of cerebral edema.

LIVER TRANSPLANTATION

Patients with acute liver failure who do not recover despite appropriate medical and supportive care should be referred as early as possible for consideration for liver transplantation. The King's College Hospital Criteria are the most commonly used criteria for the selection of patients for transplantation referral. The long-term outcome for patients undergoing transplantation for acute hepatic failure is generally not as good as outcome following liver transplantation for chronic liver diseases. The 1-, 3-, and 5-year graft survivals reported are 63%, 58%, and 56%, respectively.

CASE CORRELATION

- See also Case 21 (Acute GI Bleeding), Case 37 (Poisoning), and Case 41 (Hemorrhage and Coagulopathy).

COMPREHENSION QUESTIONS

22.1 Which of the following statements regarding acetaminophen-induced acute liver failure is most accurate?

A. The recovery/survival is <30%.

B. Hepatocytes in the portal zone are most affected.

C. It is the second most common cause of acute liver failure in the United States behind Amanita ingestion.

D. NAC therapy does not provide any benefits when delayed by more than 4 hours after ingestion.

E. Individuals with glutathione depletion have greater susceptibility to toxicity.

22.2 A 32-year-old woman with Amanita-induced acute liver failure has encephalopathy that progresses from grade I to grade III over the course of 6 hours in the ICU. She is intubated in the ICU for airway protection. Which of the following is the most appropriate next step?

    A. Initiate hemodialysis to eliminate amatoxins.

    B. Perform CT of the brain.

    C. Transfer to a liver transplantation center.

    D. Initiate broad-spectrum antibiotics.

    E. Put the patient on vasopressors to increase cerebral perfusion pressure.

22.3 A 28-year-old man develops acute fulminant hepatic failure following inadvertent ingestion of poisonous Amanita. He is currently undergoing treatment for coagulopathy and respiratory failure that is requiring mechanical ventilation. On day two in the ICU, you are notified by his nurse regarding a deterioration of his mental status and alertness level. Which of the following would be more consistent with liver-induced encephalopathy versus brain hemorrhage?

    A. Dilated pupils

    B. Asterixis

    C. Increased peripheral deep tendon reflexes

    D. Right-sided arm weakness

22.4 Which of the following treatment options has NOT been shown to benefit patients with acute hepatic failure due to Amanita poisoning?

    A. Administration of sodium bicarbonate within 2 hours of ingestion

    B. Hemodialysis with charcoal filtration

    C. Enteral nutritional support with formula with high glutamine content

    D. NG tube placement for evacuation of upper GI contents

    E. Liver transplantation

ANSWERS

22.1 E. Glutathione depletion can increase the susceptibility of individuals to acetaminophen toxicity, and this can be seen in fasting patients and patients with chronic alcohol use. Acetaminophen causes predominant injury to hepatocytes in the central zone, while sparing cells in the periportal zones. Based on this distribution, injuries to stem cells occur less frequently, resulting in good potential for recovery. Survival greater than 80% is expected with acetaminophen-induced liver injury. NAC administration has been shown to provide improved liver recovery when given as late as 16 hours after acetaminophen ingestion.

22.2 **B.** For this patient with rapid progression of encephalopathy, intracranial hypertension from increasing cerebral edema is a major concern. A CT of the brain should be obtained immediately to assess the brain. Alternatively, an intracranial pressure monitor can be placed, but this approach carries a bleeding risk of 10% to 20%. This patient ultimately may need to be referred for liver transplantation consideration, but an acute intracranial pressure increase needs to be addressed first.

22.3 **B.** This patient with acute fulminant hepatic failure is showing mental status changes. This is either due to hepatic encephalopathy or mass effect on the brain. A focal neurological sign would more likely indicate a brain lesion, whereas asterixis is more often seen in a metabolic encephalopathy such as liver failure. CT imaging is important to assess for a brain lesion.

22.4 **C.** In general, dietary glutamine intake should be limited in patients with acute liver injury, as its ingestion can increase ammonia production and worsen acute liver failure from all causes. Early evacuation of upper GI tract contents and sodium bicarbonate administration have been shown to help improve outcome of patients with acute liver failure from Amanita ingestion. Similarly, hemodialysis with charcoal filtration has been demonstrated to help eliminate the toxins associated with Amanita ingestion.

CLINICAL PEARLS

▶ Chronic alcohol ingestion stimulates cytochrome CYP2E1 activity, inhibits the rate of glutathione synthesis, and can increase toxicity to acetaminophen.

▶ The 1-, 3-, and 5-year survival following liver transplantation for acute liver failure is 10% to 20% lower than liver transplantation performed for chronic liver diseases.

▶ The MARS and bioartificial liver (BAL) are useful for the support of patients while liver recovery is occurring, and these devices can be used as a bridge to liver transplantation.

REFERENCES

Chun LJ, Tong MJ, Busuttil RW, Hiatt JR. Acetaminophen hepatotoxicity and acute liver failure. *J Clin Gastroenterol.* 2009;43:342-349.

Schilsky ML, Honiden S, Arnott L, Emre S. ICU management of acute liver failure. *Clinics Chest Med.* 2009;30:71-87.

Stravits RT. Critical management decisions in patients with acute liver failure. *Chest.* 2008;134: 1092-1102.

Trotter JF. Practical management of acute liver failure in the intensive care unit. *Curr Opin Crit Care.* 2009;15:163-167.

Wendon J. Acute liver failure. In: Hall JB, Schmidt GA, Kress JP, eds. *Principles of Critical Care.* 4th ed. New York, NY: McGraw Hill Education; 2015;1022-1026.

A 57-year-old woman with a history of type II diabetes mellitus and hypertension was admitted to the ICU 3 days ago for management of urinary tract infection-related sepsis. The patient weighs 63 kg. On the third day in the ICU, the patient's laboratory studies demonstrate an increase in serum creatinine from 1.0 mg/dL to 2.1 mg/dL. Her serum electrolytes are within normal limits. Her total urine output for the most recent 24 hours (day 2) is only 450 mL, which is significantly less than the output from the 24 hours before (day 1), recorded as 1100 mL.

▶ What is the most likely reason for her change in status?
▶ What are appropriate steps to take in the evaluation and management of this patient?

ANSWERS TO CASE 23:

Acute Kidney Injury

Summary: A 57-year-old woman is being managed in the ICU with a new diagnosis of urosepsis. On hospital day three her urine output drops significantly, and her serum creatinine increases by a factor greater than 2.

- **Most likely diagnosis:** Acute kidney injury.

- **Next steps:** Initiate immediate supportive treatment (fluid management, antibiotics directed at source-control, vasopressors, and diuretics) and obtain CBC, serum chemistry, urinalysis, and blood and urine cultures if new infection is suspected. Avoid nephrotoxic agents. Initiate consultation with the renal service for possible renal replacement therapy.

ANALYSIS

Objectives

1. Become familiar with the diagnosis, staging, and treatment of acute kidney injury (AKI).

2. List the causes of acute kidney injury in ICU patients.

3. Understand the indications for emergent renal replacement therapy.

Considerations

The patient's history indicates a known diagnosis of urinary tract related sepsis, which in itself is a potentially life-threatening condition. On her third day of hospitalization, she develops a significant difference in the serum markers of her kidney function, a decrease in urine output, and an abrupt rise in serum creatinine. These markers indicate that her kidney function is compromised, and investigation into the cause and initiation of treatment should begin. The initial decline of kidney function may be reversible with treatment; however, the underlying cause of the kidney dysfunction will need to be addressed so that ultimately the kidneys can regain normal homeostasis. It is likely that with optimal management, the kidneys' functional status may normalize; however, the possibility of further decompensation may occur, leading to the requirement of renal replacement therapy for patient survival. Her initial assessment of causes should include bilateral renal ultrasonography to rule out mechanical obstruction of the urinary tract. In addition, a careful evaluation of the patient's current and recent medications as well as possible septic sources are important to rule out medications or sepsis as potential causes of her acute kidney injury (AKI).

APPROACH TO:
Acute Kidney Injury

DEFINITIONS

OLIGURIA: Below normal level of urine output (less than 0.5 mL/kg/h).

ANURIA: No urine output for ≥ 24 hours, usually associated with poor long-term prognosis.

RENAL REPLACEMENT THERAPY (RRT): Dialysis/hemofiltration, the only FDA approved therapy for AKI.

CHRONIC KIDNEY DISEASE (CKD): An irreversible failure in the homeostasis of the renal filtration system.

SIRS: Systemic inflammatory response syndrome, comprised of abnormal body temperature (higher than 38°C or less than 36°C), heart rate >90 beats/min, respiration >20 breaths/min, or arterial partial pressure of CO_2 <32 mm Hg, and deranged white blood cell counts (greater than $12 \times 10^3/mm^3$, less than $4 \times 10^3/mm^3$, or greater than 10% bands).

SEPSIS: SIRS and an identifiable source of infection (or high level of suspicion of an identifiable source of infection).

SEPTIC SHOCK: Meeting the criteria for sepsis with low blood pressure (SBP <90 mm Hg) which is refractory to fluid resuscitation.

URINE INFECTION-RELATED SEPSIS: Sepsis caused by infection of the urinary tract and/or male genital organs (eg, prostate).

CLINICAL APPROACH

Acute kidney injury (AKI) has now replaced the term acute renal failure. It is now widely agreed that there is a spectrum of the disease extending from less severe forms of injury to that of more advanced injury. The significance of this disease is great, with up to 200,000 people each year in the United States affected, a hospital acquired prevalence of 7.1%, and reported occurrence in up to two-thirds of ICU patients. There is strong evidence that sepsis and septic shock are the most important causes of AKI in critically ill patients, accounting for 50% or more of cases of AKI in ICU patients. It is now recognized that AKI is an independent risk factor for mortality, with experimental models suggesting that AKI is associated with an upregulation of systemic inflammatory mediator release.

AKI is a clinical diagnosis characterized by rapid reduction in function resulting in an inability to maintain electrolyte, fluid and acid–base homeostasis. The mainstay for diagnosing AKI has been the measurement of urine output over a given time period, as well as a rise in specific biological markers of kidney function,

Table 23–1 • RISK, INJURY, FAILURE, LOSS, AND END-STAGE KIDNEY CLASSIFICATION (RIFLE)		
Stage/Criteria	Serum Creatinine (SCr) criteria	Urine Output Criteria
1 (**Risk**)	SCr × 1.5 from reference SCr	<0.5 mL/kg/h for >6 h
2 (**Injury**)	SCr × 2 from reference SCr	<0.5 mL/kg/h for >12 h
3 (**Failure**)	SCr × 3 from reference SCr or SCr >4 mg/dL with acute rise >0.5 mg/dL	<0.3 mL/kg/h for >24 h or anuria × 12 h
4 (**Loss**)	Complete loss of renal function for >4 weeks	
5 (**End-stage**)	End-stage kidney disease >3 months	

with the most common measurement being serum creatinine (SCr). Specifically, AKI is defined **when one of the following criteria is met:**

- SCr rises by ≥26 μmol/L within 48 h **or**

- SCr acutely rises ≥1.5-fold from the reference value (NOTE: reference SCr should be the lowest creatinine value recorded within 3 months of the event) **or**

- Urine output is <0.5 mL/kg/h for more than six consecutive hours

Staging (quantification of severity) of AKI is useful at the bedside, as AKI is considered a spectrum of severity, and the recognition of disease severity is helpful in the selection of treatments (Table 23–1).

Urine output and SCr are at present the best biomarkers for AKI. However, they are not the ideal biomarkers of AKI, as the injury to the kidney has already occurred before these values become abnormal; therefore, reliance on these markers is associated with some delays in disease recognition. This knowledge has led to the search for biomarkers that could potentially result in early diagnosis of kidney insult and earlier initiation of treatment. At present, several novel biomarkers are being investigated, and these include neutrophil gelatinase-associated lipocalin (NGAL), kidney injury molecule-1 (KIM-1), interleukin-18 (IL-18), and cystatin C. These biomarkers show early promise as tools for the early detection of AKI.

MANAGEMENT

The first step in management is to become familiar with the recognition of patients most at-risk for the development of AKI, and these include patients with age >75 years, patients with history of chronic kidney disease (CKD, eGFR <60 mL/min/1.73 m²), cardiac failure, peripheral vascular disease, or diabetes mellitus, and patients taking nephrotoxic medications. Acute medical conditions that increase the risk of AKI include reduced fluid intake or increased fluid losses (dehydration), urinary tract obstruction and/or urinary infections, sepsis, myoglobinuria, and recent drug ingestion.

A patient's urinalysis can provide useful information in determining the cause of AKI. Significant proteinuria (+3 or +4) suggests intrinsic glomerular disease. Hematuria in association with proteinuria may indicate a diagnosis of glomerular disease. Hematuria may also indicate the presence of a tumor in the lower urinary tract. Myoglobinuria produces a positive reagent strip reaction (dipstick) without traces of RBC in the urine. The presence of >5 WBC per high power field in a patient with AKI suggests the presence of infections, acute interstitial nephritis, or glomerulonephritis. Urine microscopy can also provide useful information regarding AKI causes. Urinary crystals are identified in patients with glycol poisoning or tumor lysis syndrome, and they are associated with drug exposures (sulfonamides, acyclovir, and triamterene). Other diagnostic tests for patients with AKI include urine osmolality, urine/plasma creatinine and urea ratios, urinary sodium, fractional excretion of sodium (FE_{Na}), fractional excretion of urea, free water clearance, and creatinine clearance. Calculation of FE_{Na} is commonly applied for differentiation between prerenal azotemia and AKI when patients exhibit low urine output. Patients who are prerenal have increased urinary sodium reabsorption and increased urinary urea reabsorption; therefore, they would exhibit low (<1%) FE_{Na} and FE_{Urea}. However, patients with AKI generally have dysfunction in renal sodium excretion and elevated fractional excretion of sodium ($FE_{Na} > 1\%$). It is important to recognize that there are limitations to an AKI diagnosis based on FE_{Na} measurements; for instance, the FE_{Na} can be falsely low in patients with AKI and co-existing cirrhosis, heart failure, or severe sepsis. Conversely, the FE_{Na} can be falsely elevated in patients with preexisting chronic kidney disease, on diuretic therapy, or with glucosuria.

Ultrasound is the most useful imaging modality to assess for the possibility of upper urinary tract obstruction. It is important to recognize that hydronephrosis may not be present in patients with urinary tract obstruction and hypovolemia; therefore, patients suspected of obstructive uropathy should undergo a repeat study after repletion of intravascular volumes.

Acute kidney injury can be a potentially reversible disorder if treated in a timely and appropriate manner. Early recognition is important and may improve the chances for full recovery of kidney functions. A patient's supportive measures must be optimized to include appropriate fluid therapy, administration of vasopressor and/or inotropic medications as indicated, and treatment of the underlying illness, particularly sepsis. Accurate measurements of all intake, including oral, intravenous rates and boluses, as well as all output (urine, emesis, etc.) must be accurately recorded to give the clinician the most complete and accurate assessment of the patient's volume status. This may require the use of an indwelling urine catheter for precise urine output measurement. All medications administered should be interrogated for potential nephrotoxic effects and stopped accordingly. Avoidance of intravenous radiographic contrast will help avoid further injury to the kidneys.

Generally accepted indications for renal replacement therapy (RRT) include profound **acidemia, electrolyte imbalances (eg, hyperkalemia), ingestion or idiopathic overload of toxins/metabolites, symptomatic fluid overload**, and **symptomatic uremia** (eg, increased bleeding from platelet dysfunction, pericardial tamponade, and severe mental status change). Ideally, RRT is to be initiated once the diagnosis of AKI is certain and unavoidable, but prior to terminal organ complications.

Venous access for RRT requires planning that takes into consideration the level of irreversible kidney damage and the anticipated duration of therapy. When short-term (temporary) dialysis is anticipated, veno-venous access is the preferred route. Veno-venous access is established with ultrasound-guided placement of a double lumen catheter into a large central vein (preferably internal jugular or femoral veins). This access may be used for weeks until the patient's physiologic homeostasis recovery occurs or if prolonged RRT is required. For patients in whom long-term dialysis is anticipated, planning should be initiated for the placement of arterio-venous access. In comparison to intermittent dialysis, continuous renal replacement therapy may have the advantage of achieving better control of uremia, preventing hypotension during dialysis, and improving clearance of inflammatory mediators; however, there is no convincing evidence to indicate that continuous RRT provides additional advantages over intermittent RRT. Similarly, clinical evidence does not support the use of high-dose RRT over standard-dose RRT.

All patients who survive AKI but whose kidney function does not return to normal will need planning for CKD management, including but not limited to long-term RRT access. A center for RRT will need to accept the patient and subsequently the practice of a renal physician. Kidney transplantation is the definitive treatment for those with failed kidneys.

LONG-TERM PROGNOSIS

Despite advances in the supportive care of patients with AKI in the ICU, prognostication of renal recovery continues to be a difficult challenge. Several urinary biomarkers are being investigated for their prognostication value for AKI recovery. These include urinary neutrophil gelatinase-associated lipocalin (uN-GAL), urinary hepatocyte growth factor (uHGF), urinary cystatin C (uCystatin C), and IL-18. Recent clinical studies suggest that patterns of change in these urinary markers may be valuable in predicting recovery in AKI patients.

CASE CORRELATION

- See also Case 19 (Sepsis) and Case 33 (Multi-organ Dysfunction).

COMPREHENSION QUESTIONS

23.1 A 58-year-old man with diabetes mellitus presents to the hospital with left lower quadrant pain for 2 days. He has had nausea and vomiting with subjective fevers and anorexia. His vital signs are temperature of 100.4°F, pulse of 112 beats/min, BP of 100/68 mm Hg, respiratory rate of 20 breaths/min, and 99% oxygen saturation on room air. His eyes are sunken, and his abdomen is tender in the left lower quadrant. Laboratory studies are significant for WBC of 15,000 cells/mm^3 and SCr of 1.68 mg/dL (reference value is 0.95). What is the initial best treatment to prevent further kidney injury?

A. Obtain immediate blood and urine cultures and then start empiric antibiotics.

B. Admit to hospital and keep NPO.

C. Obtain CT scan to rule out intraabdominal abscess.

D. Insert two large-bore IV's and then bolus with 1 to 2 L crystalloid.

E. Insert foley catheter to measure urine output.

23.2 A 24-year-old man weighing 80 kg is admitted to the intensive care unit following an exploratory laparotomy after a gunshot wound (GSW) to his lower right hemithorax and abdomen. Intraoperative exploration showed a 1 cm laceration on the dome of the liver, right diaphragmatic injury, and transverse colon injury requiring partial colectomy with primary anastomosis. He was also found to have a laceration of the left kidney. During the night, his urine output is measured at 60 mL/h for the first 3 hours, 50 mL/h for the fourth hour, and 20 mL/h for the fifth and sixth hours, and the urine appears dark. His heart rate and blood pressure have not changed. What is the next step in his management?

A. Place a central venous catheter for CVP monitoring.

B. Bring the patient back into the operating room for re-exploration.

C. Obtain CT imaging of the abdomen and pelvis.

D. Transfuse packed red blood cells.

23.3 You are managing patients in the intensive care unit, and you are concerned that one of your patients with sepsis due to a lung infection has developed fluid overload secondary to stage 3 AKI and may not recover her normal kidney function. What is the best plan for instituting appropriate care for this patient?

A. Obtain urinary electrolyte measurement.

B. Obtain measurement of the patient's platelet count.

C. Insert a veno-venous access catheter for RRT.

D. Refer patient for renal transplantation consideration.

E. Increase the dose of her loop diuretic medication.

23.4 A 43-year-old man with AKI had a veno-venous catheter placed for urgent RRT. He is now in his hospital bed, and his wound bandages are saturated with blood. You notice that he is also bleeding from his peripheral IV sites. What is the definitive treatment?

A. Transfusion of red blood cells

B. Transfusion of platelets

C. Initiate RRT

D. Administer DDAVP

E. Give intravenous calcium

ANSWERS

23.1 **D.** This patient is presenting with signs and symptoms concerning for the diagnosis of acute diverticulitis and septic shock. His presenting SCr of 1.68 is >1.5 that of his baseline and thus meets the criteria of AKI. This patient has intravascular volume depletion from his illness. Fluid resuscitation is the first step in early goal-directed therapy of sepsis and will subsequently yield benefit to the hypoperfusion state of his kidneys. Oxygen therapy should be given along with fluid resuscitation, followed with blood cultures and the appropriate antibiotic initiated for his presumed intraabdominal sepsis. Imaging may be helpful to guide therapy, but only after the patient is hemodynamically stable. A Foley catheter should be placed to determine fluid volume status and guide the clinician on management of fluid therapy.

23.2 **A.** This patient does not meet the definitions of AKI but is in danger of its development. One criterion for AKI is UOP <0.5 mL/kg/h for greater than 6 hours. This patient would be of concern for AKI if his UOP is <40 mL/h, which he has had for the last 2 hours. Given his injuries and recent operation, his low urine output is likely secondary to intravascular volume depletion. The next step in management would therefore be to confirm this diagnosis and then to replete his volume as necessary.

23.3 **C.** Studies have demonstrated that for acute RRT, veno-venous access is the modality of choice, especially given that this patient is fluid overloaded at this time. Urinary electrolytes are not helpful at this time to further define the patient's kidney function. Referral for renal transplantation is premature, as the patient's renal functions may eventually recover from her stage 3 AKI. Increasing the dose of her loop diuretics is an option; however, given the patient's fluid status and ongoing pulmonary problem, dialysis may be the more effective strategy for this patient at this time.

23.4 **C.** This patient has platelet dysfunction due to uremia from kidney failure. The definitive treatment is RRT. Administering blood products will not achieve the desired hemostasis that is required. Calcium is often needed as a replacement for patients receiving red blood cell transfusions, as calcium is sequestered by the high amounts of citrate in the fluid. DDAVP, also known as vasopressin arginine, can improve the binding of platelets in clot formation. It can be used as a temporizing first-line treatment for uremic bleeding if there is a delay before the patient can receive RRT.

CLINICAL PEARLS

▶ Urine output and serum creatinine are the best biomarkers for acute kidney injury.

▶ AKI is potentially reversible with the appropriate measures if performed early; however, some patients may evolve to have CKD.

▶ Renal replacement therapy (RRT) may be needed for both short- and long-term therapy with kidney injury.

REFERENCES

Chuasuwan A, Kellum JA. Acute kidney injury and its management. *Contrib Nephrol*. 2011;171: 218-225.

Hannon C, Murray PT. Acute kidney injury. In: Hall JB, Schmidt GA, Kress JP, eds. *Principles of Critical Care*. 4th ed. New York, NY: McGraw Hill Education; 2015:916-932.

Liu KD, Brakeman PR. Renal repair and recovery. *Crit Care Med*. 2008;36(4 Suppl):S187-S192.

Srisawat N, Wen X, Lee M, et al. Urinary biomarkers predict renal recovery in critically ill patients with renal support. *Clin J Am Soc Nephrol*. 2011;6:doi: 10.2215/CJN.11261210.

Waxman K. Acute kidney failure. In: Cameron JL, Cameron AM, eds. *Current Surgical Therapy*. 11th ed. Philadelphia, PA: Elsevier Saunders; 2014:1242-1247.

An 18-year-old diabetic man was brought into the ICU with a 3-day history of nausea, vomiting, and vague abdominal pain. Because of recent gastroenteritis, he had stopped both oral intake and insulin intake. On physical examination, the patient was noted to have dry mucous membranes and deep, shallow breathing with fruity breath. His blood pressure (BP) when supine was 120/60 mm Hg and pulse rate was 95 beats/min compared to a BP of 80/50 mm Hg and pulse of 120 beats/min when seated. Laboratory results are as follows:

Serum Laboratory Studies (Normal range)	
Sodium (Na^+)	130 mEq/L (136-144 mEq/L)
Potassium (K^+)	5.2 mEq/L (3.7-5.2 mEq/L)
Chloride (Cl^-)	90 mEq/L (101-111 mEq/L)
Bicarbonate (HCO_3^-)	10 mEq/L (22-26 mEq/L)
Blood Glucose	450 mg/dL (100 mg/dL)
Arterial Blood Gas Studies	
pH	7.20 (7.35-7.45)
$Paco_2$	22 mm Hg (35-45 mm Hg)
PaO_2 (on room air)	98 mm Hg (75-100 mm Hg)

▶ What is the most likely diagnosis?
▶ What is the major acid–base abnormality?
▶ What preexisting acid–base abnormality did the patient have?
▶ What is the best initial therapy for this disorder?

ANSWERS TO CASE 24:
Acid–Base Disorder

Summary: An 18-year-old man was admitted to the ICU with an anion gap metabolic acidosis.

- **Most Likely Diagnosis:** Positive gap metabolic acidosis (likely due to diabetic ketoacidosis) with respiratory compensation, and with a preexisting nongap metabolic acidosis.

- **Patient's Major Acid–Base disorder:** Metabolic acidosis with a positive anion gap with an appropriate respiratory compensation.

- **Pre-existing acid–base disorder:** Pre-existing non–anion-gap metabolic acidosis.

- **Initial Therapy:** First, correct dehydration with normal saline (0.9%). Then, once the patient is hydrated, correct hyperglycemia with IV infusion of normal insulin.

ANALYSIS

Objectives

1. Describe normal pH, and be able to characterize abnormal acid–base conditions as acidosis or alkalosis, or a combined process.

2. Be able to discern respiratory versus metabolic acid–base disorders, and whether there is appropriate compensation.

3. Describe the diagnosis and treatment of diabetic ketoacidosis (DKA).

Considerations

The patient has DKA most likely precipitated by his gastroenteritis and stoppage of food and insulin. In most cases, DKA occurs in young patients with Type 1 diabetes mellitus, but DKA may occur in older patients with Type 2 diabetes mellitus as well. It is commonly precipitated by stressors such as infection, inadequate insulin therapy and alcohol abuse. The physical findings of increased urinary frequency, excessive thirst, and deep shallow breathing (Kussmaul breathing) in response to the metabolic acidosis are very suggestive of DKA. A finger stick glucose can establish the diagnosis in seconds and should be done immediately. Additional tests should be ordered to confirm diagnosis. These tests include a full chemistry panel with electrolytes, a complete blood count (CBC), and an arterial blood gas (ABG).

APPROACH TO:

Acid–Base Disorders (Part I)

DEFINITIONS

ACIDEMIA: Condition leading to excessive hydrogen cations, pH <7.35 (7.35)

ALKALEMIA: Condition leading to insufficient hydrogen cations or excessive base, pH >7.50.

ANION GAP: Calculation to characterize metabolic acidosis. Anion Gap = $Na - (Cl + HCO_3)$, with normal being 12 +/− 2 mEq/L, assuming a normal albumin level of 4 g/L.

CLINICAL APPROACH

An easy method to determining acid–base alterations is by using a stepwise approach outline in the following order:

1. Is the pH normal, alkalemic or acidemic?

2. Is the $Paco_2$ normal, alkalemic or acidemic?

3. Is the HCO_3 normal, alkalemic or acidemic?

4. Is the primary acid–base disorder properly compensated? Yes or No? Refer to expected compensation for each acid–base disorder in Table 24–1.
   If the measured pH is higher than the expected compensation range, then another process producing alkalosis is present; however, if the calculated pH is below the measured pH, there is likely an additional acidosis condition present.

5. If a metabolic acidosis exists, what is the anion-gap, the calculated initial HCO_3, and osmolality, if given? (Refer to acid–base formulas in Table 24–1.)

Application of Principles to Patient in Case Scenario

1. Is the pH normal, alkalemic or acidemic? **Ans:** Acidemic; pH is 7.20 (7.35-7.45)

2. Is the $Paco_2$ normal, alkalotic or acidotic? **Ans:** Alkalotic; $Paco_2$ is 22 mm Hg (35-45 mm Hg)

3. Is the HCO_3 normal, alkalotic or acidotic? **Ans:** Acidotic; HCO_3 is 10 mEq/L (22-26 mEq/L)

4. Is the acid–base disorder properly compensated? **Ans:** Yes. In metabolic acidosis, use Winter's formula to predict the expected $Paco_2$, $(HCO_3 \times 1.5) + 8 = Paco_2$ (±2) or in this case, $(10 \times 1.5) + 8 = 23(\pm2)$ $Paco_2$. Since our patient's value = 22, this is an appropriate response.

5. If a metabolic acidosis exists, what is the anion gap? **Ans:** Abnormally elevated at 20 mEq/L. The anion gap calculated by the formula: $Na - (HCO_3 + Cl)$ is

Table 24–1 • ACID–BASE TERMINOLOGY, FORMULAS, AND DISORDERS	
Alkalemia: pH >7.45	**Acidemia:** pH <7.35
Hypocapnia: $Paco_2$ <35 mm Hg Respiratory Alkalosis Acute or Chronic	**Hypercapnia:** $Paco_2$ >45 mm Hg Respiratory Acidosis Acute or Chronic
Elevated Bicarbonate: HCO_3 >26 mEq/L Metabolic Alkalosis	**Decreased Bicarbonate:** HCO_3 <22 mEq/L Metabolic Acidosis
Metabolic Acidosis: A primary physiologic process that causes a decrease in the serum HCO_3, and when not complicated by other acid–base disorders, lowers the pH.	
Metabolic Alkalosis: A primary physiologic process that causes an increase in the serum HCO_3, and when not complicated by other acid–base disorders, raises the pH.	
Respiratory Acidosis: A primary physiologic process that leads to an increased $Paco_2$, and when not complicated by other acid–base disorders, lowers the pH.	
Respiratory Alkalosis: A primary physiologic process that leads to a decreased $Paco_2$, and when not complicated by other acid–base disorders, raises the pH.	
Compensatory Process: The normal expected physiological change that follows a primary acid–base disorder that attempts to restore the pH towards normal expected ranges. If the expected compensatory response is absent, consider another acidosis or alkalosis process.	
Primary Acid–Base Disorder and Normal Compensation Response	
Metabolic Acidosis	Hyperventilation = Reduce $Paco_2$ (winter's formula) $(HCO_3 \times 1.5) + 8 = Paco_2$ (±2)
Metabolic Alkalosis	Hypoventilation – Increase $Paco_2$ $(HCO_3 \times 0.9) + 15 = Paco_2$ (±2)
Respiratory Acidosis *Acute*: $Paco_2\Delta10$ from 40 → $pH\Delta0.08$ (±0.02) *Chronic*: $Paco_2\Delta10$ from 40 → $HCO_3\Delta 0.03$ (±0.02)	**Causes:** Renal HCO_3 Retention *Acute*: $Paco_2\Delta10$ from 40 → $HCO_3\Delta1$ *Chronic*: $Paco_2\Delta10$ from 40 → $HCO_3\Delta3$
Respiratory Alkalosis *Acute*: $Paco_2\Delta10$ from 40 → $pH\Delta0.08$ (±0.02) *Chronic*: $Paco_2\Delta 10$ from 40 → $pH\Delta0.03$ (±0.02)	**Causes:** Renal HCO_3 Elimination *Acute*: $Paco_2\Delta10$ from 40 → $HCO_3\Delta2$ *Chronic*: $Paco_2\Delta10$ from 40 → $HCO_3\Delta5$
Acid–Base Formulas	
Normal Anion Gap (with 4 g of Albumin)	$(Na^+) - (Cl^- + HCO_3^-) = 12$ (±2)
Calculated Initial HCO_3	(Measured HCO_3^-) + (Measured Anion Gap – 12) = 22-26 (normal)
Calculated Osmolarity	$(Na^+ \times 2) + (Glucose \div 18) + (BUN \div 2.8)$
Osmolal Gap	Measured Osmolality – Calculated Osmolality = >10 gap

Kasper DL, et al. *Harrison's Principles of Internal Medicine*. 18th ed. New York: McGraw-Hill Education, 2012. Table 40–1.

elevated at 20 mEq/L in this case: $(130^+) - (90^- + 10^-) = 20$. This is higher than the normal threshold of 14 mEq/L and indicates a positive anion gap.

6. If an anion gap exists, calculate the corrected initial HCO_3 to determine if there is a pre-existing acid–base condition? **Ans:** Yes, nongap metabolic acidosis. (Measured HCO_3^-) + (Measured Anion Gap – 12) = normally 22-26, thus 10 + (20 – 12) = 18. This starting HCO_3 of 18 mEq/L is below normal and indicates that the patient started with a (preexisiting) nongap metabolic acidosis.

extreme Acidosis & pH < 7.2 (<6.95 in DKA)
= indic. for giving HCO₃⁻

Diabetic Ketoacidosis

DKA is a life-threatening complication of diabetes leading to hyperglycemia, volume depletion, production of ketones (organic acids), metabolic acidosis, and electrolyte derangements.

In order to diagnose DKA, the following three criteria must be met:

1. Blood glucose levels >250 mg/dL

2. pH <7.30 or low serum bicarbonate (HCO_3 <15-20 mmol/L)

3. Detection of plasma ketones

The main management for DKA primarily involves restoring intravascular volume with normal saline (0.9%), correcting the hyperglycemia with regular IV insulin, correcting any other electrolyte imbalance, and treating the underlying precipitating factors.

In DKA, the underlying cause of acidosis is principally due to the formation of both of aceto-acetic acid and β-hydroxybutyric acid, both of which are ketones produced by the liver. The formations of these ketones are mainly driven by an upregulation of glucagon activity compared to insulin activity. The presence of these ketoacids decreases the serum bicarbonate concentration and increases the anion gap. Treatment of anion gap metabolic acidosis requires reversing the underlying condition that led to excess acid production. Treatment with bicarbonate is unnecessary, except in extreme cases of acidosis when the pH is less than 7.20 and less than 6.95 in DKA, a level at which dysrhythmia becomes likely and cardiac contractility and responsiveness to catecholamines and medications are impaired.

Metabolic Acidosis

When the primary disturbance is a metabolic acidosis, the anion gap helps narrow the diagnostic possibilities to an anion-gap acidosis or a non–anion-gap acidosis. Healthy individuals have an anion gap of 12 ± 2 mEq/L. The normal anion gap of 12 is represented by the negative charge of the normal 4 g albumin (−3 anions per gram of albumin). The compensatory response to a primary disturbance is predictable and tries to bring the pH back towards normal.

The process for diagnosing a coexisting metabolic disturbance involves calculating the "corrected or initial HCO_3." If the corrected HCO_3 is <24 ±5 mEq/L, a coexisting preexisting non–anion-gap metabolic acidosis is present. If the corrected HCO_3 is >24 ±5 mEq/L, a coexisting preexisting metabolic alkalosis is present. This formula is based upon the assumption that the measured anion gap represents in part the HCO_3 that was consumed compensating for the acidosis. If the anion gap is added to the measured HCO_3 concentration and the "normal" anion gap of 12 is subtracted, the result represents the HCO_3 concentration if the anion gap acidosis were not present. This formula gives the same information as the delta gap/delta HCO_3.

Anion-Gap Metabolic Acidosis

Anion-gap metabolic acidosis exists when acids associated with an unmeasured anion (such as lactate) are produced or gained from an exogenous source.

Table 24–2 • CAUSES OF HIGH ANION-GAP ACIDOSIS
Lactic acidosis
Ketoacidosis (diabetes, alcohol, starvation)
Toxins (ethylene glycol, salicylates, methanol, propylene glycol)
Renal failure

Common causes of high anion-gap metabolic acidosis include lactic acidosis, keto-acidosis (ie, ethanol, starvation, and diabetes), uremia, methanol, ethylene glycol and ASA poisoning. A decrease in bicarbonate concentration and resultant anion-gap metabolic acidosis occurs when lactic acid accumulates, as seen in states of tissue hypoperfusion. Drug-induced mitochondrial dysfunction, associated with nucleo-side therapy in the treatment of AIDS, can lead to lactic acidosis in the absence of obvious tissue hypoxia (called Type-2 lactic acidosis). Tonic-clonic seizures, which are associated with an increased metabolic rate, result in a lactic acidosis that quickly reverses; thus, administration of HCO_3 is not needed.

Ethylene glycol poisoning causes an anion-gap acidosis and acute renal failure. Clues to ethylene glycol poisoning include an osmolar gap (>10 difference between measured and calculated osmolality) and the presence of urinary calcium oxalate crystals, which are the cause of the renal failure. Methanol poisoning also causes an anion-gap acidosis with a positive osmolar gap, and optic nerve damage secondary to formic acid toxicity. Isopropyl alcohol (rubbing alcohol) poisoning causes an osmolar gap but without a metabolic acidosis (Table 24–2).

Non–Anion-Gap Metabolic Acidosis

Non–anion-gap metabolic acidosis is also called hyperchloremic metabolic acido-sis. This develops because fluids containing sodium bicarbonate are lost or hydro-gen chloride (or potential hydrogen chloride) is added to the extracellular fluid. The ensuing hyperchloremic metabolic acidosis will not change the anion gap because the reduction in the bicarbonate concentration is offset by the increase in chlo-ride. The most common cause of non–anion-gap metabolic acidosis is diarrhea. Diarrhea leads to loss of bicarbonate because the intestinal fluid beyond the liga-ment of Treitz is relatively alkaline. All types of renal tubular acidosis (RTA) cause a hyperchloremic non–anion-gap metabolic acidosis. **Proximal RTA (type 2)** is caused by a reduced capacity of the kidney to reabsorb bicarbonate. In **Distal RTA (type 1)**, the renal tubules cannot generate a normal pH gradient (nor-mal urinary pH <5.5) due to an inability to excrete hydrogen ions. **RTA type 4**, commonly associated with diabetes, is a hyperkalemic hyperchloremic metabolic acidosis that is due to hypoaldosteronism or an inadequate renal tubular response to aldosterone. This leads to a reduction in the urinary excretion of potassium, resulting in hyperkalemia, which interferes with the renal production of NH_4^+. The inhibition of renal hydrogen ion excretion caused by aldosterone deficiency leads to a non–anion-gap metabolic acidosis. Bicarbonate therapy is generally indi-cated in a non–anion-gap metabolic acidosis, whereas correction of the underlying cause is the primary concern in anion-gap acidosis. Oral bicarbonate (ie, oral citrate solution) is the preferred agent for chronic therapy of non–anion-gap metabolic acidosis. The preferred bicarbonate salt for treating hypokalemic RTA is potassium bicarbonate or potassium citrate.

Example 1: A 47-year-old man with a 3-day history of severe diarrhea is evaluated because of muscle weakness and dizziness. Laboratory studies show sodium 140 mEq/L, potassium 3.2 mEq/L, chloride 120 mEq/L and bicarbonate 14 mEq/L. Arterial blood gas studies on room air show a pH of 7.27, $Paco_2$ of 27 mm Hg and a PaO_2 of 77 mm Hg.

What is the acid–base derangement?

1. Is the pH normal, alkalemic or acidemic? **Acidemic** (pH = 7.27)

2. Is the $Paco_2$ normal, alkalotic or acidotic? **ALKALOTIC** ($Paco_2$ = 27 mm Hg)

3. Is the HCO_3 normal, alkalotic or acidotic? **Acidotic** (HCO_3 = 14 mEq/L)

4. Is the acid–base disorder properly compensated? **Yes.** Using Winter's formula, the predicted $Paco_2$ for HCO_3 of 14 is 29 ± 2 ($Paco_2$ =14 × 1.5 + 8). The $Paco_2$ (27 mm Hg) falls within the calculated compensated $Paco_2$ range of 27 to 31, indicating proper respiratory compensation.

5. If a metabolic acidosis exists, what is the anion gap and corrected bicarbonate? Anion gap = 140 − (120 + 14) = 6 (normal anion gap). Normal anion gap acidosis points toward RTA type 1, 2 or 4, with RTA type 4 having a markedly elevated high potassium level.

Answer: This patient has a non–anion-gap metabolic acidosis with proper respiratory compensation secondary to the loss of HCO_3 in diarrhea with reabsorption of chloride, thus a nongap acidosis.

Example 2: A 36-year-old woman is evaluated because of generalized weakness. Serum laboratories studies show a BUN of 40 mg/dL, Cr of 1.9 mg/dL, Na^+ of 130 mEq/L, K^+ of 3.0 mEq/L, Cl^- of 85 mEq/L and HCO_3 of 36 mEq/L. Arterial blood gas on room air shows a pH of 7.58, a $Paco_2$ of 42 mm Hg and a PaO_2 of 90 mm Hg. Urinary electrolytes show Na^+ 50 mEq/L, a K^+ of 30 mEq/L and a Cl^- of 10 mEq/L.

What is the acid–base abnormality?

1. Is the pH normal, alkalemic, or acidemic? **Alkalemic** (pH = 7.58)

2. Is the $Paco_2$ normal, alkalotic or acidotic? **Acidotic** (Pco_2 = 42 mm Hg)

3. Is the HCO_3 normal, alkalotic or acidotic? **Alkalotic** (HCO_3 = 36 mEq/L)

4. Is the acid–base disorder properly compensated? **No.** The predicted $Paco_2$ for this metabolic alkalosis should fall in the range of 45 to 49 ([36 × 0.9] + 15 = 47 ± 2). However, the actual $Paco_2$ is 42 and below the predicted range; thus, there is an accompanying respiratory alkalosis, even though the pOC_2 is 42.

5. If a metabolic acidosis exists, what is the anion gap and corrected bicarbonate? There is no metabolic acidosis, hence no need to calculate the anion gap or corrected bicarbonate.

Answer: Combined metabolic and respiratory alkalosis.

Metabolic Alkalosis

A primary increase in HCO_3 concentration can result from a loss of hydrogen chloride or less commonly, the addition of bicarbonate. This metabolic alkalosis is corrected through urinary excretion of excess bicarbonate. Increased reabsorption of bicarbonate in the renal tubule is caused by a contraction of extracellular fluid (ECF), chloride depletion, hypokalemia, or elevated mineralocorticoid activity. The most common causes of metabolic alkalosis are vomiting, nasogastric suction, and diuretic therapy. A patient with a low urine chloride level (kidneys appropriately resorbing chloride) is considered chloride responsive; in these individuals, the administration of sodium chloride reverses the alkalosis by expanding the intravascular volume and reducing the activity of the renin-angiotensin-aldosterone axis. The very low urinary chloride concentration in Example 2 suggests vomiting or remote diuretic ingestion that is correctable by sodium chloride secondary to volume expansion.

Patients with metabolic alkalosis who do not have volume depletion and a high urinary chloride level (>20 mEq/L) likely have an elevated mineralocorticoid effect on the kidney. Consequently, these disorders are also called chloride unresponsive or chloride-resistant metabolic alkalosis since repletion of vascular volume with NaCl will not help. H_2 blockers and proton pump inhibitors (PPI) may help to decrease losses of hydrogen ions in patients with prolonged gastric suction or chronic vomiting. Potassium chloride is almost always indicated for the treatment of hypokalemia. In very severe metabolic alkalosis (pH >7.6), hemodialysis is the preferred treatment. Infusion of acidic solutions is rarely indicated.

CLINICAL CASE CORRELATION

- See also Case 25 (Acid–Base Abnormalities II) and Case 37 (Poisoning).

COMPREHENSION QUESTIONS

24.1 A 60-year-old woman is admitted to the ICU for severe *Clostridium difficile* colitis. The patient has had nonstop watery diarrhea and severe dehydration. She denies any blood in her stools. Physical examination is positive for hyperactive bowel sounds. Following laboratory workup, she was noted to have the following serum chemistry: Na^+ 138 mEq/L, K^+ of 4.3 mEq/L, Cl^- of 114 mEq/L and HCO_3^- of 16 mEq/L and albumin of 4 g. Arterial blood gas shows the following pH of 7.31 and $Paco_2$ of 32 mm Hg and a PaO_2 of 87 mm Hg. What is the acid–base disorder in this patient?

A. Normal anion-gap metabolic acidosis with proper respiratory compensation

B. Chronic respiratory acidosis with metabolic alkalosis

C. Acute respiratory acidosis, uncompensated

D. Acute respiratory acidosis, compensated

24.2 A 14-year-old adolescent was admitted to the emergency department following ingestion of an unknown substance. The adolescent was slightly confused and complained of abdominal pain. On physical examination, temperature was $37°C$ ($98°F$), blood pressure 102/60 mm Hg, pulse 102 beats/min, and respiratory rate 20 breaths/min. Serum laboratory studies show Na^+ 140 mEq/L, K^+ 3.7 mEq/L, Cl^- 110 mEq/L, HCO_3^- 14 mEq/L, BUN 30 mEq/L, creatinine 2.1 mEq/L, glucose 212 mg/dL and serum osmolality 320 mEq/L. His friends state that they were experimenting by drinking different concentrations of anti-freeze. Arterial blood gas shows a pH of 7.20, $Paco_2$ of 30 mm Hg, and PaO_2 of 77 on 40% FIO_2. Which of the following acid–base conditions is most likely present?

A. Anion-gap metabolic acidosis

B. Anion-gap metabolic acidosis with hyperosmolar state, with compensation

C. Mixed anion-gap metabolic acidosis and respiratory alkalosis

D. Mixed non–anion-gap metabolic acidosis and respiratory acidosis

E. Mixed non–anion-gap metabolic acidosis and respiratory alkalosis

ANSWERS

24.1 **A.** This patient has normal anion-gap metabolic acidosis with proper respiratory compensation.

1. Is the pH normal, alkalemic, or acidemic? **Acidemic** (pH = 7.31)

2. Is the $Paco_2$ normal, Alkalotic or acidotic? **Alkalotic** ($Paco_2$ = 32 mm Hg)

3. Is the HCO_3 normal, alkalotic or acidotic? **Acidotic** (HCO_3 = 16 mEq/L)

4. Is the acid–base disorder properly compensated? **Yes.** Using Winter's formula, the predicted $Paco_2$ for HCO_3 of 16 is 32 ± 2. [(16 × 1.5 + 8 ±20) = 8]. The $Paco_2$ (32 mm Hg) falls within the calculated compensated $Paco_2$ range of 30 to 34, indicating proper respiratory compensation.

5. If a metabolic acidosis exists, what is the anion gap and the corrected bicarbonate? Anion gap = 138 – (114 + 16) = 8 (normal anion gap). Since the anion gap is within normal range, no need to calculate the corrected bicarbonate.

   The patient is complaining of watery diarrhea, which is a common cause of nongap metabolic acidosis due to losses of bicarbonate in the GI tract. The next step in a metabolic acidosis is to check if an anion gap exists or not. In this case, the anion gap is normal [(138 – (114 + 16) = 8]. It is important to establish if the metabolic acidosis is properly compensated; the predicted $Paco_2$ for HCO_3 of 16 is 32 ± 2. The $Paco_2$ (32 mm Hg) falls within the calculated compensated $Paco_2$ range of 30 to 34, indicating proper respiratory compensation.

24.2 **B.** This patient has anion-gap metabolic acidosis with hyperosmolar state with compensation.

1. Is the pH normal, alkalemic or acidemic? **Acidemic** (pH = 7.20)

2. Is the $Paco_2$ normal, alkalemic, or acidemic? **Alkalemic** ($Paco_2$ = 30 mm Hg)

3. Is the HCO_3 normal, alkalotic or acidotic? **Acidotic** (HCO_3 = 14 mEq/L)

4. Is the acid–base disorder properly compensated? **Yes.** Using Winter's formula, the predicted $Paco_2$ for HCO_3 of 14 is 29 ± 2 [14 × 1.5 + 8 = 29 ±2). The $Paco_2$ (30 mm Hg) falls within the calculated compensated $Paco_2$ range of 27 to 31 mm Hg, indicating proper respiratory compensation.

5. If a metabolic acidosis exists, what is the anion gap and corrected bicarbonate? Anion gap = 140 − (110 + 14) = 16, indicating a positive anion-gap metabolic acidosis. The corrected HCO_3 is 18, indicating a preexisting nongap metabolic acidosis.

6. Is there an osmolal gap? Measured osmolality = 320 mEq/L; calculated osmolality = (2 × 140) + (212/18) + (4.2/2.8) = 293 mEq/L; osmolal gap = 320 mEq/L − 293 mEq/L = 26 mEq/L.

The calculated osmolal gap is 26 mEq/L, which is >10 mEq/L difference, significant for unmeasured osmoles. Methanol poisoning is known to cause a positive anion-gap metabolic acidosis with a hyperosmolar state. Furthermore, the calculated anion gap of 16 confirms a positive anion-gap metabolic acidosis with a preexisiting nongap metabolic acidosis, confirmed by the corrected bicarbonate of 18. Using Winter's formula, the predicted $Paco_2$ for HCO_3 of 14 falls within the range of 27 to 31 mm Hg, indicating proper respiratory compensation. Treatment with fomepizole or ethanol is used for methanol and ethylene glycol toxicity. Both drugs reduce the action of alcohol dehydrogenase, thus decreasing the toxic metabolites of the offending drug.

CLINICAL PEARLS

▶ In metabolic acidosis, the difference of an anion-gap acidosis from a nongap acidosis directs the treatment and cause of low HCO_3.

▶ The treatment of positive-gap acidosis requires a reversal of the underlying condition.

▶ The treatment of nongap metabolic acidosis is replenishing the HCO_3 loss.

▶ In type 1 RTA, the distal tubule inability to excrete H^+ ions causes loss of urinary HCO_3.

▶ Type 2 RTA affects the proximal tubule, where HCO_3^- fails to be reabsorbed.

▶ Osmolal gaps >10 Osm, consider ethanol, methanol, ethylene glycol, and isopropyl alcohol.

▶ Methanol causes anion-gap hyperosmolar metabolic acidosis and blindness by formic acid.

▶ Ethylene glycol causes anion-gap hyperosmolar metabolic acidosis, renal failure, and calcium oxalate stones.

▶ Isopropyl or rubbing alcohol causes a hyperosmolar state but without acidosis.

REFERENCES

Adrogué HJ, Madias NE. Management of life-threatening acid–base disorders. Part I. *N Engl J Med.* 1998;338:26-34.

American College of Physicians. *Medical Knowledge Self-Assessment Program 17.* Philadelphia, PA: American College of Physicians; 2006.

Loscalzo J. *Harrison's Pulmonary and Critical Care Medicine.* New York, NY: McGrawHill; 2013.

A 34-year-old male airline pilot who regularly flies overseas fractured his left hip in a flag-football game. At home the patient developed an acute onset of dyspnea with pleuritic chest pain. The patient's left lower extremity was exquisitely tender and edematous to the level of the mid-calf. The patient was emergently transferred to the ICU. He was found to have deep venous thrombosis (DVT) and a pulmonary embolism, requiring monitoring for right-heart failure and anticoagulation therapy. On physical examination, the patient's temperature is 36°C (96.8°F), heart rate is 100 beats/min, respiration is 28 breaths/min, and blood pressure is 98/55 mm Hg. The patient's laboratory results and arterial blood gas study follows:

Serum Laboratory Studies (Normal range)	
Sodium (Na$^+$)	138 mEq/L (136-144 mEq/L)
Potassium (K$^+$)	4.0 mEq/L (3.7-5.2 mEq/L)
Chloride (Cl$^-$)	110 mEq/L (101-111 mEq/L)
Bicarbonate (HCO$_3^-$)	14 mEq/L (22-26 mEq/L)
Arterial Blood Gas Studies	
pH	7.47 (7.35-7.45)
Pa$_{CO_2}$	20 mm Hg (36-44 mm Hg)
Pa$_{O_2}$ (on room air)	92 mm Hg (75-100 mm Hg)

▶ What is this patient's acid–base disorder?
▶ What is the best treatment for this patient?

ANSWERS TO CASE 25:

Acid–Base Abnormalities Part II

Summary: This is a 34-year-old man with DVT and pulmonary embolism.

- **Acid–Base Disorder:** Chronic respiratory alkalosis with appropriate metabolic compensation

- **Treatment Options:** The pulmonary embolism protocol should be enacted (refer to Case 13) to ensure anticoagulation and hemodynamic stability. BiPAP, or another noninvasive form of ventilation, may be indicated to address any respiratory distress.

ANALYSIS

Objectives

1. To use a common stepwise approach to acid–base evaluations (as discussed in Case 24).

2. To understand the respiratory and metabolic effects on acid–base disorders.

3. To understand the most common causes of respiratory disorders related to acid–base imbalances.

Considerations

This patient has a pulmonary embolism (PE) with concomitant deep venous thrombosis. The classical presentation of a PE includes shortness of breath, tachypnea, and pleuritic chest pain. This leads to an increased minute ventilation rate (V_E), which yields a lessened $Paco_2$ level and thus the chronic respiratory alkalosis.

- Is the pH normal, alkalemic, or acidemic? **Ans:** Alkalemia; pH at 7.48 (7.35-7.45)

- Is the $Paco_2$ normal, alkalemic, or acidemic? Ans: Alkalemia; $Paco_2$ at 20 mm Hg (36-44 mm Hg), indicating a respiratory alkalosis

- Is the HCO_3 normal, alkalotic, or acidotic? Ans: **Acidotic;** HCO_3 at 14 mEq/L (22-26 mEq/L), indicating an appropriate metabolic compensation

- Is the compensation for the primary disorder appropriate, alkalosis, or acidosis? **Ans:** In a chronic respiratory alkalosis, the normal compensatory response can be calculated based on the change in $Paco_2$ from the normal value of 40 mm Hg. For each 10 mm Hg change in the $Paco_2$, the HCO_3 should decrease by 5 mEq/L ($Paco_2\Delta10 \rightarrow HCO_3\Delta5$). As such, the decreased $Paco_2$ by 20 mm Hg is appropriately compensated with the expected 10 mEq/L decrease in HCO_3, corroborating the measured value of 14 mEq/L.

- If a metabolic acidosis exists, what is the anion-gap and the corrected bicarbonate? **Ans:** This is not applicable since a metabolic acidosis does not exist.

APPROACH TO:
Acid-Base Disorders II

Introduction

Having an arterial blood gas (ABG) and concurrent serum basic metabolic panel (electrolytes, BUN, glucose) allows for an accurate evaluation of acid–base disturbances with a systematic, stepwise approach through a series of answered questions (as introduced in Case 24). In acid-base disorders, the $Paco_2$ and HCO_3 move in the same direction. If the $Paco_2$ decreases, so too will the HCO_3; and similarly if the $Paco_2$ increases, so too will the HCO_3 (reference Table 24–1). In metabolic acid–base disorders, the pH, $Paco_2$, and HCO_3 will all trend in the same direction. When the $Paco_2$ and HCO_3 trend in opposite directions of the pH, there is a mixed respiratory and metabolic component responsible for the acid–base disorder.

If the primary cause of the acid–base disorder is due to an acute respiratory cause, then the HCO_3 should trend in parallel coordination to the change in $Paco_2$. In acute respiratory alkalosis disorders, for each decrease of 10 mm Hg of $Paco_2$, there should be a compensatory decrease of 1 mEq/L of the HCO_3 concentration (refer to Table 24–1). If the change in HCO_3 measured is less than the anticipated compensation (calculated HCO_3), then a metabolic acidosis accompanies the respiratory alkalosis. In contrast, if the measured HCO_3 is greater than the anticipated compensation, then a concomitant metabolic alkalosis would also be present.

Respiratory Acidosis

Respiratory acidosis is due to a primary increase in arterial $Paco_2$, which accumulates when ventilation is inadequate. Hypoventilation can be secondary to neurological disorders (such as cerebrovascular accident [CVA] or stroke) or due to medications (such as narcotics) that affect the respiratory center of the central nervous system (CNS). Additionally, hypoventilation can be secondary to an obstruction of the airway (such as in COPD), respiratory muscle weaknesses (such as in Myasthenia Gravis or Guillain-Barré Syndrome), or chest wall deformities (such as kyphoscoliosis, obesity, and obstructive sleep apnea). The treatment of the respiratory acidosis should focus on resolving the underlying cause of the disorder. In patients with acute respiratory acidosis accompanied by measured hypoxemia (by oxygen saturation), supplemental O_2 should be administered with caution in order to maintain the O_2 saturation at, or around, 90% to avoid blocking any hypoxic drive present. Aerosolized bronchodilators such as albuterol should be administered under controlled Fio_2 or compressed ambient air (that has an Fio_2 of 21%) to increase oxygenation and decrease the $Paco_2$. Additionally, the adjunctive use of BiPAP, noninvasive ventilation, or endotracheal intubation with full mechanical ventilation may be needed for adequate ventilation.

Example 1: An 84-year-old woman is admitted to the ICU for monitoring after presenting to the ED with hemiplegia and weakness secondary to an embolic CVA. The patient appears frail with pronounced kyphoscoliosis secondary to osteoporosis. The patient is bradycardic at 52 beats/min and hypoventilating at 8 breaths/min with shallow, unlabored breaths. Serum laboratory studies show Na^+ of 144 mEq/L, K^+ of 4.7 mEq/L, Cl^- of 108 mEq/L, and HCO_3^- of 30 mEq/L. Arterial blood gas studies (on room air) show a pH of 7.34, a $Paco_2$ of 55 mm Hg, and a PaO_2 of 75.

What is the acid–base abnormality? *(normal values noted for each)*

- Is the patient acidemic or alkalemic? **Ans:** Acidemic; pH = 7.34 (7.35-7.45)

- Is the $Paco_2$ normal, alkalotic, or acidotic? **Ans:** Acidotic; $Paco_2$ = 55 mm Hg (35-45 mm Hg)

- Is the HCO_3 normal, alkalotic, or acidotic? **Ans:** Alkalotic; HCO_3^- = 30 mEq/L (22-26 mEq/L)

- Is the compensation for the primary disorder appropriate, alkalosis, or acidosis? **Ans:** Appropriate. For a chronic respiratory acidosis, the expected changes are as follows: $Paco_2 \Delta 10 \rightarrow HCO_3 \Delta 3$. As the change in $Paco_2$ is 15 mm Hg from normal, the expected bicarbonate can be calculated as $(1.5 \times 3) + 24$, which is approximately 29 (within the estimated ±2), which approximates the measured bicarbonate.

- If a metabolic acidosis present, what is the anion gap, what is the calculated bicarbonate and what is the osmolality? **Ans:** Anion gaps are evaluated in metabolic acidosis cases only.

Conclusion: This patient has a chronic respiratory acidosis with metabolic compensation.

Respiratory Alkalosis

Hyperventilation reduces the $Paco_2$, which in turn increases the pH, producing a respiratory alkalosis (refer to Table 24–1). Common causes of respiratory alkalosis include conditions involving the pulmonary vasculature (such as pulmonary hypertension and venous thromboembolism), the pulmonary parenchyma (such as pulmonary fibrosis, heart failure, and pneumonia), and the pulmonary airways (such as COPD and asthma). Other causes include conditions that impact ventilatory control mechanisms (such as anxiety, salicylate toxicity, sepsis, hypoxia, and pregnancy). The expected compensatory mechanisms for both acute and chronic respiratory alkalosis are various forms of metabolic compensation. Patients with restrictive lung diseases can only increase minute ventilation by increasing the respiratory rate and not the tidal volume (V_T). Some of these conditions include CHF, pneumonia, pulmonary fibrosis, obesity, ascites, chest bellows restriction, chest wall abnormalities, chest pain, trauma, and contusions. For example, patients experiencing psychogenic hyperventilation, such as in an anxiety disorder, would benefit from rebreathing into a paper bag, which will increase the systemic $Paco_2$ and, in turn, will correct the pH avoiding transient hypocalcemia. The only acid–base disorder that can return to a normal pH without an accompanying secondary disorder is a chronic respiratory alkalosis (e.g., pregnancy). A respiratory alkalosis often presents with parasthesias of the extremities and perioral region, shortness of breath accompanied by band-like pressure of the chest, and rarely, tetany by deionizing calcium (Ca^{2+}) via the alkalosis. Likewise, the hypocapnia causes a vasoconstriction, which can give neurological manifestations such as changes in mentation, dizziness, tremors, and possible syncopal episodes.

Example 2: A 24-year-old primagravida woman who is at 34-weeks gestation and has a history of severe generalized anxiety disorder presents to the emergency department with a panic attack. The patient is tachycardic at 125 beats/min, diaphoretic, and hyperventilating at 34 breaths/min. She was experiencing extremity and perioral paresthesia. While in the ED she had a witnessed a grand mal seizure. She was admitted to the ICU for monitoring. Serum laboratory studies show Na^+ of 140 mEq/L, K^+ of 5 mEq/L, Cl^- of 110 mEq/L, and HCO_3^- of 21 mEq/L. Arterial blood gas studies show a pH of 7.54, $Paco_2$ of 25 mm Hg, and PaO_2 of 77 mm Hg on 40% Fio_2.

What is the acid–base abnormality? (*Normal range*)

- Is the patient acidemic or alkalemic? **Ans:** Alkalemic; pH = 7.54 (7.35-7.45)

- Is the $Paco_2$ normal, alkalotic, or acidotic? **Ans:** Alkalotic; $Paco_2$ = 25 mm Hg (35-45 mm Hg)

- Is the HCO_3 normal, alkalotic, or acidotic? **Ans:** Acidotic; HCO_3 = 21 mEq/L (22-26 mEq/L)

- Is the compensation for the primary disorder appropriate, alkalosis, or acidosis? **Ans:** Appropriate. For an acute respiratory alkalosis, the expected changes are as follows: $Paco_2 \Delta 10 \rightarrow HCO_3 \Delta 2$. As the change in $Paco_2$ is 15 mm Hg from normal, the expected bicarbonate can be calculated as $24 - (1.5 \times 2) = 21 \pm 2$

- If a metabolic acidosis is present, what is the anion gap, what is the calculated bicarbonate and what is the osmolality? **Ans:** Anion gaps are evaluated in metabolic acidosis cases.

Conclusion: This patient has an acute respiratory alkalosis with metabolic compensation.

CLINICAL CASE CORRELATION

- See also Case 22 (Acute Liver Failure) and Case 24 (Acid–Base Disorder I).

COMPREHENSION QUESTIONS

25.1 A 28-year-old woman was transferred to the ICU after experiencing postsurgical respiratory decline after an emergency Cesarean section for the delivery of a preterm baby boy. The pregnancy was complicated by acute fatty liver of pregnancy. She otherwise has no medical problems nor takes any medications. The patient was started on a morphine IV infusion at 5 mg/h after the surgery and was receiving oxygen at 2 L by nasal cannula. Upon arrival to the ICU, the patient was hypoventilating at 8 breaths/min. Serum laboratory studies show glucose of 122 mg/dL, BUN of 16 mg/dL, Na^+ of 145 mEq/L, K^+ of 4.2, Cl^- of 110 mEq/L, and HCO_3^- of 20 mEq/L. Arterial blood gas studies show the following: pH 7.16, $Paco_2$ 60 mm Hg, PaO_2 60 mm Hg, and HCO_3 of 22 mEq/L. Which of the following best describes the patient's acid–base disorder?

A. Metabolic acidosis

B. Respiratory alkalosis

C. Acute respiratory acidosis with metabolic acidosis

D. Acute respiratory acidosis with metabolic alkalosis

E. Chronic respiratory acidosis with metabolic alkalosis

25.2 A 14-year-old adolescent was admitted to the ICU after being found in a semi-comatose state. The patient was described as being "very agitated" earlier in the day while studying for an upcoming biology examination. The patient has a history of well-controlled Type 1 diabetes mellitus. On physical examination the patient's heart rate was 145 beats/min, respirations were 28 breaths/min, and blood pressure was 90/60 mm Hg. Serum laboratory studies show glucose of 114 mg/dL, BUN of 14 mg/dL, Na^+ of 142 mEq/L, K^+ of 3.6 mEq/L, Cl^- of 112 mEq/L, HCO_3^- of 14 mEq/L, and an osmolarity of 290 mosm/kg H_2O. Arterial blood gas studies show a pH of 7.30, $Paco_2$ of 20 mm Hg, and a PaO_2 of 94 mm Hg. Which of the following is the likely cause of the patient's acid–base abnormality?

A. Alcoholic ketoacidosis

B. Diabetic ketoacidosis

C. Ethylene glycol toxicity

D. Methanol toxicity

E. Salicylate toxicity

ANSWERS

25.1 **C.** The patient's postsurgical pain control with opioids and marked respiratory depression is suggestive of opioid toxicity. The fatty liver may have also impacted liver function, maintaining opioid levels. The stepwise evaluation of acid-base disorders follows:

1. Is the patient normal, alkalotic, or acidotic? **Acidotic**; pH = 7.19 (7.35-7.45)

2. Is the $Paco_2$ normal, alkalotic, or acidotic? **Acidotic**; $Paco_2$ = 60 mm Hg (35-45 mm Hg)

3. Is the HCO_3 normal, alkalotic, or acidotic? **Acidotic**; HCO_3 = 22 mEq/L (22-26 mEq/L)

4. What is the primary cause of the disorder? A mixed respiratory acidosis and metabolic acidosis exists. Based on the respiratory acidosis, the expected calculated HCO_3 would be approximately 24 + 2 = 26 mEq/L in an acute situation. However, this is not the case, leading to the conclusion that the patient's disorder is a mixed acute respiratory acidosis with metabolic acidosis.

25.2 **E**. The combination of an anion-gap metabolic acidosis and respiratory alkalosis is suggestive of salicylate toxicity. This patient most likely has ingested salicylates. Metabolic acidosis is indicated by the low serum bicarbonate level and the increased anion gap of 16, which can be calculated using the formula $(Na^+) - (Cl^- + HCO3^-)$, where normal is 12 ± 2. This patient's expected Pco_2 is 29 ± 2 mm Hg, which can be calculated using Winters formula: Expected Pco_2 = 1.5 × $[HCO_3^-]$ + 8 ± 2 mm Hg. However, the patient's measured $Paco_2$ of 20 mm Hg is lower than expected for the degree of metabolic acidosis present, which confirms the presence of a concurrent respiratory alkalosis. If the toxicity were due to alcohol, there would have been an osmolar gap present and/or a measurable EtOH level. Similarly, if the cause were due to DKA or hyperosmolar state (HOS), there would have been a markedly elevated glucose. An osmolar gap would indicate potential methanol or ethylene glycol toxicity. Isopropyl alcohol toxicity gives an anion gap without an acidosis.

CLINICAL PEARLS

▶ The only acid–base disorder that returns to a normal pH without another acid–base disorder cause being present is chronic respiratory alkalosis.

▶ Changes in $Paco_2$ and HCO_3 move in the same direction.

▶ Acute respiratory alkalosis with significant elevation in pH can deionize calcium and induce a seizure via a relative hypocalcemia.

REFERENCES

American College of Physicians and the Clerkship Directors in Internal Medicine. *Internal Medicine Essentials for Clerkship Students*. Philadelphia, PA: ACP Press; 2007-2008.

Kraut JA, Nagami GT. The serum anion gap in the evaluation of acid-base disorders: what are its limitations and can its effectiveness be improved? *Clin J Am Soc Nephrol*. 2013;8(11):2018-2024.

Loscalzo J. *Harrison's Pulmonary and Critical Care Medicine*, New York, NY: McGraw-Hill, 2013.

A 66-year-old man was hospitalized two days ago following an acute hemorrhagic stroke. His CT findings demonstrated a left intracerebral hemorrhage with subarachnoid hemorrhage (SAH). The patient's Glasgow coma score (GCS) is 13. He was admitted to the ICU for monitoring and management of his hypertension. Today, on hospital day two, you receive a call from the ICU nurse because the patient appears to be more somnolent. The examination reveals that the patient has the same right extremity weakness as before and no new focal neurological findings. He is lethargic, answers slowly to commands, and appears confused. A review of medications shows nothing significant. A repeat brain CT demonstrates no changes from his initial CT. Laboratory findings reveal WBC 8000 cells/mm^3, hemoglobin/hematocrit 13.4 g/dL and 42%, sodium 124 mmol/L, and serum osmolality 288 mOsm/kg (normal: 278-305 mOsm/kg).

► What is the most likely cause of the patient's mental status changes?
► What is the likely underlying mechanism for this condition?
► What is the best treatment for this patient?

ANSWERS TO CASE 26:
Fluid/Electrolyte Abnormalities

Summary: A 66-year-old man with intracerebral and subarachnoid hemorrhage develops hyponatremia and mental status changes two days after admission to the ICU.

- **Likely cause of mental status change:** Acute hyponatremia.

- **Likely underlying mechanism:** Most likely due to cerebral salt wasting.

- **Treatment:** Correct hyponatremia with normal saline infusion. Recheck serum electrolytes every 2 to 4 hours, and carefully monitor mental status and neurological examination.

ANALYSIS

Objectives

1. To learn to identify the patients "at-risk" for the development of fluid/electrolyte abnormalities.

2. To learn the detrimental effects of fluid and electrolyte abnormalities and replacement strategies.

Considerations

This 66-year-old patient was admitted to the ICU for management of hemorrhagic stroke, hypertension, and SAH. Acute changes in mental status necessitate immediate repeat CT of the brain to rule out cerebral vasospasm as the etiology. He had no focal neurological findings. In this case, the repeat head CT returns with no interval changes. However, laboratory testing reveals an electrolyte abnormality, namely hyponatremia, which may explain the newly altered mental status. Hyponatremia is a common problem in patients with CNS disease because the brain's ability to regulate sodium and water homeostasis is often altered. It is the most common electrolyte abnormality after an aneurysmal SAH, occurring in 34% of patients after SAH. It usually occurs between the second and tenth post-bleed day, closely paralleling the period of cerebral vasospasm. It is likely due to cerebral salt wasting, but the trigger is unknown. Natriuresis and volume depletion from cerebral salt wasting may contribute to severe vasospasm in SAH. The diagnosis and management of other fluid and electrolyte abnormalities is paramount.

APPROACH TO:
Fluid/Electrolyte Abnormalities

DEFINITIONS

HYPONATREMIA: Serum sodium concentration <135 mmol/L. Hyponatremia is usually asymptomatic unless the absolute level is <120 mmol/L or the change in sodium concentration is very rapid (within hours).

OSMOTIC DEMYELINATION SYNDROME (ODS): Also known as central pontine myelinolysis, this is a neurological disorder associated with significant nerve cell damage in the pons of the brain stem. The myelin sheath is characteristically damaged, leading to acute motor dysfunction and dysphagia. This condition is associated with profound hyponatremia that is untreated, or rapid correction of chronic severe hyponatremia.

TOTAL BODY WATER (TBW): The amount of water in the body, estimated as 60% of a person's weight for men, or 50% of a person's weight for women. One-third of the total body water is located in the extracellular fluid (ECF) compartment, whereas two-thirds of the total body water is located in the intracellular fluid (ICF) compartment.

OSMOLALITY: The concentration of solute particles in a solution is referred to as osmotic activity, expressed in osmoles (Osm). *Osmolality* is the osmotic activity *per volume of water* and is expressed in mOsm/kg H_2O.

PLASMA OSMOLALITY: The primary extracellular solutes are sodium and its anions, chloride and bicarbonate, glucose, and urea. Plasma osmolality can be calculated with the following formula:

$$\text{Serum osmolality} = [Na] \times 2 + [glucose]/18 + BUN/2.8.$$

TONICITY: A measure of the *relative* osmotic activity in two solutions separated by a membrane that is permeable to water but not solutes. Tonicity is also referred to as *effective osmolality*.

PLASMA TONICITY: The cell membrane is permeable to water, but some solutes are unable to move across the cell membrane passively. These are called "effective" solutes because they create osmotic gradients across cell membranes. These osmotic gradients affect water movement between the ICF and ECF compartments. Because water moves freely between the ICF and ECF, osmolality will always be equivalent in both of these compartments. The effective solutes in the ECF include sodium and its anions, as well as glucose. Urea is able to move freely through the cell membrane. However, it makes up a very small portion of the plasma osmolality. As such, the plasma osmolality can often be considered equivalent to the plasma tonicity, also known as the *effective plasma osmolality*.

CLINICAL APPROACH

Patients "at-risk" for the development fluid/electrolyte abnormalities include those with pulmonary or mediastinal disease and CNS diseases. Hyponatremia, which manifests as vague constitutional or mental status changes, can be found in up to 15% to 30% of hospitalized patients. Hyponatremia has the potential to cause substantial morbidity and mortality and has been identified as an independent risk factor for mortality in hospitalized patients. Moreover, overly rapid correction of chronic hyponatremia can cause severe neurological deficits and death.

Sodium homeostasis: Abnormalities of plasma sodium concentration usually reflect an abnormality in total body water rather than a problem with sodium balance. Total body water and its composition are tightly regulated by both osmotic and nonosmotic processes. Under normal circumstances, plasma osmolality is the major determinant of water balance and is maintained at approximately 280 to 295 mOsm/kg by arginine vasopressin (AVP), otherwise known as antidiuretic hormone (ADH). Changes in plasma osmolality are monitored by the host by changes in the size of specialized neurons in the hypothalamus, called osmoreceptors. These changes in tonicity are relayed to the magnocellular neurons in the supraoptic and paraventricular nuclei of the hypothalamus, which synthesize AVP for subsequent storage and release. An increase in plasma osmolality triggers the release of AVP, which act on V2 receptors in the kidneys to increase water permeability in the distal tubule and collecting duct of the nephrons, resulting in water retention and a subsequent fall in the osmolality. At serum osmolarity levels >295 mOsm/kg, a person's thirst mechanism is also stimulated, triggering an increase in free-water consumption if the person is able to drink. On the contrary, a decrease in plasma osmolality of just 1% to 2% with water intake suppresses AVP secretion and leads to urinary excretion of excess water, thus raising the plasma osmolality back to normal.

Plasma AVP is also regulated by *nonosmotic* factors, such as blood pressure and circulating blood volume. Arterial stretch baroreceptors are located in the carotid sinus, aortic arch, cardiac atria, and pulmonary venous system. With an 8% to 10% decrease in arterial pressure, the baroreceptors signal the hypothalamus to release AVP into the plasma. The circulating AVP acts on V2 receptors in the kidney, increasing free-water reabsorption. In addition, AVP acts on V1 receptors on blood vessels, causing an increase in vascular resistance and blood pressure. When hyponatremia is associated with hypovolemia, the nonosmotic stimulation of AVP can cause an increase in water retention and worsening of hyponatremia, despite the presence of hypo-osmolality. During periods of low blood volume or blood pressure, baroreceptors in the cardiac atria stimulate the adrenal release of aldosterone, which contributes to sodium and water reabsorption via the proximal renal tubule.

Hyponatremia usually is a result of dysregulation of the tightly regulated process described earlier. As such, persons at risk of developing hyponatremia include those patients who are likely to have disrupted control over their water homeostasis. Risk factors for the development of hyponatremia include head or other traumatic injury, SAH, acute meningitis, transsphenoidal surgery, other general surgical operations, medications (ie, carbamazepine), and advancing age (due to a decline in blood flow to the kidney and glomerular filtration rate [GFR] with age).

Detrimental effects of fluid and electrolyte abnormalities can occur in the intensive care unit can evolve as the result of pathologic states or iatrogenically.

Symptomatic hyponatremia usually occurs with absolute sodium levels <120 mmol/L. However, symptoms may also arise secondary to very rapid changes in the serum sodium concentration. **Acute hyponatremia is classified as occurring within 48 hours,** whereas chronic hyponatremia takes >48 hours to develop. Initial symptoms associated with hyponatremia can be mild, including headache, nausea and vomiting, muscle cramps, aches, or generalized restlessness. With increasing severity, patients may become apathetic, lethargic, or acutely confused. If left undiagnosed and untreated, hyponatremia can progress to seizures, apnea, coma, and death. These symptoms are the manifestations of cerebral edema progression.

Hyponatremia in most cases reflects a state of relative intravascular and extravascular free-water excess, which causes water in the extracellular space to move across the cell membrane into the intracellular space, leading to cell swelling. Within the calvarium, because the skull provides a finite space for the brain to expand, cerebral edema that is left uncorrected can lead to the symptoms detailed earlier as well as eventual brain herniation and death.

Adaptive processes to cerebral edema in the brain include shifting of intracellular potassium to the extracellular fluid, thereby decreasing intracellular osmolality. As a result, brain cells lose water, and globally, the brain returns to normal volume within the skull. This occurs within hours of the onset of cerebral edema. The brain's acute adaptation helps explain why hyponatremia often remains asymptomatic except with rapid changes in sodium concentrations.

Though the brain has developed adaptive processes to deal with imbalances in body water and solute homeostasis, these adaptive processes occur at the expense of losing intracellular potassium and organic osmolytes in the brain. This becomes relevant during the treatment of hyponatremia, particularly chronic hyponatremia. Treatment for hypotonic hyponatremia causes a rise in the serum osmolality toward normal ranges, which draws water out of brain cells as the total body water equilibrates. **When the movement of water out of the neurons occurs too rapidly, brain cells that have previously adapted may not have enough time to re-accumulate the intracellular potassium and organic osmolytes that were lost.** Consequently, neurons may shrivel and become at **risk for osmotic demyelination.** For unknown reasons, the areas of the brain that are most sensitive to this process are near the **pons. Patients who are at high risk of osmotic demyelination after acutely correcting chronic hyponatremia include those with severe malnutrition, alcoholism, or advanced liver disease.**

Osmotic demyelination often presents after a period of initial improvement from the symptoms of severe hyponatremia. Several days after correction, new and progressive neurologic symptoms may develop, including spastic quadriparesis or quadriplegia, pseudobulbar palsy, and changes in levels of consciousness. This diagnosis can be established by brain MRI to assess for demyelinated regions in the brain.

Diagnosis and Management

Management of hyponatremia begins with a precise, often multistep, diagnostic algorithm that helps pinpoint the cause of hyponatremia to guide its treatment. This diagnostic process is multistep because hyponatremia can be categorized according to different etiologies that culminate in one similar clinical presentation. For example, unlike hypernatremia, which always is associated with hypertonicity, **hyponatremia can occur in the settings of hypotonicity, isotonicity, or hypertonicity. Thus, the first step in patient evaluation is to measure the serum osmolality.** *Hypertonic* hyponatremia occurs when effective solutes other than sodium, such as glucose or mannitol, accumulate in the ECF compartment. These solutes draw water from within cells into the extracellular space, resulting in a hypertonic hyponatremia as the sodium concentration is diluted. **A rise in the serum glucose of 100 mg/dL will cause a fall of ~1.6 mmol/L in serum sodium concentration.** *Isotonic* hyponatremia, **also called pseudohyponatremia, is usually produced by laboratory artifacts caused by severe hypertriglyceridemia, hypercholesterolemia, or paraproteinemia that causes measured serum sodium levels to be falsely low while serum osmolality remains normal.** Isotonic hyponatremia should trigger a search for an underlying cause of increased serum lipids or paraproteins. Treatment for hypertonic and isotonic hyponatremia centers on treating the underlying cause.

Hypotonic hyponatremia can be *dilutional* or *depletional*. Dilutional hyponatremia occurs when extracellular sodium concentrations are low *relative to* increases in total body water, and this can take place under two different scenarios: (1) The absolute sodium level may stay the same, but the total body water increases; and (2) the absolute sodium level increases, but not as much as the total body water, leading to a relative dilution of sodium concentration. Depletional hyponatremia develops when sodium loss outpaces water loss.

After establishing a patient's low serum osmolality, the diagnosis of hypotonic hyponatremia requires further investigation. The next step in diagnosis is to assess the patient's volume status. This is done using a combination of clinical and laboratory signs. Examination of the patient should include assessment of weight changes, orthostatic variations in vital signs, skin turgor (less useful in elderly patients), jugular venous pressure, central venous pressure if central access is available, and an echocardiogram to assess cardiac filling and inferior vena cava engorgement or compressibility. Laboratory measures of fluid status include hemoconcentration or dilution and the BUN/Cr ratio. Evaluating volume status allows for the placement of a patient's hypotonic hyponatremia into three categories: hypovolemia, euvolemia, and hypervolemia.

Hypovolemic hyponatremia is depletional and can be caused by either renal or extrarenal loss of sodium. Causes of renal sodium loss include diuretic use, cerebral salt-wasting syndrome, mineralocorticoid deficiency, and salt-wasting nephropathy. Causes of extrarenal loss of sodium include gastrointestinal losses via vomiting or diarrhea, third space losses from bowel obstruction, pancreatitis, burns, or sweat losses from endurance exercises. Differentiating between renal and extrarenal sodium loss is done by measuring urine sodium excretion. If the kidney is the site of sodium loss, a spot urine sodium concentration will be >20 mmol/L. On the contrary, a urine sodium concentration of <20 mmol/L points to an extrarenal etiology of sodium loss.

Euvolemic hyponatremia **has many causes, the most common being** syndrome of inappropriate antidiuretic hormone secretion (**SIADH**). The diagnosis of SIADH remains a diagnosis of exclusion and requires a demonstration of (1) hyponatremia, (2) low serum osmolality, (3) inappropriately concentrated urine (U_{Osm} >100 mOsm/kg), (4) persistent urinary sodium excretion (U_{Na} >20 mmol/L), and (5) exclusion of hypothyroidism or hypoadrenalism. There must also be an absence of any stimuli that might explain an increased secretion of AVP, such as hypovolemia and hypotension. If a measure of the urine osmolality returns with appropriately dilute urine (U_{Osm} <100 mOsm/kg), the cause of hyponatremia can be explained by excessive water intake (primary polydipsia or beer potomania).

Hypervolemic hyponatremia is caused by clinical entities of volume overload, such as congestive heart failure (CHF), cirrhosis, nephrotic syndrome, and other renal failure.

Distinguishing between SIADH and cerebral salt wasting is important in the management of patients with CNS injury. The biggest distinction between the two pathological entities is that SIADH is a *volume-expanded state*, whereas cerebral salt wasting is a *volume-depleted state*. In SIADH, despite low serum osmolality, increased expression of AVP leads to an ongoing dilutional hyponatremia. However, patients are not clinically hypervolemic because only one-third of the total retained water remains in the extracellular space. Cerebral salt wasting, on the contrary, is a state characterized by hypovolemia secondary to primary natriuresis. As such, patients have a negative sodium balance. Though the pathogenesis of cerebral salt wasting is not definitive, it is theorized that impaired sodium reabsorption occurs in the proximal nephron. Reduced sympathetic tone may explain the failure of renin and aldosterone levels to rise despite volume depletion. Volume depletion will ultimately trigger AVP release despite the low serum osmolality, often causing confusion between a diagnosis of SIADH and Cerebral Salt-Wasting Syndrome (CSW). However, CSW is always associated with an initial presentation of volume contraction and negative sodium balance.

The goals of treating hyponatremia are (1) to achieve euvolemia and (2) to correct low sodium levels to a safe, but not necessarily normal, range in a controlled manner to avoid the potential of osmotic demyelination. In the case of hypovolemic hypotonic hyponatremia, including cerebral salt wasting seen in SAH, volume replacement with normal saline (0.9% NaCl in water) to euvolemia generally is enough to correct the low sodium level. With volume expansion, the trigger for nonosmotic AVP release is taken away, and the kidneys will then excrete excess free water and correct the serum sodium concentration toward normal. For symptomatic hyponatremia in euvolemic or hypervolemic contexts, correction of sodium levels should take place with hypertonic saline (3% NaCl in water). Because of the risk of osmotic demyelination, this should happen in a controlled manner. **Osmotic demyelination can be avoided by limiting correction of hyponatremia to ≤10 to 12 mmol/L in 24 hours and to <18 mmol/L in 48 hours. Rate of correction should be even slower in patients with risk factors such as severe malnutrition, alcoholism, or advanced liver disease.** Acute treatment should be stopped once the patient's symptoms resolve, a safe serum sodium level (≥ 120 mmol/L) is achieved, or a total magnitude of correction of 18 mmol/L is achieved. During this acute treatment phase, serum sodium levels should be monitored at frequent intervals (every 2-4 hours).

How does one estimate the amount of infusion of hypertonic saline needed to stay within the safe rates of correction? Adrogué and Madias in 2000 published a seminal article on hyponatremia that included a formula that can be used to calculate the effect of 1 L of infusate on the serum sodium.

$$\text{Change in serum Na}^+ = (\text{Infusate Na}^+ - \text{serum Na}^+)/(\text{TBW} + 1)$$

Along with acute reversal of symptomatic hyponatremia, fluid restriction is warranted for euvolemic and hypervolemic hyponatremia. All fluids, not only water, need to be restricted. Nonfood fluids should be limited to 500 mL/d below the average daily urine volume. Several days of restriction are needed to make a significant change in the plasma osmolality. Alternative therapy in cases of SIADH includes demeclocycline, which induces a nephrogenic form of diabetes insipidus and excretion of excess free water.

Research is currently underway for new treatments for hyponatremia. The FDA has approved conivaptan, a nonselective vasopressin receptor antagonist, for 4-day IV use to treat euvolemic and hypervolemic hyponatremia. However, the use of this medication in patients with advanced cirrhosis is cautioned, as it also antagonizes V1 receptors in the splanchnic region, thus increasing splanchnic flow and further elevating portal pressures in patients with liver disease; this predisposes to esophageal bleeding. Because of these concerns, selective V2 receptor antagonists are currently being tested in phase III clinical studies.

OTHER ELECTROLYTE ABNORMALITIES

Beyond disturbances in body water and sodium homeostasis, other electrolyte abnormalities in critically ill patients are also common and associated with poor patient outcomes. The following is a discussion on three electrolytes that are commonly measured daily in the intensive care unit: **potassium**, **magnesium**, and **phosphorus**. For a summary of causes of abnormalities in these three electrolytes, please refer to Table 26–1.

Potassium

Potassium is the body's predominant intracellular cation. The importance of potassium lies in the fact that **potassium is the primary determinant of a cell's resting membrane potential.** However, only 2% of the body's total potassium stores are found in the ECF, making plasma potassium concentration an insensitive marker of changes in the total body potassium level. Furthermore, the plasma potassium concentration is regulated by a variety of signals, including catecholamines, the renin-angiotensin-aldosterone system, glucose and insulin metabolism, and direct release from exercising or injured muscle. Nevertheless, because potassium is essential for cellular functions, it is important to maintain the potassium level in the normal range (3.5-5 mEq/L).

Table 26–1 • COMMON CAUSES OF ELECTROLYTE ABNORMALITIES IN THE ICU	
Electrolyte Abnormality	Etiology
Hypokalemia	*Transcellular Shift* • β-Adrenergic activity • Insulin • Alkalemia • Hypothermia *Increased Losses* • Extra-renal (diarrhea, enterocutaneous fistula, ostomies) • Renal (diuretics, renal tubal acidosis [RTA], metabolic alkalosis, hypomagnesemia) • Hyperaldosteronism *Decreased Intake* • Anorexia • Malnutrition/malabsorption
Hyperkalemia	• Acidosis (transcellular shift) • Renal insufficiency • Adrenal insufficiency • Rhabdomyolysis • Drugs (β-antagonists, ACE inhibitors, spironolactone, heparin, β-blockers, Bactrim, pentamidine) • Blood transfusions
Hypomagnesemia	*Renal Losses* • Diuretics • Volume expansion and increased tubular flow • Hyperaldosteronism *Extra-renal Losses* • Diarrhea • Malabsorption/malnutrition (short gut, alcoholism) • Inflammatory bowel disease • Gastric suction • Chronic pancreatitis • Burns
Hypophosphatemia	*Transcellular Shift* • Carbohydrate infusion/refeeding syndrome • Calcitonin • Catecholamines • Insulin and glucose loading • Respiratory alkalosis *Decreased Intake* • Dietary insufficiency • Malabsorption • Phosphate binders • Vitamin D deficiency *Increased Renal Excretion* • Diuretics • Hyperaldosteronism • SIADH • Glucocorticoid use • Metabolic acidosis • Hypercalcemia

Hypokalemia: [K] <3.5 mEq/L can be caused by transcellular shifts or total body potassium depletion. Transcellular shifts occur when potassium moves between the ICF and the ECF. Despite the low measured serum potassium, these states do not represent true depletion. Factors that shift potassium into cells include β-agonists (such as albuterol), insulin, alkalosis, and hypothermia. Hypokalemia due to potassium depletion, on the other hand, represents a decrease in total body potassium stores and can be caused by either renal or extra-renal etiologies. For example, diuretics increase sodium delivery to the renal collecting ducts by blocking more proximal tubular sodium reabsorption; this produces a rise in the electrochemical gradient in the collecting ducts favoring sodium reabsorption at the expense of potassium secretion. Hypokalemia can occur from extra-renal sources such as gastrointestinal losses. In patients with excess GI secretion losses, the chloride loss activates the renin-angiotensin-aldosterone system, resulting in renal potassium wasting.

Hypokalemia is generally asymptomatic; however, **severe hypokalemia can present as diffuse muscle weakness, EKG changes (U waves, flat or inverted T waves, prolonged QT interval), ileus, and constipation.** Although hypokalemia usually does not produce serious arrhythmias, this condition can potentiate arrhythmias. The first goal of potassium replacement is to eliminate or treat the condition underlying a transcellular shift. The second goal is to replace the serum potassium to a concentration of 4 mEq/L, which can be accomplished with an IV or PO dose of potassium chloride. It should be noted that magnesium depletion impairs potassium reabsorption across the renal tubules, and hypomagnesemia (see the next section) can be a cause of refractory hypokalemia. As such, magnesium also must be replaced to a normal level when replacing serum potassium.

Hyperkalemia: [K] >5.5 mEq/L is often more clinically apparent in comparison to hypokalemia. It is **associated with slowing of cardiac electrical conduction and manifests with classic ECG findings.** These include peaked T waves, decreased amplitude or complete loss of the P waves, increased PR interval, and eventually QRS prolongation that can lead to asystole if left untreated. However, hyperkalemia can often be spurious due to traumatic venipuncture and subsequent potassium release or specimen hemolysis. Thus, unexpected hyperkalemia should be validated with repeat blood draw if possible.

The causes of hyperkalemia can also be categorized as **transcellular shifts versus impaired renal excretion.** Impaired renal excretion in critical care patients is mostly due to renal insufficiency. Adrenal insufficiency can also be a cause of hyperkalemia, but this is not commonly seen in ICU patients. Furthermore, many drugs, such as sulfamethoxazole (Bactrim), subcutaneous heparin, and pentamidine can cause hyperkalemia by inhibiting the renin-angiotensin-aldosterone system. Lastly, blood transfusions can contribute to hyperkalemia, as the potassium in stored erythrocytes leaks out slowly. The accumulation of extracellular potassium in stored blood is usually cleared renally in patients receiving transfusions, but this may become a problem in patients with acute renal failure or hemodynamic shock.

There are three ways of managing hyperkalemia. First, to **inhibit the arrhythmogenic nature of hyperkalemia, calcium infusions are used to stabilize** the myocardium. These infusions are temporary, lasting 20 to 30 minutes, and will temporize the condition until the effects of definitive measures take place. Second, medications that **shift potassium from the ECF to the ICF are employed to temporarily decrease the plasma potassium concentrations.** These include insulin and glucose, albuterol, and bicarbonate. Note, however, that bicarbonate actually has little clinical value because it binds to calcium in the plasma, which would render our calcium infusion ineffective if given together. **Third, more definitive measures should be undertaken to remove excess potassium from the body.** These include sodium polystyrene (Kayexalate), a cation exchange resin, furosemide, a loop diuretic that enhances urinary potassium excretion, and dialysis, the most effective method in patients with acute renal failure.

Magnesium

As the body's second most abundant cation, magnesium serves as an important cofactor in a multitude of enzyme reactions. One such magnesium-dependent system is the membrane pump that generates a cell's resting membrane potential. Magnesium is also responsible for regulating calcium movement into smooth muscle cells. As such, it is essential in helping the body maintain cardiac contractility and peripheral vascular tone. These functions make it important for magnesium levels in the plasma to be maintained at normal values.

Hypomagnesemia, defined as a serum magnesium concentration <2 mEq/L, occurs in 20% of hospitalized patients and 65% of ICU patients. Diuretics can cause hypomagnesemia, as inhibition of sodium reabsorption interferes with magnesium reabsorption. The gastrointestinal tract can also be a direct source of magnesium depletion. Diarrhea leads to a loss of magnesium; therefore, short gut syndrome and other malabsorptive states are associated with decreased magnesium absorption. Furthermore, in patients with chronic and heavy alcohol use, hypomagnesemia in the ICU may be exacerbated by depleted total body stores produced by chronic malnutrition, diarrhea, and thiamine deficiency associated with chronic alcohol abuse.

Similar to potassium, deficiencies in plasma magnesium are largely asymptomatic. However, when manifested, symptoms include weakness, tetany, and seizures. Beyond its essential role in many of the body's enzymatic reactions, magnesium replacement is important because hypomagnesemia is usually associated with other electrolyte abnormalities that will be refractory to treatment unless the magnesium level is normal. Magnesium replacement is accomplished with IV infusions of magnesium sulfate in normal saline.

Phosphorus

Phosphorus is an important electrolyte because of its participation in aerobic energy production. The presentation of phosphorus abnormalities is usually subclinical, though impaired cellular energy production may develop secondary to hypophosphatemia and can be detrimental to systemic oxygen delivery. Decreased energy production in the heart can cause decreased inotropy and cardiac output. Hypophosphatemia is also associated with reduced deformability of red blood cells, leading to hemolytic anemia. Lastly, low phosphate levels are associated with low levels of 2,3-diphosphoglycerate (2,3-DPG), which shifts the oxygen-hemoglobin dissociation curve to the left and reduces the release of oxygen to tissues.

Hypophosphatemia is defined as a plasma phosphate concentration of <2.5 mg/dL and can be caused by many factors. Glucose loads can decrease ECF phosphate, as phosphate enters cells along with glucose. The use of phosphate binders, such as sucralfate, can iatrogenically lower the phosphate level in the serum. The reintroduction of nutrition in patients with prolonged periods of nonfeeding can cause low phosphate levels via the refeeding syndrome. Hypophosphatemia is also commonly seen in patients with respiratory alkalosis, sepsis, and DKA. Phosphate replacement is accomplished with IV or PO preparations of potassium phosphate or sodium phosphate.

CLINICAL CASE CORRELATION

- See also Case 23 (Acute Kidney Injury), Cases 24 and 25 (Acid–Base Abnormalities I and II), and Case 27 (Traumatic Brain Injury).

COMPREHENSION QUESTIONS

26.1 A 53-year-old woman with a history of uncontrolled hypertension is admitted to the ICU with subarachnoid hemorrhage. She underwent an endovascular coiling procedure of an anterior communicating artery aneurysm. On post-procedure day 4, she becomes acutely confused and lethargic. On evaluation of the patient, you find her vital signs to be the following: temperature 37.5°C, HR 110 beats/min, BP 150/90 mm Hg, RR 16 breaths/min, and O_2 saturation 98% on 2 L/min oxygen by nasal cannula. She is somnolent, oriented only to person, and has a GCS of E3, V4, M6 (13). She has no focal neurologic deficits. Her mucous membranes are dry, her urine output has been 25 mL/h in the past 2 hours, and her CVP is 5. While awaiting a repeat CT scan of the head, laboratory values return and reveal serum sodium of 128 mmol/L and serum osmolarity of 260 mOsm/kg water. What is your next step in management of this patient?

A. Fluid bolus with 3% NS.

B. Fluid bolus with 0.9% NS.

C. Fluid restriction.

D. Give demeclocycline.

E. Give the patient salt tabs to take PO.

F. Urgent hemodialysis.

26.2 An otherwise healthy 40-year-old woman with a history of remote appendectomy is postoperative day 5 after an exploratory laparotomy and adhesiolysis
for complete bowel obstruction. Yesterday, her nasogastric tube was removed
and she was started on a clear liquid diet. You are notified by her nurse to
evaluate her for altered mental status. Upon your evaluation, she is confused
and agitated. Her vital signs are stable and normal. She is clinically euvolemic
and weighs 60 kg. Laboratory testing reveals a serum sodium concentration
of 122 mmol/L and serum osmolarity of 240 mOsm/kg water. You decide to
correct her hyponatremia using IV infusion of 3% saline. At what rate will
you run your infusion for the next 12 to 24 hours?

A. 33 mL/h

B. 66 mL/h

C. 100 mL/h

D. 133 mL/h

E. 250 mL/h

26.3 An 18-year-old gentleman is intubated and sedated in your ICU following an
exploratory laparotomy for multiple gunshot wounds to the abdomen. On
postoperative day 1, morning labs reveal a serum potassium concentration of
6.2 mmol/L. Which of the following is the LEAST IMPORTANT part of
your initial evaluation and management of this patient?

A. Repeat potassium measurement

B. 12-lead ECG

C. Infusion of calcium gluconate

D. Treatment with insulin and glucose

E. Fluid bolus with 0.9% saline

ANSWERS

26.1 **B.** The patient in question has had coiling of an intracerebral aneurysm.
She most likely presents with altered mental status due to hyponatremia
secondary to cerebral salt wasting syndrome. Several clues in the vignette
help you decide that she is clinically hypovolemic (mild tachycardia, low
urine output, dry mucous membranes, and low CVP). **The first goal of
treating symptomatic hyponatremia is to achieve euvolemia.** As such, this
woman should receive an IV fluid infusion with an isotonic solution, such
as normal saline. Once euvolemia is achieved, the impetus for nonosmotic
AVP release is resolved. If the patient still remains symptomatic at that time,
considerations should then be made for correction with hypertonic saline,
which carries some risk for complications such as fluid overload and/or cerebral edema.

26.2 **A.** The patient in question weighs 60 kg, and as such, her TBW is estimated at 30 L (0.5 × 60). Using the equation from Adrogue et al, infusion of a liter of 3% saline will change the serum concentration by 12.7 mmol. The calculation is done below:

$$3\% \text{ Saline} = 513 \text{ mmol/L of sodium}$$
$$\text{Patient's serum sodium} = 122 \text{ mmol/L}$$
$$\text{TBW} = 30$$
$$\text{Change in serum [Na]} = (513 - 122)/(30 + 1) = 12.7 \text{ mmol}$$

A safe target for correction of serum sodium is 10 mmol in 24 hours. For this patient, a correction of 10 mmol would take 790 mL (10/12.7 = 0.79). Infusion of 790 mL over 24 hours would take a rate of 33 mL/h.

26.3 **E.** The evaluation and treatment of hyperkalemia involves all of the aforementioned answers except for fluid boluses. Repeat measurements should be pursued to confirm a true hyperkalemia. An ECG should be performed to assess for myocardial instability. A calcium infusion should be given to stabilize the myocardium. Temporary correction of hyperkalemia can be done with albuterol or insulin. More definitive treatment includes giving polystyrene (Kayexalate), furosemide, or undergoing hemodialysis if the patient is in acute renal failure. There is no role for fluid boluses in the management of hyperkalemia.

CLINICAL PEARLS

▶ High-risk patients for osmotic demyelination after acutely correcting chronic hyponatremia include those with severe malnutrition, alcoholism, or advanced liver disease.

▶ Osmotic demyelination associated with hyponatremia treatment can be avoided by limiting correction of hyponatremia to ≤10 to 12 mmol/L in 24 hours and to <18 mmol/L in 48 hours.

▶ Treatment of hyperkalemia includes several categories: **temporary—** insulin + glucose, sodium bicarbonate; **membrane stabilization—** calcium infusion; **elimination (definitive)** —sodium polysty rene (Kayexelate), loop diuretics, and hemodyalsis.

▶ Clinical manifestations and the aggressiveness of treatment depend on the absolute level of derangement and time course of the abnormality.

REFERENCES

Adrogué HJ, Madias NE. Hyponatremia. *N Engl J Med*. 2000;342:1581-1589.

Diringer MN, Zazulia AR. Hyponatremia in neurologic patients: consequences and approaches to treatment. *The Neurologist*. 2006;12(3):117-126.

Marino PL. *The ICU Book*. 4th ed. Philadelphia, PA: Lippincott, Williams & Wilkins; 2013.

Rabinstein AA, Wijdicks EFM. Hyponatremia in critically ill neurological patients. *Neurologist*. 2003;9(6):290-300.

Sterns RH. Disorders of plasma sodium—causes, consequences, and correction. *New Engl J Med*. 2015;372:55-65.

Schrier RW, Bansal S. Diagnosis and management of hyponatremia in acute illness. *Curr Opin Crit Care*. 2008;14:627-634.

Tisdall M, Crocker M, Watkiss J, Smith M. Disturbances in sodium in critically ill adult neurologic patients: a clinical review. *J Neurosurg Anesthesiol*. 2006;18:57-63.

Topf JM, Rankin S, Murray P. Electrolyte disorders in critical care. In: Hall JB, Schmidt GA, Kress J, eds. *Principles Critical Care*. 4th ed. New York, NY: McGraw-Hill; 2015;99:943-967.

Verbalis JG, Goldsmith SR, Greenberg A, et al. Diagnosis, evaluation, and treatment of Hyponatremia: expert panel recommendations. *Am J Med*. 2013;126(10):S1-S42.

An 18-year-old man had an unintentional fall from a second story balcony. He had a Glasgow coma score (GCS) of 5 (E1, V1, M3), normal blood pressure and pulse rate, and evidence of scalp lacerations and skull deformity during his initial evaluation in the emergency department. The patient was immediately intubated, and a brain CT scan revealed linear skull fractures, bilateral frontal lobe contusions, intraparenchymal hematoma, and diffuse cerebral swelling. The neurosurgeon determined that these injuries did not warrant surgical treatment at the time. A ventriculostomy drain was placed in the ICU for monitoring and revealed intracranial pressure (ICP) of 26 mm Hg.

▶ What is the primary goal in the management of this patient?
▶ What are next appropriate management steps?

ANSWERS TO CASE 27:
Traumatic Brain Injury

Summary: An 18-year-old man has fallen from 20 feet and has severe traumatic brain injury (TBI). His CT scan shows intraparenchymal hemorrhage and diffuse swelling. Placement of the ventriculostomy shows that he has intracranial hypertension.

- **Primary goal in management:** The primary goal in the treatment of this patient is to support his airway, breathing, and circulation (ABCs) and prevent secondary brain injury.

- **Next appropriate management steps:** This patient has a TBI and an elevated ICP. After appropriately ruling out or addressing extracranial traumatic and potentially life-threatening injuries, the next steps need to include measures to reduce the ICP and maintain the cerebral perfusion pressure (CPP). These measures may include elevation of the head of bed (if possible), maintaining the head in midline position, removal of cerebrospinal fluid (CSF), the use of mannitol, vasopressors, and/or hypertonic saline and brief hyperventilation. If these measures do not work, surgical intervention may be necessary.

ANALYSIS

Objectives

1. Learn the prognostic factors for traumatic brain injuries.

2. Learn the optimal supportive strategies (ventilation, fluid/electrolyte, and hemodynamic strategies) for patients with severe brain injuries and intracranial hypertension.

3. Learn the factors that contribute to secondary brain injury.

Considerations

This patient suffered a significant fall from height and presented with a Glasgow coma scale (GCS) of 5 that is indicative of severe intracranial injury. His CT scan has shown that he has skull fractures and severe injury to the brain. The ability to minimize swelling and maintain adequate perfusion to the brain is of the utmost importance, as secondary injury to the brain significantly worsens the outcome. Special attention needs to be paid to **avoid any episodes of hypotension and/or hypoxia.** A ventriculostomy is helpful in the diagnosis and treatment of TBI. This device can be used not only for ICP measurements but also to remove CSF for temporary relief of intractable intracranial hypertension.

APPROACH TO:

Traumatic Brain Injury

DEFINITIONS

COUP INJURY: Brain injury occurring at the site of the impact.

CONTRE COUP INJURY: Brain injury occurring on the opposite side of the impact.

TRAUMATIC BRAIN INJURY: Injury to the brain as a result of an external force leading to disruption of brain tissue and blood vessels. The injury can consist of skull fractures, intracranial bleeding (subdural, epidural, intraparenchymal), cerebral contusions, and diffuse axonal injury.

MONRO-KELLIE DOCTRINE: Doctrine that describes cerebral compliance. The major structures within the cranial vault include brain tissue, CSF, and intracranial blood. As the volume of one of these increases, the skull does not allow for space expansion, so there is a mandatory increase in ICP. Only with the reduction of one of these (skull restrictions, tissue, fluid, or blood) can there be a reduction in ICP.

CEREBRAL PERFUSION PRESSURE (CPP): CPP = MAP − ICP: Under normal circumstances, the cerebral blood flow remains constant over a wide range of CPP. This is often referred to as the zone of autoregulation. Normally, CPP below 50 mm Hg causes ischemic damage, while CPP above 150 mm Hg can cause hyperperfusion injury. Acute disease processes can alter the range of the zone of autoregulation, leading to increased risk of cerebral damage.

CLINICAL APPROACH

Prognostic Factors for Traumatic Brain Injuries

Traumatic Brain Injury (TBI) remains one of the major causes of morbidity and mortality. In the United States, brain injury was only recently surpassed by gunshot wounds as the number one cause of death in trauma patients. There is a significant amount of post-injury care that is needed in this population, as many patients require rehabilitation or suffer from post-traumatic stress disorder (PTSD) or other mental illnesses. The goal in treating patients with TBI is to minimize the risk for developing secondary brain injury. Identifying those factors which tend toward a worse prognosis is not as clear, however. The prognosis for TBI is dependent on a multitude of factors, including the type and severity of the injury, the time to treatment, and physiologic occurrences after the injury. There have been models based on large numbers of retrospective analyses that have identified some prognostic factors for TBI.

The most commonly identified factors in almost all models that identify risk factors for poor outcomes are **older age, low initial motor score in the GCS**, and **decreased pupillary reactivity** at admission. Additional prognostic information is provided by the initial CT scan. The inclusion of other clinical information, such as secondary insults (hypotension and hypoxia) and laboratory parameters (glucose and hemoglobin), appears to strengthen the prognostic indication.

Table 27-1 • GLASGOW COMA SCALE SCORE					
Motor Response		Verbal Response		Eye-Opening Response	
Obeys commands	6	Oriented	5	Opens spontaneously	4
Localizes to pain	5	Confused	4	Opens to speech	3
Withdraws from pain	4	Inappropriate words	3	Opens to pain	2
Flexor posturing	3	Unintelligible sounds	2	No eye opening	1
Extensor posturing	2	No sounds	1		
No movement	1				

The GCS (Table 27–1) was introduced to help improve uniformity, reproducibility, and communication of patients' neurological conditions between different care providers. The routine use of the GCS allows stratification of patients for initial therapy. The GCS measures the patient's consciousness in three separate components. They are scored for their eye opening response, their verbal response, and their motor response, with a minimum score of 3 and maximum of 15. The patient is awarded the best score possible for each category. For example, a patient who is a new paraplegic but can follow commands with their arms is given a score of 6 on the motor scale (not a 1 because he does not move his legs). A low score for the motor component of the GCS has been identified as the most important predictor of poor outcome.

The pupillary examination is an essential component of the initial examination for all trauma patients. Detection of pupil asymmetry, dilation or loss of light reflex in an unconscious patient is concerning for ipsilateral intracranial pressure increase. The mass effect of intracranial injuries increases the intracranial pressure, and this is reflected by compression of the cranial nerves and pupillary changes. Patients who have concerns for intracranial injury and have unequal or nonreactive pupils should have rapid lowering of their ICP.

The type of injury seen on the CT scan appears to indicate the likelihood of poor outcome. Direct lacerations of epidural arteries produce epidural hematomas, while the disruption of bridging subdural veins causes subdural hematomas. Intracerebral contusions are most likely the result of tissue disruption from the direct force of the injury. Contre-coup injuries are common and can be the more severely injured side. A subarachnoid hemorrhage has been reported to double the mortality. Conversely, an epidural hematoma is associated with a better outcome, and good outcomes are heavily dependent on early recognition and evacuation of the hematoma. The brain damage caused by an epidural hematoma is mostly produced by compression, instead of intrinsic brain injury. Early relief of this pressure likely results in full recovery for most patients. Diffuse axonal injury (DAI) may not be seen on initial CT scan but often results in poor long-term outcome. Small punctate lesions seen on initial CT scan may hint toward DAI, but MRI is the definitive imaging for diagnosis. The MRI for diagnosis of DAI does not need to be done in the early treatment stages. CT findings can also correlate with increased intracranial pressures. The loss or compression of the basilar cisterns can occur from the elevated ICP and is a predictor of poor outcome. With improved transport and rapid access to CT scans, there is new risk for underestimating early intracranial injuries seen on the initial CT scan. Therefore, any patient with TBI who has intracranial pathology should have an early (4-6 hours) follow-up CT image and early neurosurgical consultation.

Supportive Strategies for Severe Brain Injuries and Intracranial Hypertension

Aggressive restoration of intravascular volume, maintenance of adequate CPP, and avoidance of hypoxia are the primary endpoints in the supportive therapy for patients with intracranial hypertension. There are several different therapies and maneuvers that can be utilized to achieve these goals. Cerebrospinal fluid drainage, controlled hyperventilation, mannitol, hypertonic saline, and barbiturates are among the most commonly used therapies to alleviate intracranial hypertension. Maneuvers directed at improving cerebral perfusion requires that patients have appropriate continuous monitoring with intracranial pressure monitors, central venous catheters (CVP monitoring), and arterial lines (MAP monitoring). Patients with increased intracranial pressures should be positioned to optimize venous drainage from the brain; this can be accomplished with elevation of the head of the bed and positioning the head in a neutral, midline position.

The monitoring of ICP is essential for all patients with severe head injury. The concern for herniation from elevated ICP is the impetus for placement of ICP monitoring. The range for when to treat elevated ICP is not as clear, but interventions are usually recommended at ICPs greater than 20 to 25 mm Hg. Increased intracranial pressure may have a direct injurious effect on the brain tissue, but the greatest harm associated with increased ICP is the increase in resistance to cerebral blood flow, which produces additional secondary brain injury.

Maintaining adequate blood flow to the brain is important treatment therapy, but it is not as easy as it would seem. Under normal circumstances, cerebral pressure autoregulation maintains a stable cerebral blood flow (CBF) over a wide range of CPP (approximately 50-150 mm Hg). However, this zone of autoregulation is disrupted in patients with TBIs, resulting in an increased reliance on raised MAP to maintain sufficient cerebral perfusion. Previously, a CPP of greater than 70 mm Hg was the goal for patients with TBI. However, data from the National Institutes of Health (NIH) sponsored North American Brain Injury Study on Hypothermia suggested that transient decreases in CPP <60 mm Hg was not associated with worse outcome than CPP >60 mm Hg. The recent data seem to question the utility of maintaining the MAP artificially high to improve CPP, and this practice in fact may increase the duration of intracranial hypertension. It appears that attention to CPP is important though the best strategy for management is not clear. However, it is accepted that routinely artificially driving the CPP to values above 60 mm Hg is not associated with improved outcome and is not currently recommended.

As it is the support of the metabolism of the cells and not necessarily the total blood flow that is important, methods have been introduced to monitor cerebral cellular metabolism. The two cerebral perfusion monitoring methods are the oxygen saturation in the internal jugular vein ($JVSo_2$) and the tissue oxygen tension in the brain ($Ptio_2$). These methods have obvious limitations. The $JVSo_2$ is a measurement of entire brain oxygen utilization, which may not help when there is a focal lesion. Conversely, the brain tissue oxygenation measures only focal area of tissue and may not be representative of other areas of injury. Currently, no device can be singled out as an ideal monitor.

Avoidance of hypotensive episodes is important and is accomplished by use of plasma expansion (crystalloids, colloids, blood products) and vasopressors. It is important to recognize that while patients with TBI may have hypotension as a result of their TBI, this is an uncommon occurrence; therefore, any hypotension in a patient with a TBI should be considered to be hypovolemic in nature. The achievement of euvolemia is necessary prior to the addition of vasopressors, as the constriction of cerebral blood vessels in a hypovolemic patient can contribute to worsening ischemia. Crystalloid administration is best accomplished by use of normal saline. This is different from patients who need volume resuscitation as the result of hemorrhage. The normal saline can aid in expanding the intravascular volume and is associated with less brain tissue swelling than with the use of lactated Ringers or other hypotonic solutions. For similar reason, fluids containing dextrose and water should not be given to patients with TBI, as the free water may infuse into the brain tissue and thereby increase brain swelling. Vasopressor use usually involves an α-agonist that has focused activity on the vasculature. Treatment of hypertension is rarely indicated in the patient with head injury. There is no evidence that hypertension promotes continued intracranial hemorrhage.

Patients with severe brain injury (GCS <8) require early intubation for protection of their airway. This also allows for the provision of increased oxygen administration to reduce hypoxia. Additionally, the minute ventilation can be controlled and the patient can be **hyperventilated** to decrease the $Paco_2$ and thus cause vasoconstriction. This will decrease both the cerebral blood flow and cerebral blood volume. The decrease in blood volume can aid in the acute decrease in elevated ICP. Potential benefits of controlled hyperventilation are probably most prominent in the first 24 to 48 hours after injury, so hyperventilation to decrease ICP should be used with extreme caution and only for short periods of time. Thereafter, if intracranial hypertension persists, controlled hyperventilation to $Paco_2$ values of 30 to 35 mm Hg may be considered, but again for only short time periods. For the majority of individuals, controlled ventilation to maintain $Paco_2$ between 35 to 40 mm Hg is optimal.

Cerebral edema in patients with TBI can result from both direct cellular injuries from the traumatic event or later from vasogenic edema during the recovery phase. Currently, the strategies for removing cerebral edema are limited to osmotic agents, usually mannitol or hypertonic saline. **Mannitol increases the osmotic gradient and by Starling forces, draws fluid from the interstitial compartment of the brain into the plasma, thereby decreasing the brain volume and ICP.** Mannitol can have adverse consequences, as it is a potent diuretic and can significantly decrease the intravascular volume and consequently decrease the CBF. As such, it should only be given to patients who have documented euvolemia and ongoing continuous monitoring to avoid treatment-related hypotension. Hypertonic saline also creates a steep osmotic gradient to draw fluid into the vascular compartment; however, it is not a diuretic and can be used in patients with hypotension. The use of hypertonic saline is not widespread, likely due to the lack of robust literature supporting its efficacy.

Painful and noxious stimuli in patients with TBI can contribute to an increase in ICP. Adequate pain control and sedation is critical when caring for these patients. However, the use of such agents can limit the neurologic examination; therefore, short-acting agents are preferred. Barbiturate comas have also been utilized to aid in the decrease of cerebral metabolism, but these should be limited to situations where sedation alone is insufficient to maintain patient comfort. Neuromuscular blockade may be added if further ICP control is needed, but again, it interferes with the ability for neurological examination.

Factors Contributing to Secondary Brain Injury

Secondary brain injury refers to the injurious events that occur after the initial injury. Other than public safety intervention measures (ie, requirement of helmet wearing, etc.), there is little that can be done to prevent the primary injury. It is the severity of the secondary insult that often determines the overall outcome of patients with TBI and as such has become the major goal in the treatment of patients with TBI. The two factors that are most injurious are hypotension and hypoxia. Another significant factor that can contribute to secondary brain injury is secondary hemorrhage, often referred to as "blossoming" of the initial hemorrhage.

The pathophysiology behind the cause of secondary injury lies within a variety of biochemical processes and injury to the "supporting cells" in the brain, including microglia, astrocytes, oligodendrocytes, and endothelial cells that are critical to the survival of neurons. The goal of the numerous clinical trials involving treatment of patients with brain trauma with various pharmacologic agents is to determine means by which these processes may be mitigated. However, to date, there has been limited success demonstrated in these investigations.

With a lack of pharmacologic interventions that can be used to prevent or reverse secondary injury, the primary goals are to minimize hypotension and hypoxia. **A single episode of systolic blood pressure of ≤90 mm Hg that occurs during the period from injury through resuscitation doubles the mortality and significantly increases the morbidity of TBI patients.** This reinforces the priority of avoiding hypovolemia and early consideration for vasopressor initiation when hypotension is refractory to fluid management.

Hypoxia is also known as a significant contributor to poor outcomes in patients with TBI. The incidence of hypoxic episodes has decreased with the practice of early intubation and mechanical ventilatory support. The avoidance of decreased oxygen carrying capacity (anemia) is often cited in the literature as a need to maintain a hematocrit of above 30. Currently, this level of hematocrit is not substantiated by the literature, and the adverse effects of blood transfusions are well known. However, it is generally accepted that patients with TBI should avoid significant anemia, and the need for transfusion is left to the judgment of individual critical care provider.

Secondary hemorrhage is certainly one of the most devastating forms of secondary injury. The additional blood volume increases the mass effect and ICP, limiting the ability to maintain adequate CBF. Additionally, the increased bleeding initiates oxidative stress, inflammation, and edema resulting in cell death. Reducing secondary hemorrhage after CNS trauma may have profound effects on overall outcome.

Monitoring the patient's coagulation status, especially in those who have undergone significant blood transfusions, is critical since coagulopathies will contribute to further bleeding and increased mass effects.

Another important source of secondary injury is continued fever. It is not clear as to how or why continued fever increases secondary brain injury, but it is thought that the increased metabolic requirement of the cells is the cause. Patients with severe brain injuries and fevers should be treated aggressively with medications and mechanical cooling devices to reduce their core temperatures.

> ## CASE CORRELATION
>
> - See also Case 17 (Meningitis/Encephalitis), Case 28 (Blunt Trauma), and Case 32 (Stroke).

COMPREHENSION QUESTIONS

27.1 An 18-year-old man was riding his motorcycle when he crashes into a light pole. On presentation to the trauma bay, his eyes are open to pain, he is mumbling, and he has flexor posturing. What is his GCS?

A. 6

B. 10

C. 9

D. 8

E. 7

27.2 A 35-year-old woman is the passenger in a car involved in roll over. When she arrives at the trauma bay, her GCS is 5 (E1, V1, M3), and she is intubated. She is hypotensive with a systolic blood pressure of 80 mm Hg that is not responsive to fluid resuscitation. Her FAST shows free fluid in the abdomen. The initial management should be:

A. Immediately place a ventriculostomy in the trauma bay.

B. Take the patient to the CT scanner to image her brain and cervical spine.

C. Take the patient immediately to the operating room.

D. Admit to the ICU, start fluid boluses and blood transfusions.

E. Take patient to the angiography suite for aortic angiography and embolization.

27.3 A 21-year-old man had a bicycle crash with subsequent intracerebral hemorrhage and ventriculostomy placement. Later that day, his ICP rises to 35 mm Hg, and he is given 100 g of mannitol. Over the next hour, his blood pressure decreases from 120/80 mm Hg to 90/60 mm Hg. The most likely cause of his hypotension is:

   A. Increased intracerebral pressure

   B. New intracranial bleeding

   C. Spinal shock

   D. Decreased intravascular volume

   E. Myocardial depression

27.4 A 19-year-old man is hit in the head with a baseball bat and is brought to the hospital by his friends 5 minutes after being assaulted. His GCS is 10 and blood pressure is 150/90 mm Hg. He has a CT scan of his brain, which shows a small area with intraparenchymal hemorrhage (~3 cm in diameter). He is taken to the ICU for monitoring. His treatment should include which of the following?

   A. Mannitol administration, repeat CT scan in 24 to 48 hours, and monitoring on the ward

   B. Ventriculostomy placement and admission to the ICU for monitoring

   C. Intubation, fluid administration, vasopressors, and repeat CT in 6 hours

   D. Admission to the ICU for monitoring and repeat CT in 6 hours

   E. Emergent craniectomy and evacuation of the intracerebral hematoma

ANSWERS

27.1 **E.** His GCS is 7. Using the Glasgow coma scale, he receives 2 points for opening his eyes to pain, 2 points for incoherent speech, and 3 points for flexor posturing.

27.2 **C.** This patient was involved in a significant trauma and presents to the trauma bay with a decreased GCS. She is intubated for airway protection. She is receiving fluid for her hypotension, but it does not respond to fluid administration and her FAST examination shows that there is free fluid in the abdomen. The two most injurious events in a patient with a TBI are hypotension and hypoxia. It appears that the patient has continued bleeding in her abdomen as seen by free fluid in the abdomen and a blood pressure that does not respond to fluids. **The key issue in this case is severe hypotension despite IV fluids, most likely due to ongoing intra-abdominal bleeding. The surgical team will need to be prepared for a multitude of possible causes for hemorrhage with the appropriate consultants on stand-by.** Controlling the bleeding in the operating room is the best method to decrease the likelihood of hypotensive episodes.

27.3 **D.** Mannitol works to decrease cerebral edema by increasing the osmotic gradient from brain tissue to the plasma, thereby drawing the fluid out of the brain tissue. However, mannitol also acts as a significant diuretic and can deplete the total intravascular volume. This can lead to hypotension and increase the risk of secondary brain injury. It should only be used in patients who are known to be euvolemic.

27.4 **D.** This patient has a moderate head injury as indicated by his GCS. He has a small intraparenchymal bleed, but because of his rapid presentation to the emergency department, this bleed may "blossom" later. His injury is not severe enough at the moment to warrant intubation, ventriculostomy placement, vasopressors, or surgical decompression. However, because of the risk of increased bleeding, he does need to be monitored in the ICU with frequent neurologic examinations and a repeat head CT in about 6 hours.

CLINICAL PEARLS

▶ Early supportive therapy in patients with TBI includes restoration of intravascular volume, maintenance of adequate cerebral perfusion pressure, and avoidance of hypoxia.

▶ Hypotension in a patient with TBI should be considered to be hypovolemic first, and efforts should concentrate on identifying and correcting the source of hypovolemia.

▶ Reducing the ICP can be accomplished with elevation of the head of bed, neutral head position, osmotic diuresis, and brief hyperventilation.

▶ Reduction of secondary brain injury is the primary goal in treating patients with TBI.

REFERENCES

Clifton GL, Drever P, Valadka A, Zygun D, Okonkwo D. Multicenter trial of early hypothermia in severe brain injury. *J Neurotrauma*. 2009 Mar;26(3):393-397.

Mariano GS, Fink ME, Hoffman C, Rosengart A. Intracranial pressure: monitoring and management. In: Hall JB, Schmidt GA, Kress JP, eds. *Principles of Critical Care*. 4th ed. New York, NY: McGraw Hill Education; 2015:786-820.

Oropello JM, Mistry N, Ullman JS. Head injury. In: Hall JB, Schmidt GA, Kress JP, eds. *Principles of Critical Care*. 4th ed. New York, NY: McGraw Hill Education; 2015:1121-1137.

Weingart JD. The management of traumatic brain injury. In: Cameron JL, Cameron AM, eds. *Current Surgical Therapy*. 11th ed. Philadelphia, PA: Elsevier Saunders; 2014:1001-1005.

A 48-year-old man was an unrestrained driver who fell asleep at the wheel while driving on a highway. His car struck the highway divider, resulting in vehicle roll-over and ejection of the patient from the vehicle. He was evaluated in the emergency department (ED), and various injuries were identified by CT imaging. The patient had bi-frontal cerebral contusions, facial fractures, left-sided rib fractures, left pulmonary contusion, non-displaced bilateral pubic rami fracture, left mid-shaft femur fracture, and a grade II splenic laceration. In the ED, the patient received 2 L of crystalloid and had a blood pressure of 100/80 mm Hg, pulse of 98 beats/min, respiratory rate of 24 breaths/min, and Glasgow coma scale (GCS) of 13. He is transferred to the ICU for monitoring and further care.

▶ How should this patient be monitored?
▶ What are the priorities in the management of this patient?

ANSWERS TO CASE 28:
Blunt Trauma

Summary: A 48-year-old man has been in a high-speed motor vehicle collision sustaining blunt mechanism polytrauma. His injuries include traumatic brain injury, pulmonary contusion with multiple rib fractures, pelvic fracture, grade II splenic laceration, and a femur fracture. He is hemodynamically stable with a GCS of 13 and is now in the ICU.

- **Monitoring:** This patient will need to be monitored for signs of deterioration in his pulmonary status, hemodynamic status, and neurological status. Pulse-oximetry will be helpful for continuous monitoring of oxygenation. Respiratory rate and respiratory effort are important to monitor given his pulmonary contusion and chest wall injuries. Hemodynamic monitoring with CVP catheters and/or intra-arterial pressure monitors, as well as serial hemoglobin and hematocrit measurements for evidence of continued blood loss from his multiple injuries, will be important during the initial 24 to 36 hours. Close follow-up of his neurological functions with serial GCS evaluation will be important to monitor his intracranial injury. In addition, a repeat brain CT 8 to 12 hours following the initial CT can be helpful.

- **Priorities in management from the organ standpoint:** Breathing concerns (chest wall and lungs) first, bleeding sources (spleen and pelvis) are next, followed by brain injury, and lastly non–life-threatening orthopedic injuries.

ANALYSIS

Objectives

1. Learn common injuries produced by blunt trauma.

2. Learn to prioritize and coordinate the management of patients with multiple injuries, including intra-abdominal injuries, blunt chest injuries, orthopedic injuries, and brain injuries.

3. Learn the criteria for the selection of nonoperative management of solid organ intra-abdominal injuries.

Considerations

This patient is a 48-year-old man who has been in a high energy mechanism motor vehicle crash, with significant mechanism for potential major injuries. He has undergone radiographic imaging, and his identified injuries include a brain injury, thoracic injuries, pelvic fracture, splenic laceration, and a femur fracture. He is currently in the ICU for observation of his head injury, optimization of his pulmonary status, and monitoring of potential bleeding from his splenic laceration and pelvic fracture. He is at risk for deterioration of his mental status secondary to his brain injury and/or from developing hemorrhagic shock due to splenic or pelvic hemorrhage. Additionally, his respiratory status may deteriorate, requiring potential intubation to maintain adequate oxygenation and ventilation.

Two factors have been consistently identified as leading to worse outcomes in head injury patients: **hypotension and hypoxemia.** It is imperative that these be prevented and/or addressed aggressively in this patient.

CLINICAL APPROACH

Common Injuries Produced by Blunt Injury

Blunt mechanism of injury is the most common type encountered in trauma patients. However, different types of blunt mechanisms produce different types of injuries. For example, high-speed motor vehicle crash, falls from a roof, and falls from standing all produce different injury patterns. Blunt trauma patients are often quite challenging to treat due to the fact that with a severe mechanism, multiple organ systems may be involved. In these patients, the prioritization of care is important to optimize outcomes.

Commonly affected organ systems in blunt trauma patients include the central nervous system (brain and spine), respiratory system (chest wall and lung), solid intra-abdominal organs (liver and spleen), gastrointestinal system (intestines and the mesentery), urologic system (kidneys and bladder), and musculoskeletal system (long bone and bony pelvis).

Central nervous system injuries will include skull fractures and brain injuries. The main issue with skull fractures is that there is often underlying associated brain injury. Brain injuries include cerebral contusion/hematoma, epidural hematoma, subdural hematoma, and subarachnoid hemorrhage. These injuries clinically manifest as altered mental status (confusion) or depressed level of consciousness as reflected in a decreased GCS score. A brain injury or skull fracture mandates neurosurgical consultation, although the majority of these injuries are treated by observation and serial neurological examinations.

Respiratory system injuries include rib fractures, pulmonary contusion, pneumothorax, and hemothorax. Rib fractures contribute to significant morbidity and even mortality, particularly with two or more fractures and/or patients over the age of 45. Rib fractures cause significant pain that can lead to splinted respirations and compromised inspiratory effort. The sequelae of this may be pneumonia and respiratory failure requiring mechanical ventilatory support, which carries its own set of complications. The most common cause of a pulmonary contusion is a significant deceleration force, leading to direct impact of the lung parenchyma against the chest wall. The contused lung does not exchange gas effectively but is still perfused, leading to a physiological shunt and hypoxemia. **Unfortunately, pulmonary contusions often worsen post injury secondary to the sequestration of intravenous fluids within the injured lung parenchyma.** Pneumothorax may occur as a result of a bone fragment from a broken rib lacerating the pulmonary parenchyma, causing air to accumulate in the pleural space. At its extreme it may lead to enough air occupying the thorax that the mediastinum shifts and impedes venous return to the heart. This may result in circulatory collapse and is termed "tension pneumothorax."

Prompt recognition and treatment with tube thoracostomy is a life-saving procedure in these patients. Hemothorax is the result of bleeding into the pleural space, most often from the chest wall or lung parenchyma. Besides the risk of exsanguination, accumulated blood in the thorax may lead to late infection, resulting in empyema and sepsis that would require operative drainage.

Solid abdominal organ injuries (liver and spleen) are associated with hemorrhagic risks during the initial hours and up to 1 to 2 days post-injury. Intervention in the form of angiography/embolization or operations may be necessary to control hemorrhage. Most clinically significant bleeding will be manifested as drops in blood pressure or hemoglobin and hematocrit within the first 24 hours following the injury. Patients with severe liver injuries may develop bile leaks; these patients may present with bile peritonitis, which may be amenable to nonoperative treatments such as CT-guided drain placement and biliary decompression by ERCP with endoscopic stent placement.

One of the more recent trends in the management of blunt trauma patients with visible "blushes" in the liver or spleen seen on CT scans is prophylactic embolization to prevent on-going bleeding. This practice has evolved in many centers with the development of better micro-embolization techniques and with greater availability of expertise.

Hollow viscus injury may result in the development of peritonitis if enteric contents irritate the peritoneal cavity. Clinically, the patients will often exhibit a hyperdynamic picture associated with leukocytosis. This will result in a profound inflammatory/septic response and requires operation and possible bowel resection for therapy. Mesenteric injuries may result in exsanguinating hemorrhage or bowel ischemia with delayed presentation of peritonitis. These injuries are best treated operatively.

Renal injuries from a blunt mechanism may result in parenchymal laceration or renovascular injuries. Renal lacerations result in hemorrhage and perinephric hematoma. In extremely rare circumstances, particularly if the renal pelvis is involved, these injuries may result in the development of an urinoma and sepsis, which would require drainage either operatively or percutaneously. Renovascular injuries occur as a result of the kidney's retroperitoneal location. The forces involved in a high energy mechanism in effect cause a "stretch" of the renal artery from its origin at the aorta. This causes an intimal injury to the renal artery which will lead to renal artery thrombosis and renal ischemia. Unfortunately, success with revascularization of the kidney following blunt traumatic injury has been extremely limited. An ischemic kidney may result in the development of persistent hypertension or chronic flank pain requiring subsequent nephrectomy.

Pelvic fractures can result in life-threatening hemorrhage. The pelvis can be thought of as a "ring." When this ring is disrupted by fracture, two potential problems may develop. First, the pelvis is well vascularized, so hemorrhage from veins and arteries may develop. Additionally, the disrupted "ring" leads to an increase in pelvic volume. As a result, hemorrhage can occur unimpeded since there is no tamponade effect normally present with an intact pelvic ring. Additionally, bone fragments from the pelvis may lacerate pelvic organs such as the rectum, the vagina, and the urethra. Pelvic fractures in and of themselves may be fatal, and unfortunately they are frequently associated with other life-threatening injuries.

Management of Patients with Multiple Injuries

Mortality from trauma demonstrates a temporal relationship. Immediate deaths generally occur from devastating brain injury or massive exsanguination from aortic ruptures. Fatality that occurs in minutes may be a result of airway issues, overwhelming brain injury, or hemorrhage. Fatality that occurs from a few hours up to the first two days after injury is often caused by hemorrhage or from sequelae of traumatic brain injury. Mortality that occurs after the initial week is usually due to multi-system organ dysfunction or sepsis/infection. As a result, the key to triaging injury is recognizing this temporal pattern of mortality. These principles guide the Advanced Trauma Life Support guidelines for resuscitation. In brief, these principles are:

A-Airway

B-Breathing

C-Circulation

D-Disability

E-Exposure/Environment

Inability to maintain the airway leads to rapid demise of the patient. Airway problems are most often due to inability of the patient to protect his/her airway secondary to diminished level of consciousness due to brain injury or shock. If a patient is not alert or responsive, it is important that the airway is secured, ideally via orotracheal intubation. This is the first priority in trauma patients with a blunt mechanism. In the scenario described, the patient has a GCS of 13, which implies adequate mentation/sensorium to protect his airway. As a result, he does not require emergent intubation in the ER or in the ICU. If, however, his condition deteriorates, there should be no hesitation in establishing a definitive airway. A GCS of 8 or less is defined as coma and would mandate intubation for securing an airway.

Patients with GCS >9 who are believed to have intact airways can be monitored without intubation in the ICU with frequent neuro/mental status checks. If the patient's mental status worsens as represented by a decrease in GCS, it would be appropriate to notify the neurosurgical consultant and obtain a repeat head CT to evaluate for possible progression of brain injury (see Figure 28-1). Additionally, if the GCS drops significantly, it would be prudent to intubate the patient urgently in order to prevent hypoxia from an inability to maintain an airway secondary to diminished consciousness.

If, on presentation, the patient's GCS was 8 or less, a level II recommendation from the American Association of Neurological Surgeons suggests that intracranial pressure monitoring is warranted. This requires an invasive procedure performed by a neurosurgeon at the patient's bedside (Figure 28–1).

Patients with multiple rib fractures and pulmonary contusion need to undergo close observation, preferably with cardiac monitoring and pulse oximetry. Management of patients with significant pulmonary contusion can become more challenging when

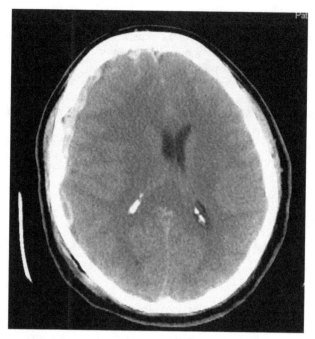

Figure 28–1. This brain CT demonstrates a subdural hemorrhage of the right side with midline shift. Hemorrhage on a non-contrast head CT is demonstrated by white density. (Used, with permission, from Javid Sadjadi, MD.).

associated with other injuries with a large amount of blood loss. This is because fluid and blood products administered to resuscitate the patient from hemorrhagic shock can aggravate the pulmonary contusion-related oxygenation defects. The process can be even further complicated if the patient also has a severe brain injury because any further hypoxic and hypotensive insult will cause secondary brain injuries and worsen the neurologic outcome. Awareness of these complications is important to help balance the resuscitation of patients with multi-system trauma.

Splenic injuries cause concerns for further bleeding. A computed tomography (CT) scan scale for grading splenic injuries has been developed (Table 28–1). The majority of splenic injuries may be observed. The presence of the following indicates risk of failure of nonoperative management:

1. Lower hematocrit at admission

2. Lower blood pressure at admission

3. Higher CT grade of injury

4. Higher injury severity score

5. Lower Glasgow coma scale

6. Larger volume of hemoperitoneum

Table 28–1 • SPLENIC INJURY CLASSIFICATION		
Grade	Hematoma	Laceration
I	Subcapsular; <10% area	Capsular tear; <1 cm, nonbleeding
II	Subcapsular; 10%-50% area	Intraparenchymal; 1-3 cm in diameter >3 cm or involving trabecular vessels
III	Subcapsular >50% area Intraparenchymal >2 cm	>3 cm or involving trabecular vessels
IV	Ruptured hematoma with active bleeding	Hilar vessel or segmental vessel involvement, or >25% devascularization of spleen
V	Completely shattered	Devascularization

Data from retrospective reviews has suggested that the addition of angioembolization may lead to increased rates of successful nonoperative management of spleen injuries.

Pelvic fractures may also lead to clinically significant hemorrhage. The disruption of the bony ring causes injury to the venous plexus of the pelvis and also to the branches of the internal iliac artery. Additionally, bleeding occurs from the fractured bone edges themselves. Bleeding is most pronounced in pubic rami and symphysis fractures. Acetabular and iliac wing fractures tend not to bleed but may result in early onset osteoarthritis. Pelvic hemorrhage can most often be controlled by placing a pelvic binder, which reduces the potential volume bleeding that can occur and can help reduce pelvic bleeding. If a binder does not control the hemorrhage as demonstrated by continued hemodynamic instability, hemorrhage may be controlled by angiography with embolization and preperitoneal pelvic packing performed in the operating room (Figure 28–2).

Femur fractures may result in bleeding of up to 1 L within the soft tissue in the thigh. However, it may be unwise to perform early definitive operative fixation of most patients' femur fractures until it is clear that there are no immediately

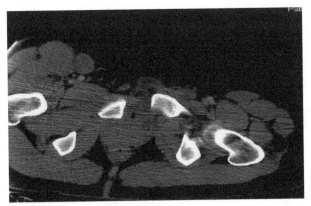

Figure 28–2. The image demonstrates an "open book" pelvic fracture with disruption of the pubic symphysis. This injury is prone to bleeding and requires binder placement. (Used, with permission, from Javid Sadjadi, MD.).

life-threatening issues from solid organ or brain injuries. Most orthopedic traumatologists will apply damage control orthopedic surgery for patients with multiple blunt trauma. An example of this practice is to realign a patient's femur to control hemorrhage and reduce pulmonary complications by placing a Steinman pin and traction at the bedside. This weighted traction would reduce his femur fracture to length until the patient's physiologic status is optimized prior to definitive operative femur fixation.

In summary, patients with multiple blunt traumatic injuries from high-energy mechanisms are best managed by being monitored in the ICU. Prioritization of the management of various injuries is essential to optimize outcome. The intensive care provider must communicate and coordinate care for these patients to optimize outcome.

Criteria for the Selection of Nonoperative Management of Solid Organ Intra-Abdominal Injuries

The management of spleen and liver injuries in blunt trauma patients has shifted toward a nonoperative paradigm. The focused abdominal sonogram for trauma (FAST) has changed the method of diagnosis of intraperitoneal hemorrhage following blunt trauma. Traditionally, physical examination and the invasive adjunct of diagnostic peritoneal lavage were the main tools used to diagnose intra-abdominal hemorrhage. The FAST examination is noninvasive, rapid and can readily identify intra-abdominal free fluid, which in a hemodynamically unstable patient is presumed to be blood and mandates an operative exploration.

If a patient is hemodynamically stable, the next step even with a positive FAST examination is CT of the abdomen/pelvis. This allows the physician to identify injuries and plan therapy.

A large multicenter database review identified several risk factors for failed nonoperative spleen injury management. These risk factors were:

1. Increased age

2. Increased injury severity score

3. Decreased hematocrit

4. Increased grade of injury

5. Increased amount of hemoperitoneum

Additionally, the study identified the following probabilities of failed nonoperative management by the grades of injury (Table 28–2).

Table 28–2 • GRADE OF SPLENIC INJURY AND NEED FOR SPLENECTOMY	
Grade	% Requiring Splenectomy
I	4.8
II	9.5
III	19.6
IV	33.7
V	75

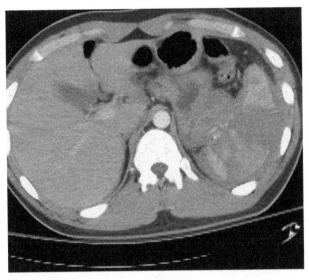

Figure 28–3. The image above demonstrates a Grade IV spleen injury with two large fractures affecting the splenic hilum with a small vascular blush and some hemoperitoneum. This patient was successfully treated nonoperatively with angioembolization. (Used, with permission, from Javid Sadjadi, MD.).

Any development of hemodynamic instability mandates exploration and likely splenectomy.

Liver lacerations can behave somewhat differently then spleen lacerations. Patients who present with CT-demonstrated blunt hepatic injury and are hemodynamically stable rarely require operative treatments. The necessity of operation for blunt liver injury is dictated by clinical findings, not radiographic findings (Figure 28–3). Some patients with a "blush" demonstrated by CT can benefit from angioembolization.

CASE CORRELATION

- See also Case 27 (Traumatic brain injury) and Case 29 (Trauma and Burns).

COMPREHENSION QUESTIONS

28.1 Which of the following patients may benefit from placement of an intracranial pressure monitor?

A. A 24-year-old man who fell from 10 ft and presented with a GCS of 7 but a normal head CT scan

B. A 28-year-old man involved in a high-speed motor vehicle collision with a GCS of 8 who is receiving propofol and has a right-sided subdural hematoma

C. A 19-year-old woman who fell from standing and had a witnessed seizure but has a GCS of 9 and a small subarachnoid hemorrhage

D. An 82-year-old man who fell from his bed, is confused, and cannot move his left side

E. A 17-year-old teenager with an epidural hematoma based on CT and GCS of 15

28.2 A 35-year-old woman is in a high-speed motor vehicle crash. On presentation, she is complaining of abdominal pain. Her pulse is 136 beats/min, blood pressure is 76/40 mm Hg. A FAST examination is positive for fluid. The best next step is:

A. Intubation

B. CT scan of the abdomen/pelvis

C. Exploratory laparotomy

D. Admission to the intensive care unit

E. Mesenteric angiography and embolization of bleeding vessels

28.3 A 23-year-old man is involved in a 10 ft fall from a ladder. He complains of pelvic pain. On arrival his heart rate is 120 beats/min and blood pressure is 90/65 mm Hg. On examination he has ecchymoses of his buttocks. X-rays identify pelvic fracture with a widened pubic symphysis. FAST examination is normal. The best next step is:

A. Placement of pelvic binder in emergency room

B. Angiography

C. Exploratory laparotomy

D. CT of the abdomen/pelvis

E. Open reduction and internal fixation of the pelvis

28.4 A 47-year-old man with bi-frontal cerebral contusion, mandibular fracture, bilateral pulmonary contusion, splenic laceration, liver laceration associated with a "blush," and a right femur fracture is transported to the ICU following his initial evaluation. His pulse rate is 105 beats/min, blood pressure is 105/80 mm Hg, respiratory rate is 24 breaths/min, GCS is 11, and oxygen saturation is 94% on 2 L O_2 nasal cannula. Which of the following is the best management option?

A. Transfusion of PRBC and FFP to maintain normal hemoglobin and coagulation profile

B. Angioembolization of the liver laceration associated with the "blush"

C. Early operative intramedullary rod placement for his femur fracture

D. Intubation and mechanical ventilation

E. Operative intervention for his liver injury and operative fixation of his femur

ANSWERS

28.1 **B.** Although there is insufficient data to make Level I recommendations, patient B does fulfill the criteria of the American Association of Neurological Surgeons for possible intracranial pressure monitoring. These criteria are: CT confirmed intracranial hemorrhage, GCS of 8 or less, and receiving sedation.

28.2 **C.** This scenario describes a patient who was involved in a high-speed motor vehicle collision and is hemodynamically unstable. Her FAST examination is positive, suggesting intra-abdominal hemorrhage. She requires exploratory laparotomy. Bleeding takes priority in this instance, as without control of hemorrhage she is likely to die; she is already hemodynamically unstable, suggesting that she is in Class IV shock. Angiography and embolization are options for relatively stable patients with solid organ injuries, and early embolization can help avoid surgical interventions in some of the patients. If this patient stabilizes with resuscitation and a CT demonstrates such injuries, then angiography and embolization can be viable options.

28.3 **A.** This patient has a pelvic fracture with a pattern known to result in bleeding. Additionally, he is hemodynamically unstable. A normal FAST examination has ruled out intra-abdominal hemorrhage. It must be assumed that his hemodynamic instability is secondary to bleeding from his pelvic fracture. The first step is to place a pelvic binder to reduce the potential pelvic space where bleeding can occur. If his hemodynamic status improves, he would not need angiography. If he continues to deteriorate despite placement of the binder and transfusion, he would next require angiography and possible embolization of branches of the internal iliac artery that may be bleeding.

28.4 **B.** This patient has a TBI, bilateral pulmonary contusions, liver injury with a "blush," and femur fracture. He is hemodynamically stable with these injuries. Of all the choices listed, the most appropriate treatment is angioembolization of the liver injury. This approach may stop the active bleeding and minimize fluid/blood product administration, which can worsen his oxygenation from the pulmonary contusions. Worsening of the pulmonary contusion can lead to intubation, which may make it more difficult to monitor his neurologic status. In addition, positive pressure ventilation can worsen his pulmonary contusions.

CLINICAL PEARLS

▶ Patients who have suffered blunt polytrauma can have multiple potentially lethal injuries. It is the physician's responsibility to triage the patient's injuries.

▶ The great majority of mild head injuries (GCS 13-15) can be monitored and do not require intervention.

▶ A positive FAST examination in a hypotensive patient mandates exploration.

▶ Several radiographic findings can help predict success of nonoperative management of spleen injuries.

▶ Liver injury management (operative versus nonoperative) is dictated by the patient's clinical status.

REFERENCES

Ali J. Priorities in multisystem trauma. In: Hall JB, Schmidt GA, Kress JP, eds. *Principles of Critical Care.* 4th ed. New York, NY. McGraw Hill Education; 2015:1116-1121.

Bratton SL, Chestnut RM, Ghajar J, et al. Guidelines for the management of severe traumatic brain injury. VI. Indications for intracranial pressure monitoring. *J Neurotrauma.* 2007;24 Suppl 1: S37-S44.

Moore EE, et al. Organ injury scaling: spleen and liver (1994 revision). *J Trauma.* 1995;38:323-324.

Peitzman AB, et al. Blunt splenic injury in adults: multi-institutional study of the Eastern Association for the Surgery of Trauma. *J Trauma.* 2000;49:177-189.

A 30-year-old man is admitted to the ICU. The patient is a fire fighter who was inside a burning building when the floor collapsed, causing him to fall into the basement. The patient was trapped under a large amount of debris and was rescued after approximately 35 minutes. On examination at the scene, he had a pulse of 112 beats/min, blood pressure of 90/70 mm Hg, and bilateral thigh deformities with accompanying soft tissue swelling. He has burn wounds involving the entire anterior chest and abdomen, as well as circumferential burns involving both upper arms. The burn wounds on his legs appear to extend down to the muscles. His Glasgow coma score (GCS) in the emergency center was 10, and the patient was intubated. His carboxyhemoglobin level was 27%. Dark, tea-colored urine returned after the insertion of the urinary catheter. A CT scan of the abdomen and pelvis was done and revealed a laceration of the liver with minimal amount of free fluid in the abdomen. Fracture of the right iliac crest was also noted.

▶ What are your priorities for this patient's care in the ICU?
▶ How do you manage his fluid resuscitation?
▶ What are measures that you would take to prevent organ injuries that may develop as a result of his burns?

ANSWERS TO CASE 29:

Trauma and Burns

Summary: This patient is a 30-year-old man with severe burns on his trunk and upper extremities in association with multiple other traumatic injuries. His presentation to the emergency department is consistent with shock and inhalation injury.

- **Priorities:** Orotracheal intubation to secure the airway. Place the patient on 100% oxygen to minimize injuries from his carbon monoxide inhalation. Large-bore secured intravenous access should be placed for ongoing fluid resuscitation and for central venous pressure monitoring. His thigh deformities likely indicate femur fractures that should be verified by x-rays, followed by reduction and stabilization. The burn wounds should be gently cleaned and covered with silver sulfadiazine and gauze dressing.

- **Fluid Resuscitation:** Initial fluid resuscitation can begin using either the Parkland formula or the modified Brooke formula. Endpoints of resuscitation include urine output >0.5 to 1.0 mL/kg/h and adequate central venous pressures. The initial fluid administration may need to be greater in this patient because of the other associated injuries (liver, pelvis, and long bones) and his myoglobinuria. Similarly, because of these potential bleeding sources, the patient's hemoglobin, hematocrit, coagulation profile, and platelet counts need to be closely monitored and normalized if necessary during the early resuscitation period.

- **Strategies to prevent organ injuries:** Large burns produce cardiac depression from circulating systemic inflammatory mediators. Pulmonary injuries may result from direct burn effects or acute lung injury (ALI), and acute kidney injury may develop as the result of insufficient fluid resuscitation and myoglobin-induced injuries. Primary prevention begins with timely and appropriate fluid resuscitation based on hemodynamic monitoring and responses to resuscitation (urine output, lactate, and base deficits). Early and timely wound management is also important in the prevention of distant organ dysfunction. For example, early burn wound excision has been demonstrated to produce fewer burn wound-associated septic complications and improved survival.

ANALYSIS

Objectives

1. Learn the management of thermal-related injuries (inhalation injuries, infections, acute kidney injuries, pain management, metabolic and nutritional support).

2. Learn to recognize and prioritize the care of burn patients with other associated injuries.

Considerations

This patient suffered from severe burn injuries as evidenced by the extent of his wounds, which involve the entire circumference of his trunk and upper extremities. Because he was trapped in a burning building for quite some time, he was exposed to the toxic byproducts of fire, mainly carbon monoxide and cyanide. Inhalation of these toxins, along with direct heat and the steam of the flames, can cause edema and severe damage to the airway. Hence, early intubation is warranted. The patient's carboxyhemoglobin (COHgb) of 27% is concerning and indicates significant carbon monoxide (CO) inhalation; COHgb levels of 30% are often associated with permanent central nervous system dysfunction, and COHgb levels greater than 60% often produce coma and death. Carbon monoxide has a 240-fold greater affinity for hemoglobin than oxygen; consequently, the half-life of CO in blood in room air is prolonged at 250 minutes. The half-life of COHgb can be reduced to 40 to 60 minutes by placing the patient on 100% O_2. This patient's history of having fallen several stories to the basement resulting in severe bone injuries and subsequent immobility is of concern for the occurrence of muscle degradation and rhabdomyolysis; therefore, precautions should be taken to identify and treat this potential complication.

In this patient with a pelvic fracture, bilateral femur abnormalities and a liver laceration, the associated injuries are critical. He needs diagnostic studies to ensure there is no active retroperitoneal bleeding (ie, angiography or CT angiography). Additionally, urgent orthopedics consultation is necessary for early skeletal stabilization. The grade of the liver laceration can be determined based on the CT findings, and serial hemoglobin and hematocrit levels can be helpful to determine if operative or angiographic interventions are needed.

CLINICAL APPROACH

Management of Thermal Injuries

Burns are a major cause of trauma in the United States, as over one million cases occur annually. Burn injuries can be produced by heat, chemicals, electricity or radiation, with thermal injuries being the most common. Thermal injuries are a significant cause of morbidity and mortality because of the profound inflammatory response generated both locally and systemically.

Skin Biology and Pathophysiology

The epidermis and dermis are two distinct layers which make up the skin. The epidermis is the outermost layer and has the unique responsibility of protecting the host from infection, fluid loss, and ultraviolet light. It is also the site of vitamin D absorption, and it provides much of our thermal regulation. It is derived from ectoderm and hence is capable of regeneration. In contrast, the dermis lies underneath the epidermis and provides the structural framework of skin. Collagen is the principal structural molecule found in this layer. It is the dermis that gives skin its durability and elasticity.

Burns can cause significant damage to the structure and function of the skin. Jackson's classification of the burn wound outlines the pathophysiology resulting from thermal injury. There are three physical zones of tissue injury resulting from a burn: the zone of coagulation, the zone of stasis, and the zone of hyperemia. The zone of coagulation is in the center and constitutes the most severely injured tissue. The cells in this zone are coagulated and necrotic. The zone of stasis is immediately beyond the zone of coagulation and is characterized by ischemia and vasoconstriction. The zone of stasis is important, as it oftentimes is initially viable but can progress to the zone of coagulation when exposed to severe edema and/or hypoperfusion (consequences of inappropriate initial fluid management and support of tissue perfusion). Beyond the zone of stasis is the zone of hyperemia. In this zone the tissue is viable but often involved in profound inflammatory changes from surrounding cells.

Clinical Assessment

A burn patient should be treated as would any other trauma patient, meaning the initial assessment should focus on the patient's airway, breathing, and circulatory systems. Assessment of the extent of the burns and other major injuries should also take place at this time. Inspection of the airway includes evaluation of the mouth, nose, oropharynx, and trachea. Facial burns, cinched nose hairs, the presence of soot, foamy oral secretions, and mucosal edema should alarm the provider of possible inhalation injury, and early intubation should take place. Additionally, labored breathing with shallow breaths, use of accessory muscles, stridor or diminished neurologic function also warrants intubation. A significant portion of initial deaths from fires occur secondary to hypoxia from oxygen deprivation or toxin inhalation.

Perhaps one of the biggest advances in managing severely burned patients is the use of early aggressive fluid resuscitation. The Parkland formula, named after the hospital in Dallas, Texas, is a guide to volume repletion. For adults with affected total body surface area (TBSA%) greater than 15 or children with affected TBSA% greater than 10, it is recommended that supportive care, continued monitoring, and aggressive fluid resuscitation be given. The Parkland formula calculates the amount of volume that should be given in a 24-hour period by measuring the affected (TBSA%) × (4 mL of lactated Ringers solution) × (weight of the patient in kilograms). Half of the calculated amount should be given in the first 8 hours following the injury, and the remaining half should be given in the subsequent 16 hours. This is only a guide for resuscitation and should be used in conjunction with other information (eg, urine output, central venous pressure, clinical response, etc.) to determine volume status. The modified Brooke formula is an alternative resuscitation approach using lactated Ringers at 2 mL/kg/% TBSA, with one-half given in the first 2 hours and second half in the subsequent 16 hours; for the next 24 hours, colloid is given at (0.3 to 0.5 mL/kg)/% TBSA burn + D_5W to maintain urine output >0.5 mL/kg/h.

Calculating TBSA can be tricky. Usually only second- and third-degree burns are included in estimating TBSA. Wallace's rule of nines is a way of estimating the extent of burn injury in adults. The body is divided into sections and given a percentage (a fraction or multiple of 9) of body surface area. In this schema the anterior chest, posterior chest, abdomen, buttocks, unilateral anterior lower extremities, unilateral posterior extremities, circumferential unilateral arm, and

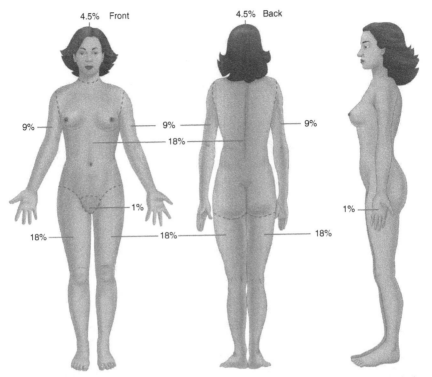

Figure 29–1. Rule of nines to estimate patient's burn size by dividing the body into regions in which the body total surface area can be calculated by multiples of nine. (Reproduced, with permission, from Brunicardi FC, Andersen DK, Billiar TR, et al. *Schwartz's Principles of Surgery.* 9th ed. New York: McGraw-Hill Education, 2010. Figure 8–1).

circumferential head each equal 9%. The perineum equals 1%. In total, the entire body is 100% (Figure 29–1). The rule of nines does not apply to children, as they are proportionately different from adults. Hence, an adaptation of the rule of nines estimates a larger surface area for the circumferential head and less for the extremities. In our patient, the calculated TBSA equals 36%.

Management of Burn Wounds

Determining the depth of the burn wound can provide some insight into the direction of management. First-degree burns are superficial and only involve the epidermis. They appear erythematous in color and do not have any blisters. Usually they heal within a few days but can take up to 2 weeks. Treatment usually is the application of a topical cream for barrier and symptom relief.

Partial thickness burns (formerly known as second-degree burns) extend beyond the epidermis and are further classified as superficial or deep. Superficial partial thickness burns are characterized by painful blisters, usually pink in color. Topical agents such as silver sulfadiazine can be used for management of these burns, which usually heal within 2 weeks without much residual impairment and

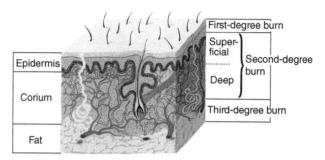

Figure 29–2. Layers of the skin showing depth of first-degree, second-degree, and third-degree burns. (Reproduced, with permission, from Doherty GM. *Current Diagnosis & Treatment: Surgery.* 13th ed, McGraw-Hill Education, 2010. Figure 14–1).

minimal scarring. On the other hand, deep partial thickness burns are dry, mottled, and variably painful. Silver sulfadiazine can also be used in their management; however, surgical excision and skin grafting may be necessary for wounds that do not heal within 3 weeks. Severe scarring, subsequent functional impairment and contracture are associated with chronic deep partial thickness burn wounds.

Third-degree burns are full-thickness burns that involve the entire epidermis and dermis. Usually this burn is painless, as the nerve endings have also been damaged. These burns appear white or black with eschar formation. Spontaneous healing of these wounds can only occur by contraction, since the precursors for skin regeneration have been damaged. Similarly, deep partial-thickness burns have limited regenerative capacity, where spontaneous regeneration is usually prolonged. Therefore, full-thickness and deep partial-thickness burns usually benefit from operative interventions with surgical excision and skin grafting for optimal functional outcomes. Early excision of devitalized tissue also reduces the local and systemic effects of inflammatory mediators (Figure 29–2).

Multiple Organ Dysfunction Syndrome After Burns

Due to the profound local and systemic inflammatory response from thermal injury, nearly every organ system has the potential to be compromised following a severe burn. In the immediate post-injury period, the neurologic, pulmonary, and cardiovascular systems are most commonly affected. Neurologically, burn victims can have a decline in their level of alertness for a number of reasons including hypoxia, inhalation of toxins, and associated traumatic head injuries. Supplemental oxygen should be given immediately. A low GCS warrants endotracheal intubation and mechanical ventilation. In patients who are alert, it is important to be aware that superficial and partial thickness burns can cause excruciating pain and warrant careful and continuous dosing of analgesics.

A substantial percentage of severe burns is associated with inhalation injury. Direct heat and steam can cause damage to the upper and lower airways and cause significant swelling leading to airway obstruction. Carbon monoxide and hydrogen cyanide are the byproducts of fires, and these toxins lead to inflammation and pulmonary edema that prevent adequate gas exchange. Hence, early intubation and mechanical ventilation should be considered. Carbon monoxide levels should be checked, and consideration for hyperbaric oxygen therapy should be given for patients with a CO% greater than 25. In the ICU, regular tracheobronchial care (ie, deep suctioning, therapeutic bronchoscopy, use of adjuvant pharmacologic agents such as bronchodilators or N-acetylcysteine) should be provided.

Cardiovascular collapse following severe burn injury is usually caused by volume depletion from fluid loss after skin disruption and vasodilation from local and systemic inflammatory mediator releases. To combat hypovolemia, aggressive fluid resuscitation should be initiated in the emergency department and continued in the ICU. The Parkland formula provides an initial guideline for fluid resuscitation. In the ICU, continued measurements of urine output and central venous pressure should be used to determine the patient's response to fluid management. Often, the initial fluid resuscitation plans need to be adjusted to minimize the effects of under- or over-resuscitation.

One of the most devastating conditions associated with extensive burns is burn wound sepsis. Burn injuries disrupt the skin's protective barrier which, in turn, renders the host susceptible to burn wound infections. Severe thermal injuries induce a relative immunocompromised state that can lead to sepsis. Initially, burn wounds are sterile but quickly become colonized with indigenous skin flora such as *Staphylococcus*. The wounds can become subsequently colonized with gram-positive and gram-negative organisms, yeasts from the host oral-digestive flora, and contaminations from healthcare workers and the hospital environment. *Pseudomonas aeruginosa* is a common organism found in burn wounds in many U.S. hospitals. The application of digestive tract decontamination reduces hosts' GI tract colonization and has been shown to reduce the occurrence of burn wound sepsis in the ICU setting.

The metabolic demands are significantly increased after thermal injury. For severe burn patients (>20% TBSA injured), early nutritional support is critical, with the nitrogen repletion and the maintenance of nitrogen balance being the most critical aspect of therapy. Early enteral nutritional support in this patient population is associated with improved maintenance of gastrointestinal tract, physiological and immunological functions, decreased burn wound sepsis, and decreased hospital length of stay. Nutritional goals should include a high-protein diet with considerations for supplemental glutamine. Daily protein intake should be in the range of 1.5 to 2.0 g/kg/d. Avoidance of hyperglycemia is critical for minimizing infectious complications. Daily weight measurements with weekly assessment of pre-albumin levels are helpful for the determination of response and for guiding nutritional planning. Nutritional strategies are optimal when a multidisciplinary team approach is taken, including inputs from nutritionists.

MANAGING ASSOCIATED INJURIES

Burn victims oftentimes have associated traumatic injuries which can be life-threatening or compromise functional outcomes if not identified and treated in a timely manner. Burn victims should be treated as any other trauma patient. The initial assessment should begin with the ABCs of trauma but should be followed by a comprehensive secondary survey to identify other potential injuries. Radiographic imaging, such as x-rays, CT scans, and ultrasounds are useful diagnostic tools.

Severe thermal injuries are often associated with immobility and subsequent muscle degradation. The renal system can be affected by hypovolemia from capillary leak as a result of a profound systemic inflammatory response, and it can also be affected secondary to rhabdomyolysis. Urine output measurements are important in the monitoring of volume status. Serial laboratory measurements of blood urinary nitrogen, creatinine, and creatine phosphokinase (CPK) are useful in the management of rhabdomyolysis and the prevention of acute kidney injuries.

LONG-TERM CONSEQUENCES

Should a patient survive a severe thermal injury, there are still several long-term consequences of burns. Psychiatric issues may develop as the result of prolonged hospitalization, multiple surgical procedures, severe skin scarring, contracture and/ or impaired function. Long-term rehabilitation and counseling are important to improve functional recovery. Additionally, the severely injured burn patient has an increased risk of developing skin cancer. A *Marjolin's ulcer* is a squamous cell carcinoma that arises from a burn scar. Any changes in a burn scar should prompt further investigation via tissue biopsy to rule out malignancy.

> ## CASE CORRELATION
> - See also Case 27 (Traumatic brain injury) and case 28 (blunt trauma)

COMPREHENSION QUESTIONS

29.1 A patient has deep partial burn wounds involving the entire anterior chest and abdomen and circumferential burns involving both upper arms. His estimated weight is 75 kg. Based on the Parkland formula, how much IV fluid should he receive in the first 8 hours following his injury?

A. 2000 to 4000 mL LR

B. 4000 to 6000 mL LR

C. 8000 to 12,000 mL LR

D. 10,000 to 12,000 mL albumin

E. 4000 to 8000 mL albumin

29.2 A 45-year-old woman suffered a thermal injury to her dominant arm 2 years ago. It took 6 months of aggressive wound care for the initial injury to heal. She presents to her MD with itching at the scar which is irregularly bordered and has changed in shape over the past few months. Her PMD calls you to discuss the case since you cared for the patient in the ICU during her hospitalization. What do you tell him regarding the wound?

A. Observe the wound, as it does not appear to be infected.

B. Prescribe an antibiotic, as it may be infected.

C. Prescribe hydrocortisone cream, which the patient should apply daily.

D. Take a tissue biopsy of the wound to rule out malignant transformation.

E. Refer the patient to a dermatologist.

29.3 In which of the following patients is immediate intubation most appropriate?

A. A 33-year-old man found unconscious in a house fire with 20% TBS burn and COHgb level of 27%

B. A 33-year-old man found in a house fire with facial hair burns and normal COHgb level

C. A 33-year-old man with 30% TBSA truncal area burn when his clothing caught on fire at an outdoor barbecue

D. A 68-year-old man with 10% burn to his anterior chest, abdomen, and genitalia from spilling a boiling pot of water

E. A 68-year-old man with burns to both lower legs when his trousers caught on fire while burning leaves in his yard

ANSWERS

29.1 **B.** This patient has burns to the anterior chest and abdomen and both arms, so the total body surface area involvement can be estimated at 18% (abdomen and chest) + 9% × 2 (both arms) = 36%. Based on the Parkland formula that provides 4 mL/kg × percent BSA, the calculation would be 4 × 75 × 36 = 10,800 mL over 24 hours. During the first 8 hours, half of the calculated volume will be given, which is approximately 5400 mL.

29.2 **D.** Patients with chronic wounds, including burn scars, are at risk of developing malignant transformation in the chronic wounds. Squamous cell carcinoma has been known to develop, and a history of shape change or growth would mandate tissue biopsy.

29.3 **A.** This patient is unconscious and has markedly elevated COHgb value. He would benefit from early intubation and positive pressure ventilation with 100% oxygen for treatment of his carbon monoxide injuries. In answer choice B, the burns on the patient's face need to be monitored closely for potential airway-related trauma, but he does not have an absolute indication for early intubation. The other individuals described do not have concerns that would suggest the need for early intubation.

CLINICAL PEARLS

▶ A burn patient is a trauma patient. Therefore, initial assessment should begin with the ABCs of trauma with assessment of the severity of burn wounds and other traumatic injuries.

▶ A common tool used to guide fluid replacement is the Parkland formula.

▶ Every major organ system can be compromised following severe burns.

▶ Early intubation, mechanical ventilation, aggressive fluid resuscitation, infection control and enteral nutrition will reduce morbidity and mortality in the severely burned patient.

▶ Tissue biopsy is necessary for all changes in burn wound scars to rule out malignancy.

REFERENCES

Chipp E, Milner C, Blackburn A. Sepsis in burns: A review of current practice and future therapies. *Ann Plastic Surg.* 2010;65:228-236.

Church D, Elsayed S, Reid O, Winston B, Lindsay R. Burn wound infections. *Clin Microbiol Rev.* 2006 April;19(2):403-434.

Evers L, Bhavsar D, Mailander P. The biology of burn injury. *Exp Dermatol.* 2010;19:777-783.

Latenser BA. Critical care of the burn patient. In: Hall JB, Schmidt GA, Kress JP, eds. *Principles of Critical Care.* 4th ed. New York, NY: McGraw-Hill; 2015:1180-1189.

Milner SM, Asuku M. In: Cameron JL, Cameron AM, eds. *Current Surgical Therapy.* 11th ed. Philadelphia PA: Elsevier Saunders; 2014:1128-1131.

Sheridan R. Practical management of the burn patient. In: Cameron JL, Cameron AM, eds. *Current Surgical Therapy.* 11th ed. Philadelphia PA: Elsevier Saunders; 2014:1131-1138.

A 78-year-old woman with hypercholesterolemia, hypertension, and a 30-pack a year smoking history is admitted to the ICU for a non-ST segment myocardial infarction. The patient is started on aspirin, low molecular weight heparin, metoprolol, and morphine. The patient's vital signs stabilize, and she begins to improve. On ICU day three the patient becomes combative with alternating periods of lethargy and aggression. The nursing staff notes that she did not sleep the previous night. The patient's physical examination and vital signs are largely unremarkable other than some lethargy and weakness. No focal neurological deficits are noted, and cardiac, abdominal, and pulmonary examinations are all normal. Vital signs are as follows: temperature 98.1°F, BP 112/76 mm Hg, pulse 78 beats/min, respiratory rate 15 breaths/min, and O_2 saturation 97% on 2 L per nasal cannula. CT scan shows no acute intracranial pathology. Laboratory workup is below:

Serum Laboratory Studies (Normal range)		Arterial Blood Gas Study	
Sodium (Na⁺)	138 mEq/L (136-144 mEq/L)	pH	7.36 (7.35-7.45)
Potassium (K⁺)	3.9 mEq/L (3.7-5.2 mEq/L)	$Paco_2$	43 mm Hg (36-44 mm Hg)
Chloride (Cl⁻)	102 mEq/L (101-111 mEq/L)	PaO_2	87 mm Hg (75-100 mm Hg)
Blood Urea Nitrogen (BUN)	19 mg/dL (7-18 mg/dL)	CO_2	21 mmol/L (20-29 mmol/L)
Creatinine (Cr)	1.2 mg/dL (0.6-1.2 mg/dL)		
Glucose	97 mg/dL (64-100 mg/dL)		

▶ What is the most likely diagnosis?
▶ What are the best initial steps in the management of this patient?

ANSWERS TO CASE 30:
Altered Mental Status

Summary: A 78-year-old woman develops altered mental status on day three of ICU admission following an NSTEMI. The patient's vital signs and physical examination are otherwise normal.

- **Most likely diagnosis:** ICU delirium.

- **Initial management steps:** Secure the patient's safety by stabilizing her clinical status with a rapid evaluation for the most common treatable and reversible causes of altered mental status (AMS).

ANALYSIS

Objectives

1. To list the common causes of alterations in mental status.

2. To understand the methods used to evaluate AMS.

3. To understand the possible choices in the treatment of patients with delirium.

Considerations

The patient's presentation is most likely the result of ICU delirium, a common complication of ICU admissions that often goes undiagnosed. Delirium is common in elderly patients admitted to the ICU with major medical comorbidities, with as many as 80% of intubated patients and 50% of non-intubated patients experiencing this complication. Risk factors for ICU delirium include cognitive deficits, age greater than 65, alcoholism, hypertension, elevated creatinine, high illness severity, and many drugs such as benzodiazepines. This particular patient is at high risk due to her age, hypertension, long list of medications, and recent medical comorbidities. Additional items on the differential diagnosis would include medication side effects, infection, and stroke. It is important to note that medication-related adverse effects in an elderly patient are a very common cause of delirium, as polypharmacy is becoming more common in the aging population. Twelve percent of patients in the United States older than 65 years take 10 or more medications each week, and adverse drug reactions in the elderly account for 10% of emergency department visits and up to 17% of acute hospitalizations. A review of every patient's medications, particularly in the elderly, should be a part of routine care to avoid polypharmacy and potential medication-related adverse events. Additionally, infection should always be a primary consideration in elderly patients presenting with mental status changes and failure to thrive. The patient has had a recent thromboembolic event and therefore does have an increased risk for further thromboembolic disease. However, her neurologic examination is nonfocal, which would be less consistent with stroke as the underlying cause of her presentation. This observation is further supported by the negative CT of the brain. A careful differential diagnosis for neurological problems should be undertaken to assess for conditions such as meningitis, drug toxicity, electrolyte abnormalities, and stroke as a cause of altered mental status.

APPROACH TO:
Altered Mental Status

DEFINITIONS

DELIRIUM: An acute state of confusion

COMA: A sleep-like state in which the eyes are closed and the patient is unarousable even when vigorously stimulated.

CLINICAL APPROACH

In the ICU, evaluating and monitoring the mental status of patients with multiple serious disease processes is a daunting task. It is estimated that **half the patients admitted to a hospital in an acute condition will undergo some form of delirium during their admission.** Half of these cases of delirium go undiagnosed. In normal consciousness, there is a state of awareness of self and the environment and the ability to carry out activities of daily living (ADL). An intact and functioning brain stem and reticular activating system and its cortical projections are required for normal consciousness. AMS may range from an agitated, confused state (delirium) to an unarousable, unresponsive state (coma). Whether it is delirium, coma, or some state in between, each category represents a stage of the same disease process and is investigated in the same manner. The potential causes are broad and diverse; major causes include metabolic derangement, exposure to toxins, structural lesions, vascular insult, seizure, infection, and substance abuse.

Differential Diagnosis of AMS

Metabolic derangements may include disorders of temperature control, electrolyte balance, glucose or hormone levels, and vitamin insufficiency. Both hyperthermia and hypothermia can cause AMS. Electrolyte disorders include hypernatremia, hyponatremia, hyper and hypoglycemia, and hypercalcemia. Hypoglycemia occurs commonly in the treatment of diabetes mellitus and is life-threatening. Severe untreated hypothyroidism can result in a myxedema-derived coma. Thyrotoxic crisis, or "thyroid storm," is a life-threatening complication of hyperthyroidism characterized by marked agitation, restlessness, delirium, or coma. AMS is a broad term that can encompass anything from sudden confusion and agitation to impaired awareness and profound unresponsiveness, even coma. A patient's mental status is assessed by the level of consciousness (ie, attentiveness) via the reticular system, while cognition (ie, thought process) happens via the cortical projections. **Delirium is an acute altered level of consciousness described as waxing and waning with fluctuating inattentiveness and perceptual disturbances.** A patient in delirium will present in a confused and agitated state, unaware of his/her surroundings. It is common to see delirium superimposed on dementia in the elderly in up to 80% of cases.

A **patient in a comatose state is considered a medical emergency and must be assessed immediately for underlying, reversible causes.** The most common causes of coma are cerebrovascular disease or hypoxic injury, electrolyte disorders, encephalopathies, and drug toxicity. The longer the coma state lasts, the less likelihood there is of recovery. Hepatic encephalopathy needs to be investigated immediately as a possible cause of coma. The administration of D50W is standard in patients found in a comatose state since reversing hypoglycemia, if present, can be lifesaving. Coma without focal signs but with meningismus, with or without fever, suggests meningitis, meningoencephalitis, or subarachnoid hemorrhage. Coma with focal signs implies a structural lesion such as stroke, hemorrhage, tumor, or abscess formation.

Acute pituitary gland hemorrhage or infarction can lead to pituitary apoplexy. Lastly, thiamine deficiency in alcoholics or the malnourished may lead to Wernicke encephalopathy when glucose-containing fluids are administered. For this reason it is important to correct nutritional and vitamin deficiencies, most notably thiamine, before administering glucose in these patients. Toxins can arise from exogenous or endogenous sources. Exogenous sources include illicit and prescription drugs, alcohol, and noxious fumes. Endogenous sources can arise from organ system failure. Examples include ammonia secondary to liver failure (hepatic encephalopathy), uremia secondary to kidney failure (uremic encephalopathy), and cardiopulmonary insufficiency (hypoxia and/or hypercapnia).

Structural lesions can cause coma through diffuse insult to the cerebral hemispheres, damage to the reticular activating system in the brain stem, or interruption of the connections between the two. Massive hemispheric lesions result in coma either by expanding across the midline laterally to compromise both cerebral hemispheres (lateral herniation) or by impinging on the brain stem to compress the rostral reticular formation (transtentorial herniation). Mass lesions of the brain stem produce coma by directly affecting reticular formation. Because the pathways for lateral eye movements traverse the reticular activating system, impaired eye movements (doll's eye) are often an element of diagnosis. Doll's eyes are present when the patient's eyes move opposite of the direction of the head (normal intact brain stem), whereas in negative Doll's eyes the eyes are fixed and look straight ahead regardless of head movement (abnormal brain stem).

Space-occupying lesions include neoplasms (primary or metastatic), intracranial hemorrhage, and infection. Vascular insults include hemorrhagic or ischemic phenomena, inflammation, and hypertension. Subarachnoid hemorrhage and hemorrhagic stroke cause intracerebral hemorrhage, and cerebral ischemia can result from thrombotic or embolic occlusion of a major vessel. Unilateral hemispheric lesions from stroke can blunt awareness, but they do not result in coma unless edema and mass effect cause compression of the other hemisphere. Global cerebral ischemia, usually resulting from cardiac arrest or ventricular fibrillation, may cause anoxic encephalopathy and coma. Vasculitis of the central nervous system may also cause AMS, as well as other systemic signs and symptoms.

Malignant hypertension can lead to a stroke or hypertensive encephalopathy. Central nervous system infections also adversely affect mental status. Infection may also travel from a distant site to cause AMS, such as the development of septic emboli from endocarditis. Infection or fever from any source can cause delirium in the elderly. Delirium tremens is characterized by hallucinations, disorientation, tachycardia, hypertension, low-grade fever, agitation, and diaphoresis. **Most commonly, altered mental status is caused by metabolic derangements, toxin exposure, structural lesions, vascular insults, seizures, infections, and withdrawal syndromes. A mnemonic used to remember the most common causes of altered mental status is: WITCH HAT—*withdrawal, infection, toxins/drugs, CNS pathology, hypoxia, heavy metals, acute vascular insult, and trauma.***

Evaluation

Rapid identification of the cause of AMS is required to treat the patient effectively. The etiologies of AMS are various and multifactorial in most instances. Patient safety is foremost, and the ABCs of resuscitation and adequate hydration must be prioritized. Vital signs, O_2 sat levels, glucose, electrolytes, CBC, and urine analysis should be evaluated. The patient should be screened for illicit drugs and possible toxic levels of prescribed medications. Potential interactions of medications should not be ignored. When possible, a history obtained from family members can help to establish a baseline mental status and pinpoint the cause of AMS. Pertinent details of the patient's history, including the use of prescribed or over-the-counter medications, vitamin supplements, and drug abuse will aid the correct diagnosis and treatment.

The laboratory evaluation should include an arterial blood gas, complete metabolic panel, CBC with differential, ammonia, and liver enzyme level. Focused testing for ASA, acetaminophen, and tricyclic antidepressants depends upon the history and clinical suspicion. The physical examination should address three main questions: (1) Does the patient have meningitis? (2) Are signs of a mass lesion present? and (3) Is this a diffuse syndrome of exogenous or endogenous metabolic origin?

The neurological examination should focus on whether there are lateralizing signs suggesting a focal lesion or signs of meningismus and fever that would suggest an infection. The key features to be noted during the physical examination are pupil size and reactivity, ocular motility, motor activity (including posturing), and certain respiratory patterns. Coma without focal signs, fever, or meningismus suggests a diffuse brain insult such as hypoxia or a metabolic, drug-induced toxicity, an infectious or postictal state. In the case of coma after cardiac arrest, patients who lack pupillary and corneal reflexes at 24 hours and motor responses at 72 hours have a poor chance of meaningful recovery.

Patients with focal findings on examination or who exhibit unexplained coma should undergo emergent imaging to exclude hemorrhage or mass lesion. Lumbar puncture is indicated when meningitis or subarachnoid hemorrhage is suspected and when neuroimaging is normal. The possibility of nonconvulsive status epilepticus should be evaluated by emergent electroencephalogram. Delirium may predispose patients to prolonged hospitalization, frequent impairment of physical function, and increased rates of institutionalization. Therefore, rapid detection, evaluation, and intervention are essential. Diagnosis of delirium is based upon clinical information. The **confusion assessment method (CAM) algorithm** is a useful tool in diagnosing delirium. Physical examination is useful in determining the etiology of AMS. Assessing for neurologic causes may help determine the severity of damage to the CNS. Focal neurologic signs should be assessed, and a CT scan should be performed to evaluate intracranial pathology. It is important to remember that before performing a lumbar puncture in the case of suspected meningitis, CT imaging of the brain should be performed first. This will detect any structural abnormalities and possibly avoid herniation from a lumbar puncture.

Diagnosis of Delirium

It is critical to diagnose and determine the cause of delirium. To diagnose delirium, a patient must have an acute change in mental status that is fluctuating between altered levels of consciousness. Laboratory testing and physical examination can shed light on the source of the delirium. The CAM is the most accurate tool available to diagnose delirium. However, this tool may miss as many as 50% of cases. That, in addition to the fact that ICU delirium increases both risk of death and cost, makes further research into the detection of delirium imperative. This statistic elucidates just how important it is for all providers of ICU patients to maintain a high clinical suspicion for delirium. Table 30–1 outlines the CAM method allowing clinicians to evaluate delirium and to present focused questions that expedite the correct diagnosis of the delirium.

Currently, there are no laboratory tests, imaging studies, or other tests that can reliably provide greater accuracy than the CAM algorithm (sensitivity, 94%-100%; specificity, 90%-95%). Some clues that can help in identifying the etiology of the AMS include: the time course of mental status changes, the association of

Table 30–1 • CONFUSION ASSESSMENT METHOD FOR THE DIAGNOSIS OF DELIRIUM	
Feature	Comment
1. Acute onset and fluctuating course	Usually obtained from a family member or nurse and shown by positive responses to the questions, "Is there evidence of an acute change in mental status from the patient's baseline? Does the abnormal behavior fluctuate during the day, ie, tend to come and go, or increase or decrease in severity?"
2. Inattention	Shown by a positive response to the following: "Did the patient have difficulty focusing or concentrating? For example, being easily distracted or having difficulty keeping track of what was being said."
3. Disorganized thinking	Shown by positive response to the following: "Was the patient's thinking disorganized or incoherent, such as rambling or irrelevant conversation, unclear or illogical flow of ideas, or unpredictable switching from subject to subject?"
4. Altered level of consciousness	Shown by any answer other than "alert" to the following: "Overall, how would you say what the level of consciousness of the patient is?" Normal = alert; Hyperalert = vigilant; Drowsy, easily aroused = lethargy; Difficult to arouse = stupor; Unarousable = coma
Diagnosis of delirium requires the presence of the features of 1 and 2, plus either 3 or 4	

those changes with other events (eg, medication changes or development of physical symptoms), the presence of sensory deprivation (absence of glasses or hearing aids), and the presence of uncontrolled pain. A medication history with particular attention to sedative hypnotics, barbiturates, alcohol, antidepressants, anticholinergics, opioid analgesics, antipsychotics, anticonvulsants, antihistamines, and medications for Parkinson disease is very useful in including or excluding these in the list of possible etiologies of the patient's AMS. The more medications the patient is taking, the greater the likelihood that a medication is causing or contributing to the delirium. Patients and caretakers must be aware that medications include any over-the-counter medications, vitamins, supplements, elixirs, and creams.

Performance of a complete neurological and medical examination is critical in determining the patient's mental status. One should seek for signs of infection, heart failure, myocardial ischemia, dehydration, malnutrition, urinary retention, and fecal impaction. The laboratory evaluation should be tailored to the specific clinical situation. Cerebral imaging, although commonly used to rule out other pathology, is usually not helpful in the diagnosis of delirium unless there is a history of a fall or evidence of focal neurologic impairment. Targeting intervention to the individual's risk factors, such as cognitive impairment, sleep deprivation, immobility, visual and hearing impairment, and dehydration may reduce the incidence of delirium. Delirium often results from a combination of underlying vulnerability and acute precipitating factors (Table 30–2).

Table 30–2 • COMMON CAUSES OF DELIRIUM	
Category	Diseases
Autoimmune	• CNS vasculitis • Lupus cerebritis
Neoplastic	• Diffuse brain metastases • Brain tumors
Hospitalization	• ICU psychosis
Toxins	• Prescription medications (narcotics, anticholinergics, benzodiazepines) • Drugs of abuse (alcohol, illicit drugs) • Poisons (carbon monoxide, pesticides)
Metabolic	• Electrolyte abnormalities • Hypothermia and hyperthermia • Vital organ failure (liver failure, renal failure, cardiac failure) • Vitamin deficiency (B12, thiamine, folate) • Severe anemia • Severe malnutrition
Infectious	• Systemic infections • CNS infections
Endocrine	• Thyroid (hyper or hypo) • Hyperparathyroidism • Adrenal insufficiency
Cerebrovascular	• Hypoperfusion • Hypertensive encephalopathy • Focal ischemic strokes and hemorrhages

Amelioration of underlying vulnerability and prevention of acute precipitants will reduce the incidence of delirium. The use of **physical restraints** is generally **avoided** because they can increase agitation and the risk for patient injury. However, if other measures to control a patient's behavior are ineffective and it seems likely that the patient, if unrestrained, may cause personal injury or injury to others, restraints can be used with caution. The use of sedating agents may exacerbate or prolong delirium. **Antipsychotics or anxiolytics** should only be used in life-threatening circumstances such as in the ICU or when behavioral measures have been ineffective. Low-dose haloperidol, risperidone, and olanzapine are equally effective in treating agitation associated with delirium. These are associated with little respiratory depressive effect, a feature much desired in the respiratory compromised patient. One should attempt to use the lowest dose of the least toxic agent that successfully controls the agitation. Lorazepam used along with antipsychotic agents is complementary without adding undesirable side effects.

Treatment

The treatment of AMS depends upon its etiology. A significant part of the treatment of delirium is to institute preventive measures. Most notably, precipitating factors such as lack of sleep and dehydration should be addressed. Recently, a prediction model called the PRE-DELIRIC model has been introduced which has had success in predicting the likelihood of delirium in an ICU stay with a formula that utilizes 10 readily available criteria within 24 hours of ICU admission. The criteria include age, APACHE-II score, presence and type of coma, the patient's admission category (surgery, medicine, trauma, or neurosurgery), the presence of infection, the presence of metabolic acidosis, morphine use, sedation, urea level, and whether the admission was urgent. Additionally, emphasizing patient ambulation and exercise as soon as possible has been shown to decrease time spent in the ICU. Vitamin B12 and folic acid should also be administered, and patients must be hydrated adequately. A quiet, lowly lit environment during the day, an even darker environment during the evening, and sleeping hours should be maintained. The patient should be advised to avoid reversing the normal rest and sleeping pattern.

Medications

Neuroleptics should be used with caution to avoid possible undesirable side effects. Newer neuroleptics such as risperidone, olanzapine, and quetiapine have fewer adverse effects than haloperidol. The lowest effective dose should be used, and therapy should be tapered downward ASAP, especially in the elderly. Low-dose haloperidol causes less sedation and is highly effective in treating delirium, especially when used in combination with lorazepam. The combination of 5 mg of haloperidol with 1 mg of lorazepam is effective in the treatment of delirium. The use of risperidone has fewer side effects than haloperidol and should be substituted for the latter when possible. Sedatives such as lorazepam are the drugs of choice when treating delirium due to alcohol withdrawal. These agents are also useful in decreasing anxiety. Respiratory depression can be minimized by careful monitoring, especially in the elderly.

Flumazenil can be used for benzodiazepine intoxication. This can lead to rapid withdrawal symptoms including seizures, which now may be untreatable with benzodiazepines since flumazenil will block its effect. Dexmedetomidine is also a sedative that does not cause respiratory depression. Naloxone and naltrexone should also be kept in mind with narcotic drug overdose, especially opioid intoxication where they competitively inhibit opioid-binding sites. They are therefore useful in any opioid intoxication. Proper nutrition and removal of precipitating factors are essential in preventing a relapse.

CLINICAL CASE CORRELATION

- See also Case 3 (Scoring Systems and Patient Prognosis), Case 27 (Traumatic Brain Injury), Case 32 (Stroke), and Case 37 (Poisoning).

COMPREHENSION QUESTIONS

30.1 A 79-year-old woman is admitted to the ICU when she was found to have a pulmonary embolism after presenting to the ER with shortness of breath. The patient has a medical history significant for prior stroke, hypertension, hypercholesterolemia, and baseline dementia. Throughout her hospital course, the patient receives low molecular weight heparin, lisinopril, simvastatin, a daily aspirin, and a diphenhydramine at night to help her sleep. On the second day, the patient becomes agitated, and nursing staff notes that the patient has become increasingly confused and disoriented. The patient's mental status waxes and wanes, and eventually you are called to evaluate the patient. The patient's vital signs are normal other than mild tachycardia at 105 beats/min. The patient is unable to provide a recent history or review of systems due to her altered mental state, but cranial nerve examination is normal and no focal deficits are appreciated. Which of the following most likely contributed to the patient's current state?

A. Cerebrovascular accident

B. Hypoglycemia

C. Medication

D. Dementia

E. Hyponatremia

30.2 A 22-year-old man is admitted to the hospital after presenting to the ER with abdominal pain and is found to have acute appendicitis. The patient has his pain controlled and is scheduled for surgery for the following morning. However, later that evening, the patient begins to become slightly anxious. His vital signs, which had been previously within normal limits, now demonstrate mildly increased blood pressure of 138/88 mm Hg and a temperature of 100.2°F. As the day continues, the patient becomes increasingly confused and delirious. The patient's physical examination is mostly benign, including no focal neurological deficits, a benign abdomen with clean and healthy-appearing incisions, and nothing abnormal other than mild tachycardia and agitation. Upon speaking to the patient's family, it is found that the patient recently dropped out of college due to problems with alcohol and was drinking roughly 15 beers per day. Upon questioning the patient, he is agitated and difficult to direct but admits to roughly that level of consumption. What is the best management strategy for the developing pathology in this patient?

A. Aggressive hydration with D5 fluids

B. Expectant management with close monitoring for complications

C. Flumazenil

D. Oral antibiotics to cover possible wound infection

E. Benzodiazepines, hydration, and electrolyte monitoring with hydration and vitamin supplementation (especially thiamine)

ANSWERS

30.1 **C.** This patient has a number of risk factors that predispose her to delirium, including age, multiple medical comorbidities, ICU admission, and underlying neuropsychiatric conditions. However, medications are a common cause of delirium and a good place to start in the search for an underlying cause. It has been stated that as many as 12% to 39% of all cases of delirium are medication-induced; anticholinergics, pain medications, and sedatives are some of the most common causes. This patient was given a diphenhydramine for its ability to treat insomnia, which is another important concern to address in the ICU, but diphenhydramine and other first generation antihistamines have known anticholinergic effects, making them common precipitating factors for delirium. Initial management should include cessation of the offending agent and an in-depth medical reconciliation review. Additionally, measures need to be taken to prevent the patient from harming herself. Potentially, the use of haldol and lorazepam may be used in severe cases. It is important to note that lorazepam as a benzodiazepine sedative carries with it an inherent risk for progression of the delirium. Avoid "sundowning" by attempting to ensure that the patient adheres to as close to a normal circadian rhythm as possible with natural light during the day and a quiet, dark environment at night. Paying close attention to hydration status and electrolyte balances is crucial, and close communication with the patient will help facilitate the treatment.

30.2   **E.** Alcohol withdrawal is a very common and serious concern for all patients admitted to the hospital. It has been estimated that roughly 8% of all hospital admissions, 16% of surgical patients, and 31% of trauma patients will develop alcohol withdrawal. Most patients that experience alcohol withdrawal experience minor symptoms related to autonomic hyperactivity from roughly 8 to 24 hours following a rapid cessation of long-term alcohol intake. Patients experience symptoms such as sweating, tachycardia, tachypnea, and heightened blood pressure but remain neurologically intact. Respiratory alkalosis is another common laboratory finding due to the increased respiratory rate in addition to depleted levels of magnesium, phosphate, and potassium. Roughly 30% of these patient progress to alcoholic hallucinosis, which generally manifests 8 to 48 hours following cessation of alcohol. Hallucinations, both visual and tactile, have been documented during alcoholic hallucinosis; however, sensorium remains intact. Roughly 5% of individuals progress even further to delirium tremens, which is characterized by any or all of the previous symptoms with the addition of delirium. Seizures are a potential complication at any point during withdrawal; however, their presence has not been shown to be predictive of progression to delirium tremens. The best treatment for withdrawals is prevention and as such, a thorough history is critical. This history is often difficult to obtain and nearly impossible in many trauma patients, so ethanol levels are routinely ordered in many emergency rooms. Once a patient has been identified with withdrawal symptoms, early action is required. Maintenance of hydration status is key, but it is important to note that alcoholics experience multiple nutritional deficiencies. Thus, if a thiamine deficiency is present, it needs to be corrected before glucose-containing fluids are administered to prevent further depletion. Benzodiazepines are the pharmacologic mainstay of treatment, but no single medication has proven superior. As such, other factors such as duration of action, route of administration, and cost are the main factors in choosing the correct drug. What has been shown to affect outcomes, however, is the administration strategy. Symptom-based administration using the Clinical Institute Withdrawal Assessment for Alcohol (CIWA) scale, which lays out 30 signs and symptoms of withdrawal, has been shown to be superior to scheduled dosing with less medication administration being required. The CIWA scale is limited by the requirements that the patient must be able to communicate, which may exclude some patients, but it remains an extremely helpful tool for accurately identifying alcohol withdrawal.

CLINICAL PEARLS

▶ AMS is an acute change in consciousness and cognition and considered a medical emergency that must be diagnosed early and treated immediately to reach the best outcome.

▶ Polypharmacy, particularly in elderly patients with multiple comorbid medical conditions, is a frequent cause of adverse events; ongoing review of the need and appropriate dosing of medications should be a part of routine care.

▶ The most common causes for AMS are (WITCH HAT): **W**ithdrawal, **I**nfection, **T**oxins/drugs, **C**NS pathology, **H**ypoxia, **H**eavy metal, **A**cute vascular insult, **T**rauma.

▶ CAM assessment of delirium is the most accurate test available for diagnosing delirium.

▶ Differentiate dementia from delirium in the elderly, as the two may superimpose each other.

▶ Haloperidol, risperidone, and olanzapine are all effective in treating agitation with delirium.

▶ Delirium is a disturbance of consciousness and cognition over a short period of time and is associated with increased morbidity and mortality, no matter the cause.

REFERENCES

Clifford S, Deutschman MS. *Evidence Based Practice of Critical Care.* Saunders; Philadelphia; pp 535-545; 2010.

Hayes BD, Klein-Schwartz W, Barrueto F Jr. Polypharmacy and the geriatric patient. *Clin Geriatr Med.* 2007;23(2):371-390.

Loscalzo J. *Harrison's Pulmonary and Critical Care Medicine.* McGraw-Hill; pp 290-292, New York; 2010.

Toy E, Simon B, Takenaka K, Liu T, Rosh A. *Case Files: Emergency Medicine.* 2nd ed. New York, NY: McGraw-Hill Education; 2009.

A 54-year-old man is brought to the ICU for altered mental status (AMS) after police found him ambulating in the middle of the street. The patient has slurred speech with an ataxic gait, and there is a large ecchymotic, raised area on his left temporal region. It is also noted that the patient has cyanosis of his fingers. Past medical history and medications cannot be obtained, and no usable information is found on his person. Blood pressure is 185/98 mm Hg, heart rate is 100 beats/min, and respiration rate is 10 breaths/min. A computed tomography (CT) scan of the brain shows a small-to-moderate sized subdural hematoma with accompanying intraparenchymal blood in the region of the left temporal lobe. Shortly after returning from CT, the patient begins to have tonic-clonic seizure activity, which stops after 4 minutes and administration of lorazepam 2 mg IVP. The patient remains somnolent in bed, and it is found that his O_2 saturation is 84% on room air. Four minutes after the first set of convulsions stop, the patient again begins to have tonic-clonic convulsions.

▶ What is the most likely diagnosis?
▶ What is the most likely mechanism responsible for the patient's condition?
▶ What is the best immediate treatment?

ANSWERS TO CASE 31:
Status Epilepticus

Summary: This 54-year-old man has suffered a traumatic brain injury (TBI) with both subdural and intraparenchymal bleeding and presents with altered mentation and hypoxia to the ER. He subsequently suffers from two seizures without any recovery in an 8-minute period.

- **Most likely diagnosis:** Status epilepticus (SE).

- **Most likely mechanism:** TBI and hypoxia leading to decreased seizure threshold.

- **Best immediate treatment:** Intravenous benzodiazepines should be administered, followed by an antiepileptic such as phenytoin. Should seizures persist past the second dose of benzodiazepines and phenytoin, phenobarbital can be attempted. Although rarely necessary or used, general anesthesia with midazolam, propofol, and even inhaled anesthetics such as isoflurane can be used for refractory SE.

ANALYSIS

Objectives

1. To understand the most common causes for seizures.

2. To discuss the diagnosis and treatment of SE.

3. To understand the role of medications and toxins in causing seizures.

Considerations

From what can be ascertained, this 54-year-old man suffered from blunt trauma to the left temporal region resulting in a TBI, including both subdural and intraparenchymal bleeding. He is cyanotic, indicating hypoxia. After these injuries, this patient also suffers a 4-minute tonic-clonic seizure with incomplete recovery and subsequently has another tonic-clonic seizure. This is consistent with the diagnosis of SE. The most likely mechanism for the multiple seizures is the patient's TBI and hypoxia causing a decreased seizure threshold, particularly of the temporal lobe. The most important steps in the management of this patient include proper oxygenation and maintenance of his airway, full aspiration precautions (elevated head of bed at 30-45 degrees), IV access, and seizure control. The pharmacological approach to seizure control consists of early benzodiazepine use, antiseizure medications, and in extreme cases, induction using general anesthesia. Complications include aspiration of gastric secretions, trauma (best prevented with bed padding), and elevated creatine phosphokinase (CPK), which can lead to rhabdomyolysis-induced renal toxicity (best managed with adequate IV hydration). The severity of SE can be appreciated by its in-hospital mortality rates. Convulsive SE carries a 10% to 20% morality rate, nonconvulsive has a 20% to 50% rate, and refractory cases carry a 25% to 60% rate.

APPROACH TO:
Status Epilepticus

Status epilepticus has had many different definitions over the years, most recently being defined by continued seizure activity over 5 to 10 minutes without recovery, or two seizures back to back without full recovery. Although the exact pathophysiology of SE is not well understood, it is believed to occur when there is a failure of the normal inhibitory pathways present within cells which then allows for a continual excitatory loop. The refractory nature of SE increases with duration and can result in neuronal damage and impairment.

SE is a life-threatening, medical emergency that requires immediate management. Prolonged seizures can cause respiratory and circulatory dysfunction, and after 30 minutes, they begin to cause cell death at the level of the hippocampus and above. Emergency medical services should be contacted for anyone having a witnessed seizure lasting longer than 2 minutes, as multiple studies show a significant drop in the number of seizures that self terminate past this point (Table 31–1).

MANAGEMENT

Initial management consists of airway control and identifying any reversible and treatable causes. Intubation is almost always required in SE, as patients cannot protect their airway adequately during their extended seizure activity. Ventilation control allows for hyperventilation-caused hypocapnia, which can help offset the SE-associated metabolic acidosis that results from the increased muscle metabolism and lactic acidosis. Other steps include vital signs monitoring, initiating two large bore IVs for initiation of IV fluids that include thiamine and dextrose solutions, and a full neurological examination as soon as possible. A fingerstick glucose should be obtained, as well as blood counts, metabolic panels, calcium and magnesium levels, liver function tests, arterial blood gases, toxicology screening, coagulation studies, and antiseizure medication levels. These can aid in the identification of the seizure etiology. Proper management of ventilation during this time may become difficult due to high mechanical ventilation pressures during active seizures, and pharmacological paralysis may be necessary. **SE most commonly manifests itself as a series of tonic-clonic seizures but can become nonconvulsive, particularly once treatment is initiated.** Seizure control is of utmost importance in

Table 31–1 • DEFINITIONS OF SEIZURE DISORDERS	
Definitions	Comments
Status epilepticus (SE)	>30 min of continuous seizure activity or two or more seizures without full recovery of previous baseline mental status
Epilepsy	When two or more seizures occur more than 24 h apart or become recurrent
Seizure	Any event causing a change in behavior associated with alteration and erratic brain function

these patients, whether convulsive or not. A large amount of evidence shows that early seizure control improves long-term outcomes. Current guidelines mandate that seizure control should be established within 60 minutes of SE onset. The best immediate treatment includes **intravenous benzodiazepines (eg, diazepam or lorazepam), followed by an antiepileptic such as phenytoin or fosphenytoin.** Both benzodiazepines and phenytoin can be given simultaneously from the beginning of the SE management. First- and second-line medications have been shown to be successful in terminating 86% of SE cases if initiated within 20 minutes of seizure onset, but only 15% if initiated after 30 minutes (this is believed to occur due to internalization of GABA receptors at the cellular level), prompting the need for a high index of suspicion and immediate management.

Phenytoin or fosphenytoin rate of infusion will depend on whether the patient is [fos]phenytoin-naive or not. Rates for phenytoin should not exceed 50 mg/min and fosphenytoin 150 mg/min in order to prevent side effects like hypotension and bradyarrhythmias. If time permits, GI loading doses are well tolerated. Should seizures persist, phenobarbital is considered a third-line drug. **For refractory SE, which can occur in as many as a third of the patients being treated, patients may require general anesthetic dosages of midazolam, pentobarbital, propofol, or even isoflurane in order to obtain seizure control.** All of the aforementioned treatments carry a risk of causing hypotension and arrhythmias, which is why vasopressor use is often necessary.

Other considerations include investigating the etiology, obtaining seizure control and continuous electroencephalogram (EEG) monitoring and neurological consultation. A CT/MRI scan is positive in 30% of children in SE. EEG is critically important and can prevent delays or pauses in treatment in a patient who stops having tonic-clonic movements but continues seizing, as in the case of nonconvulsive SE (NSE). These delays and pauses are the reason why NSE carries such a high mortality and morbidity.

Neurological Consultation

Neurological consultations will likely be necessary in any patients diagnosed with SE, particularly if two or more antiepileptic medications fail to stop the seizure activity. Some patients may even have NSE due to continued electrical firing in the brain without outward motor activity; this is only diagnosed by continuous EEG monitoring.

CAUSES OF SEIZURES

Drug-Induced Seizures

Antiepileptic drug (AED) noncompliance is the most common cause for subsequent seizures, though it carries the best prognosis over other causes. Apart from noncompliance, there are also medications which are known to decrease seizure thresholds and can even cause seizures in otherwise healthy patients. Table 31–2 summarizes these drugs by medication class. Special attention should be paid to patients in renal insufficiency or with CNS comorbidities when determining the preferred dosage of any of these antiepileptic drugs. Phenytoin itself has multiple

Table 31–2 • MEDICATIONS KNOWN TO LOWER THE SEIZURE THRESHOLD	
Medication Class	Medications Known to Lower Seizure Threshold
Antimicrobials	Imipenem, penicillin (high dose), cefazolin, cefmetazole, fluoroquinolones, metronidazole, isoniazid, aztreonam
Psychiatric drugs	Bupropion, lithium, clozapine, flumazenil, phenothiazines
Anesthetics	Lidocaine, bupivacaine
Miscellaneous	Theophylline, cyclosporine, metrizamide (IV contrast)

side effects, including the induction of a positive antinuclear antibody (ANA) test with a lupus-like (single DNA, RNA, antihistone) syndrome, drug-induced fever, and Stevens-Johnson syndrome. The ANA in drug-induced cases is of RNA origin; ANA of DNA origin is seen in SLE.

Ethanol

Because of its effects on γ-aminobutyric acid (GABA) receptors, ethanol can be the culprit for SE in both acute intoxication and in withdrawal/delirium tremens (DT). Chronic alcohol abuse contributes to an increased risk for head trauma, stroke, and brain atrophy (and thus increased risk of subdural hematomas). All of these factors can precipitate seizures. **Alcohol withdrawal seizures carry a 5% risk of progressing to DTs,** which is a severe state of alcohol withdrawal associated with a hypermetabolic state and a high mortality. **Chronic phenytoin therapy is not effective and should not be used in seizures caused by alcohol abuse.**

Infectious Causes

Infections of the central nervous system and elsewhere can be responsible for seizures and SE. SE caused by encephalitis, whether bacterial (such as neurosyphilis from *T. pallidum* or Lyme Disease from the *Borrelia* species), viral, or parasitic (such as cerebral malaria), carries a worse prognosis. Even systemic infections, like bacterial endocarditis, can cause vegetations which can embolize and precipitate seizures and strokes. HIV/AIDS is also associated with several pathogens that can lead to convulsive states, including *Cryptococcus*, *Toxoplasma*, and *Polyomavirus*, the agent of progressive multifocal encephalopathy (PME). Amongst the childhood exanthems, measles can give rise to subacute sclerosing panencephalitis (SSPE) years after the initial infection, leading to a state of chronic recurrent seizures. Neurocysticercosis, caused by an infection with *Taeniasolium* (a porcine tapeworm), is the most common parasitic pathogen of the CNS and can lead to SE. It is the most common cause of acquired epilepsy in developing countries.

Psychogenic Nonepileptic Seizures

Psychogenic nonepileptic seizures (PNES), otherwise known as pseudoseizures, should be distinguished from SE or any other true epileptic condition. The use of anticonvulsant drugs in the treatment of pseudoseizures can contribute to iatrogenic complications. Features that raise suspicion of PNES are psychiatric comorbidities, a gradual onset of the seizures, motor activity characterized by pelvic-thrusting or head-rolling, and vocalizations (such as crying and shouting in the middle of the seizure). Physical examination often reveals geotropic eye movements (eyes moving away from the examiner with briskly reactive pupils). The absence of cyanosis and/ or seizure activity that intensifies when the patient is restrained is consistent with PNES. **The gold standard for the diagnosis of PNES is video electroencephalography**, in which no encephalographic changes would be expected while the patient has a seizure. Management of PNES must also concentrate on treating underlying psychiatric comorbidity. In situations where an EEG may not be available or the seizure was not witnessed, a prolactin level drawn within 20 minutes of seizure onset can help determine whether it was truly a seizure or a psychogenic non-epileptic seizure. A true seizure will have a small, but noticeable, increase in serum prolactin.

Causes and Prognosis

Prognosis for SE is best if the etiology is related to alcohol or AED noncompliance and is worse if due to cerebrovascular accidents, hypoxia, or some type of CNS infection or tumor. When it comes to CNS injuries, **TBI and acute subdural hemorrhages are the most common etiology for subsequent seizures 12% to 50% of the time. Acquired seizure disorders account for 8% to 35% of SE.** In hypoxic-ischemic encephalopathy, close follow-up for subsequent seizures (5%-40%) is needed since development of SE occurs 30% of the time, while in intracerebral hemorrhages (10%-30% risk of subsequent seizures, 1%-21% risk of development of SE), subarachnoid hemorrhages (4%-16%, 10%-14%), and ischemic strokes (5%, 1%-10%) carry a lower risk. **AED prophylaxis is only indicated in moderate to severe TBI.**

Electroencephalographic Studies

In asymptomatic patients with a known history of seizures, a single EEG will only reveal an abnormality in about half of the cases. EEGs provide evidence of the abnormal electrical activity seen in seizures and can be used to differentiate both the type and location of a seizure. Because a single EEG can often be normal even if performed immediately after a witnessed seizure, evidence shows that EEGs performed for extended periods (such as with video EEGs) are more sensitive for diagnosis. Indications for urgent EEG monitoring include suspicion of PNES or when there is a suspicion of NSE. There is increasing evidence showing less optimal outcomes in the treatment of SE due to a delay in the definitive diagnosis of NSE. In order to determine if pharmacological paralytics are necessary during SE stabilization—as in determining the effectiveness of the anticonvulsant therapy on the tonic-clonic seizure activity—continuous EEG monitoring should commence within 1 hour of the precipitating event and continue for optimally 48 hours to prevent NSE (recall that benzodiazepines may help with stabilization but have a short half-life).

Neuroleptic Malignant Syndrome

Neuroleptic malignant syndrome (NMS) is a life-threatening neurological disorder caused by an adverse reaction to neuroleptic or antipsychotic drugs (such as haloperidol). NMS presents with muscle rigidity, fever, autonomic instability, and delirium.

NMS causes elevation in CPK and can lead to renal failure. Antipsychotics users should be monitored for this side effect. Treatment includes removal of the drug, followed by aggressive hydration and dantrolene therapy.

> ## CLINICAL CASE CORRELATION
> - See also Case 27 (Traumatic Brain Injury), Case 30 (Altered Mental Status), and Case 32 (Stroke).

COMPREHENSION QUESTIONS

31.1 A 27-year-old woman who is a swimsuit model was found unconscious in her fitting room by her assistant. Her assistant reveals to the paramedics that the patient was found on the floor and had urinary and fecal incontinence. The assistant also reveals that the patient has recently been abusing chlorthalidone in her attempt to maintain a slim figure. When admitted to the ICU she was awake but confused and unable to provide any history. Within 20 minutes of admission, the patient begins to have tonic-clonic seizure activity. What laboratory abnormality is expected as the cause for her status epilepticus?

A. Hyperglycemia

B. Alcohol abuse

C. Anemia

D. Hyponatremia

E. Leukocytosis

31.2 A 54-year-old Caucasian woman with a past medical history of extensive psychiatric illness, including bipolar disorder, was being treated in the ICU for diverticulitis. The patient has had a prolonged course of admission, with multiple superimposed infections, recurrent fevers, and hemodynamic instability. The patient has been placed on numerous and prolonged antibiotics. The on-call physician was consulted because the patient was experiencing seizures described mainly as changes in mental status. What is the most likely cause of the patient's seizures?

A. Traumatic brain injury

B. Hypoglycemia

C. Medication side effect

D. Pseudoseizures

E. Noncompliance with medications

ANSWERS

31.1 **D.** This patient is currently in status epilepticus given the incomplete recovery from her original seizure (when found unconscious with urinary incontinence) and subsequent seizure. The most likely etiology of seizures in this patient is thiazide diuretic overuse resulting in hyponatremia. Although it can be tempting to attempt to aggressively treat the etiology in this case, we must remember that the patient is likely suffering from chronic hyponatremia, and correction should be performed slowly such as over 48 hours. This means that treatment with 3% saline can cause central pontine demyelination and cause further complications.

31.2 **C.** This patient suffered seizures due to a combination of medications which all lowered her seizure threshold. This question required you to know that diverticulitis is usually treated with a combination of metronidazole and ciprofloxacin, a fluoroquinolone. These medications, along with her lithium, caused her seizure threshold to decrease enough to where she spontaneously suffered a seizure. Although her psychiatric history may lead to the differential of pseudoseizure, there is no information other than her bipolar history given in the question to point toward pseudoseizure.

CLINICAL PEARLS

▶ Status epilepticus carries a very high mortality and morbidity.

▶ Early seizure control is of utmost importance in SE.

▶ The first drugs of choice for the control of tonic-clonic seizures are the benzodiazepines.

▶ EEG should be used, particularly in patients needing third-line medications, to prevent undiagnosed NSE and its complications.

▶ Consider neuroleptic malignant syndrome as a cause of SE in cases where fever is present and there is a known use of haloperidol and/or succinylcholine.

▶ Patients with SE may have rhabdomyolysis and acidosis, which is treated with hydration and urinary alkalinization.

▶ Consider general anesthesia for cases of intractable SE.

▶ Traumatic brain injury leads to a 12% to 50% chance of seizures and thus requires AED prophylaxis.

▶ Many commonly used drugs can decrease the seizure threshold, causing seizures in otherwise normal individuals.

▶ Prolactin elevation can be used to differentiate psychogenic non-epileptic seizures from true seizures if there is no EEG available.

▶ CNS infections as well as non-CNS infections can cause seizure states.

REFERENCES

Browne T, Holmes G. Review article. Primary care, epilepsy. *N Engl J Med.* 2001;344:1145-1151.

Clifford S, Deutschman MS. *Evidence Based Practice of Critical Care.* Philadelphia, PA: Saunders; 2010.

Loscalzo J. *Harrison's Pulmonary and Critical Care Medicine.* New York, NY: McGraw-Hill Education; 2013.

Manno EM. Status epilepticus: Current Management Strategies. *Neuro hospitalist.* 2011,Jan;1(1): 23-31.

Mazurkiewicz-Bełdzińska M, Szmuda M, Zawadzka M, et al. Current treatment of convulsive status epilepticus—a therapeutic protocol and review. *Anesthesiol Intensive Ther.* 2014;46(4):293-300.

A 52-year-old Caucasian man with a history of hypertension and smoking develops a sudden onset of difficulty speaking and drooling from the left side of his mouth and weakness in his left hand. The patient is taken to the closest hospital and admitted to the ICU. Past medical history reveals poorly controlled hypertension, and no history of migraines, seizures, or diabetes. The only medication is an ACE inhibitor. Vital signs are BP 150/80 mm Hg, pulse 89 beats/min, respirations 20 breaths/min, temperature 98.9°F, and Sao_2 95%. The physical examination reveals a well appearing, awake middle-aged male in no acute distress. Neuro: The patient is awake, responsive, and appropriate. He answers questions correctly and follows commands. The patient has a mild left facial droop, and his forehead moves symmetrically. Motor: Right arm and leg extremity with 5/5 strength. Left arm cannot resist gravity, left leg with mild drift. Sensation: Intact bilaterally to fine touch. Neglect: Mild neglect to left side. Mild to moderate dysarthria. Laboratory evaluation: CBC, renal, and ECG unremarkable; glucose 110; noncontrast head CT (Figure 32–1) shows no intracranial hemorrhage or mass lesions.

▶ What is the most likely diagnosis?
▶ What is the next step in the treatment of this patient?

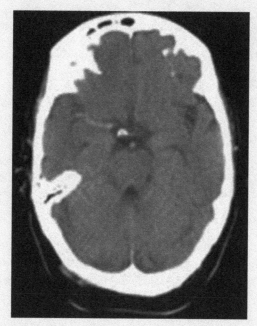

Figure 32–1. CT imaging of the brain.

ANSWERS TO CASE 32:
Stroke

Summary: A 52-year-old Caucasian man with risk factors for cerebrovascular disease has symptoms consistent with a right middle cerebral artery distribution ischemic stroke, now 2 hours from symptom onset. A CT scan without contrast is performed.

- **Most likely diagnosis:** Ischemic stroke.

- **Next step:** Intravenous thrombolysis is indicated within 3 hours (up to 4.5 h by European guidelines) of onset of ischemic stroke in patients with a measurable deficit who meet inclusion/exclusion criteria. Strict monitoring of vital signs and neurologic examination findings is required to achieve a target blood pressure less than 180/105 mm Hg and to detect signs of symptomatic intracranial hemorrhage.

ANALYSIS

Objectives

1. To understand the causes of cerebral vascular atherosclerosis and disease.

2. To understand general management of acute stroke therapy.

3. To understand the common complications of stroke therapies.

4. To understand the medications for the prophylaxis of stroke.

5. To understand how to assess stroke severity using the National Institutes of Health Stroke Scale (NIHSS).

Considerations

This is a 52-year-old previously healthy man who arrives in the hospital within 2 hours of the onset of new neurological deficits. This is very suspicious for a cerebrovascular accident (stroke). The CT scan does not show a hemorrhage, so this is likely an ischemic stroke. This patient is fortunate to have arrived to the hospital in time for intervention such as thrombolytic therapy. For most patients with ischemic stroke who arrive at the hospital beyond the treatment window for intravenous thrombolysis, oral or rectal aspirin is usually appropriate treatment; aspirin taken within 48 hours of ischemic stroke onset modestly reduces the risk of recurrent stroke at 2 weeks without significantly increasing the risk of hemorrhage. Most studies demonstrate a benefit to routine blood pressure lowering treatment in the acute phase of stroke; however, overzealous treatment can lead to hypotension and worsening cerebral ischemia.

APPROACH TO:
Stroke

Stroke can be defined as any vascular injury that reduces cerebral blood flow to a specific region of the brain, causing neurologic impairment. The onset of symptoms may be sudden or stuttering, often with transient or permanent loss of neurologic function. Approximately 87% of all strokes are ischemic in origin, caused by the occlusion of a cerebral vessel. Approximately 13% are hemorrhagic strokes caused by the rupture of a blood vessel into the parenchyma of the brain (intracerebral hemorrhage, or ICH) or into the subarachnoid space. Stroke is the third leading cause of death in the United States and a leading cause of long-term disability. On average, someone has a stroke every 40 seconds, and someone dies of a stroke every 4 minutes. There is a 5% to 10% in-hospital mortality rate for ischemic stroke and 40% to 60% for intracerebral hemorrhage. Ischemic brain injury culminates in anoxic cell death. Initially after arterial occlusion, an area of edema with structural integrity surrounds a central core of tissue death. This is the area that can recover from the first minutes to hours of the insult. No clinical deficits and findings necessarily reflect irreversible damage. Depending on the duration and severity of the ischemia, the edematous area may be incorporated into the infarct or normal tissue. Thirty-day mortality rates are in the range of 10% to 17%. Older patients do worse after stroke; poor prognosis is also noted with the coexistence of ischemic heart disease and diabetes mellitus (DM). Mortality is related to the size of the infarct; the risk of death is as low as 2.5% with lacunar infarcts and as high as 78% with space-occupying hemispheric infarcts. This is why current milestone recommendations include (measured from "door" to certain point) a time less than 10 minutes to physician, less than 15 to stroke team, less than 25 to CT start, less than 45 to CT read, less than 60 to drug, and less than 3 hours to stroke unit admission. The 45 minute and 60 minute milestones are two of the most important, as they can make or break the outcome.

SEVERITY ASSESSMENT

A complete neurologic examination is warranted in all patients with suspected stroke to localize the deficit to the central nervous system and inform prognosis. In the acute stroke setting, when time is of the essence, validated scales for measuring neurologic impairment can be rapidly performed by any healthcare provider. The NIHSS is a useful and rapid tool in the assessment of severity of stroke and can be used in determining treatment option. NIHSS scores have been shown to be reproducible and valid and to correlate well with the amount of infarcted tissue on CT scan. The baseline NIHSS score can identify patients who are appropriate candidates for fibrinolytic therapy as well as those at increased risk for hemorrhage. In addition, it has been used as a prognostic tool to predict outcome. An NIHSS score calculator can be found at http://www.mdcalc.com/nih-stroke-scale-score-nihss/.

TREATMENT

The dictum is "time is brain." Hence, as soon as a patient is diagnosed with possible stroke, acute imaging should be performed to rule out a hemorrhagic process and the patient screened for possible thrombolytic therapy (refer to milestones mentioned previously). **The primary determinant of eligibility is the time since stroke onset. IV tissue plasminogen activator (tPA) has the best outcomes if performed within 1.5 hours from symptom onset. In the United States it is also indicated up to 3 hours from symptom onset, and European guidelines go up to 4.5 hours. However, treatment in the 3 to 4.5 hour range has extended contraindications. These include age >80, NIHSS score >25, oral anticoagulation regardless of coagulation studies, or history of diabetes with previous stroke.** Thrombolysis aims to restore cerebral blood flow to the ischemic penumbra where cerebral tissue has sustained ischemic injury but has not yet progressed to infarction. The recommended rTPA dose is 0.9 mg/kg with a maximum of 90 mg, with the first 10% being given IV over a period of 1 minute, and the remaining 90% given within 1 hour. Treatment leads to a 31% to 50% favorable neurologic or functional outcome at 3 months. Headache, nausea, or worsening of neurologic examination findings are signs of intracranial bleeding and should prompt stopping the infusion and repeating the head CT. The main risk factors for symptomatic ICH are treatment beyond the time window and blood pressure above recommended targets. Blood pressure should be less than 185/110 mm Hg before thrombolysis, which can be achieved with intravenous labetalol or nicardipine, according to American Heart Association guidelines. In addition to acute intracranial hemorrhage and severe uncontrolled hypertension, there are several other absolute and relative contraindications to IV rTPA, including head trauma or stroke in the previous 3 months, thrombocytopenia, coagulopathy, patients on low-molecular-weight heparin, direct thrombin and factor Xa inhibitors, and severe hypoglycemia or hyperglycemia. Relative contraindications include advanced age, mild or improving stroke symptoms, severe stroke and coma, recent major surgery, arterial puncture of noncompressible vessel, recent gastrointestinal or genitourinary hemorrhage, seizure at onset, recent MI, CNS structural lesion and dementia.

Anticoagulation

The American Heart Association/American Stroke Association 2013 guidelines state that urgent anticoagulation is not recommended for the treatment of patients with acute ischemic stroke. Similarly, 2012 guidelines from the American College of Chest Physicians (ACCP) recommend early aspirin therapy over therapeutic parenteral anticoagulation for patients with acute ischemic stroke or transient ischemic attack (TIA). Aspirin (ASA) dosing (160-325 mg/d) initiated within 48 hours after the onset of stroke and continued for 2 weeks leads to better survival and function by reducing risk of recurrent ischemic stroke. In addition, early (within 24 hours) initiation and short-term use of dual antiplatelet therapy with **clopidogrel plus aspirin may be beneficial for patients with high-risk transient ischemic attack (TIA) or minor stroke.** The utility of other antiplatelet agents, alone or in combination with aspirin, remains to be proven in this setting. ASA should be withheld for 24 hours in patients treated with the use of IV thrombolytics to decrease the risk of bleeding. The use of unfractionated heparin (UNFH), low-molecular-weight heparins (LMWH), heparinoids, thrombin inhibitors, or oral anticoagulants in the acute phase of stroke improves functional outcomes.

Management of Cardiovascular Risk Factors

Aggressive management of cardiovascular risk factors, including smoking cessation, treatment of hypertension, and initiating statin therapy, is recommended. Aspirin (ASA) should be started after 24 hours (300 mg daily for the first 2 weeks), and extended release dipyridamole should be started for secondary prevention. Atrial fibrillation (AF) is a common arrhythmia that increases the risk of stroke. Warfarin therapy should be initiated with a goal of an international normalized ratio (INR) between 2 and 3 with appropriate heparin or LMWH bridging. Apixaban, a direct antithrombin inhibitor, does not require monitoring of the INR and is used in non-valvular AF. These agents have been more effective than ASA for the prevention of stroke in patients with AF. Although warfarin is more effective, maintaining and constant monitoring for appropriate INR levels limits its use and has been found to only be therapeutic 60% of the time, which can lead to subsequent strokes. At least a third of patients with AF who are at risk for stroke are either not started on oral anticoagulant therapy or are not compliant with therapy.

ASA reduces the risk of stroke in patients with AF by about 20% and is used to treat patients with atrial fibrillation for whom vitamin K antagonist therapy is contraindicated. Addition of clopidogrel to an ASA regimen in patients for whom vitamin K antagonist therapy is contraindicated further reduces the risk of stroke by 28%, but the combination increases the risk of major hemorrhages. There has also been an increase in Factor Xa inhibitors available on the market, such as rivaroxaban, apixaban, betrixaban, YM150, and DU-176b. The benefit of these Factor Xa inhibitors is there is no need for INR monitoring, but there have been some complications with their reversal in episodes of hemorrhages, whether cerebral or GI.

Prevention and Management of Complications

Patients with an acute stroke are at an increased risk for deep venous thrombosis (DVT) and pulmonary embolism (PE). This risk for DVT and PE increases with age and stroke severity scores. Early mobilization and rehabilitation to a level the patient can tolerate are indicated for all survivors of stroke to improve recovery and mitigate medical complications. These patients are prone to urinary tract infections from indwelling catheters, aspiration pneumonia from dysphagia, and DVT. Subcutaneously administered low-dose UNFH or LMWH is recommended for patients at high risk for DVT and PE, and for those with immobility. Heparinoids do not reduce the risk of recurrent stroke in the acute setting for either cardioembolic or noncardioembolic stroke. Acute intravenous heparin occasionally is used in patients with rare causes of stroke, such as dissection or a hypercoagulable state, or in patients with mechanical cardiac valves if the risk of hemorrhage into the infarct is low.

Large supratentorial infarcts and space-occupying edema of the brain may lead to transtentorial or uncal herniation, usually between the second and fifth day after the onset of stroke. Compared to medical therapy, surgery (hemicraniectomy, dura-plasty, a dural patch to enlarge the intradural space) in the first 48 hours of the onset of stroke reduced the case fatality rate (22% vs 71%). Patients who received care in a stroke unit were more likely to survive, regain independence, and return home than those who did not receive such specialized care.

Hypercoagulable States

Hypercoagulable conditions can lead to strokes. The most common conditions in this group include oral contraceptive use, pregnancy, Factor V Leiden deficiency, protein C and S deficiencies, antithrombin III deficiency, and lupus anticoagulant. Patients with these conditions usually present with some form of deep venous thrombosis. Procoagulant states should be suspected, especially when recurrent episodes of deep venous thrombosis are diagnosed. Arterial thrombosis should definitely increase awareness of the presence of one of these conditions. Clots can travel from the venous circulation through the heart via an atrial or ventricular septal defect to the left side of the heart and to the arterial circulation leading to the brain (paradoxical emboli). Lupus anticoagulant is a specific immunoglobulin against phospholipids that prolongs the clotting time; it does not produce bleeding but instead a paradoxical procoagulant condition. It is seen in 25% of people with systemic lupus erythematosus (SLE), but it is also seen in otherwise normal, healthy subjects. In some people it is associated with an increased risk of blood clots and may be the cause of recurrent spontaneous abortions. Risk factors are SLE and a recent use of phenothiazine medication. Specialized clotting studies and levels of the factors involved are required to make an accurate diagnosis.

Prevention of Stroke

In the long term (beyond 90 days after stroke), dual antiplatelet therapy with aspirin and clopidogrel is not recommended for stroke prevention. The MATCH trial, with over 7500 patients, found that the combined use of aspirin and clopidogrel did not offer greater benefit for stroke prevention than either agent alone but did substantially increase the risk of bleeding complications.

Prevention consists primarily of low-dose ASA and dipyridamole in patients with ischemic stroke, oral anticoagulation in patients with cardiac embolism, treatment of hypertension, statin therapy, and glucose control in patients with diabetes. Cessation of smoking and carotid endarterectomy in patients with ipsilateral carotid stenosis has been shown to be effective.

Even in the United States, only a minority of patients with acute ischemic stroke receive intravenous rTPA. The use of intravenous rTPA is currently restricted to a 3-hour time window (up to 4.5 by European guidelines) after the onset of symptoms, with potential benefit when used up to 6 hours after the onset of a stroke. Later use was improved by quantification of the ischemic penumbra with perfusion MRI/CT. The intent of thrombolysis is to recanalize occluded arteries. Complete recanalization of an occluded middle cerebral artery 2 hours after the start of thrombolysis was achieved in one-third of patients. In some cases, continuous 2-MHz transcranial Doppler ultrasonography applied for 2 hours simultaneously with rTPA augmented the rate of arterial recanalization. The addition of intravenous galactose-based micro bubbles may also increase rates of recanalization along with Doppler therapy.

Compared with intravenous thrombolysis, intra-arterial thrombolysis may increase the likelihood of recanalization. The administration of both intra-arterial recombinant pro-urokinase and intravenous heparin within 6 hours after the onset of stroke, compared with intravenous heparin alone, resulted in a higher rate of recanalization of the middle cerebral artery (66% vs 18%) and a higher rate of a favorable functional outcome at 3 months (40% vs 25%, $P = 0.04$).

Procedures required to deliver intra-arterial thrombolytic agents to the site of vascular occlusion involve more time than intravenous therapy. Thrombolytic therapy in which intravenous thrombolysis is followed by intra-arterial thrombolysis may permit more rapid treatment and improved rates of recanalization. Mechanical thrombectomy in patients with acute intracranial occlusion of the intracranial carotid artery has resulted in a higher rate of recanalization.

Elevated blood pressure, hyperglycemia, and fever in the first hours to days after ischemic stroke have all been associated with poor long-term outcomes. Antihypertensive therapy during the acute phase of stroke is held unless the diastolic blood pressure exceeds 120 mm Hg or the systolic blood pressure exceeds 220 mm Hg in patients who do not receive rTPA. Monitoring blood pressure is recommended before, during, and after rTPA therapy. Intravenous antihypertensive therapy to maintain the systolic blood pressure <185 mm Hg and the diastolic blood pressure below 110 mm Hg is recommended. Hypothermia has also improved functional outcomes in trials involving patients with global cerebral ischemia after cardiac arrest and traumatic spinal cord injury, but the improvement was not consistent among those with traumatic brain injury.

Conclusions

Patients with signs and symptoms of CVA strongly suggestive of stroke should undergo prompt brain imaging (CT or MRI). MRI is more sensitive for early ischemic changes, but either method can fully rule out hemorrhage. In the absence of bleeding or other contraindications to thrombolysis, such as spontaneous, complete clearing of the deficits, increase in BP ≥ 185/110 mm Hg, or presentation >3 hours (possibly 6 hours) after the onset of symptoms, the patient should receive therapy with intravenous rTPA. Cardiovascular risk factors should be addressed, and anticoagulation should be initiated when atrial fibrillation (AF) is present.

RECENT IMPORTANT DISCOVERIES

Compared to ASA, apixaban had superior efficacy in reducing the risk for embolic events in patients with AF. It has a 50% level of bioavailability and is partially excreted by the kidneys. Apixaban, at a dose of 2.5 mg twice daily, is effective and safe for the prevention of DVT after elective orthopedic surgery. The direct thrombin inhibitor dabigatran gained a Class I recommendation as a useful alternative to warfarin (Coumadin) for the prevention of stroke and systemic thromboembolism in patients with paroxysmal to permanent AF. Risk factors for stroke or systemic embolization are increased in patients with prosthetic heart valves, hemodynamically significant valvular disease, renal failure (creatinine clearance <15 mL/min), and advanced liver disease (impaired baseline clotting function).

Routinely switching patients who are already successfully taking warfarin to dabigatran is not recommended and remains an individual decision. Dabigatran requires a twice daily dosing and has a greater risk of nonhemorrhagic side effects; thus, patients already taking warfarin with excellent INR control have little to gain by changing to dabigatran. The patient's compliance with a twice-daily dosing is a real issue. However, management to sustain monitoring of INR is needed with warfarin, which adds to cost and compliance.

Selective serotonin reuptake inhibitors (SSRI) are effective after ischemic stroke. Some SSRIs improved motor recovery after stroke, but this has not been universally confirmed. Fewer fluoxetine recipients than placebo recipients had depression, and treatment with thrombolytic agents did not alter the findings. The SSRIs are therapeutic treatment of stroke and should be considered as an adjunct to physiotherapy in the rehabilitation of motor deficits in moderate-to-severe stroke. Reports of a decreased effect of clopidrogrel in patients taking proton pump inhibitors (PPI) did not conclude that there was an increase in the risk for a recurrence of stroke in clopidogrel/PPI users. Vitamin supplementation did not prevent major CV events in patients with previous myocardial infarction, unstable angina, or stroke.

CLINICAL CASE CORRELATION

- See also Case 3 (Scoring Systems and Patient Prognosis), Case 27 (Traumatic Brain Injury), Case 30 (Altered Mental Status), and Case 31 (Status Epilepticus).

COMPREHENSION QUESTIONS

32.1 You are evaluating a 62-year-old man with a past medical history of hypertension who presented an hour after an episode of total right eye vision loss. The patient states that in the past, he had a similar episode that resolved after 5 minutes. The patient states that he only takes hydrochlorothiazide for his HTN. BP in the ER is 185/97 mm Hg, pulse is 85 beats/min and regular, and his respirations are 14 breaths/min. Physical examination shows no focal neurological deficits. Heart rate rhythm are regular, and no murmurs, rubs, or gallops are auscultated. CT of the brain without contrast reveals no acute findings. Which diagnostic test should be performed in order to help determine the etiology of this patient's symptoms?

A. Transesophageal echocardiogram

B. CTA of the brain

C. Carotid ultrasound

D. Lipid profile

32.2 A 47-year-old woman with a past medical history of poorly controlled HTN and mechanical valve replacement presents to your ER 2 hours after experiencing right-sided facial droop and right-arm weakness and dysarthria. Her husband is at the bedside and states that she has never had symptoms like this before. On physical examination, her blood pressure is 180/100 mm Hg, pulse rate is 98 beats/min, and respirations are 16 breaths/min. A quick lab panel reveals her INR is 1.3, her blood glucose is 47, and platelets are 188,000. Which of the following is currently a contraindication to her receiving tPA?

A. Platelets

B. INR

C. Blood pressure

D. Glucose .

ANSWERS

32.1 **C.** The best course of action is to perform carotid ultrasonography (US). The patient is suffering from amaurosis fugax, which is a transient blindness in one eye due to atherosclerotic emboli from the carotid artery. Amaurosis fugax is a type of transient ischemic attack (TIA). Carotid US will reveal internal carotid artery stenosis and must be either identified or ruled out, as it can signify a high likelihood of recurrence and the need for intervention. A stenosis greater than 70% carries the highest risk for a stroke 2 weeks after a TIA. The main benefits of carotid US are it is noninvasive and has a relatively low cost while providing a large amount of useful information that can change treatment. Compared to angiography of the neck and/or brain vessels, carotid US has a much smaller cost. Transesophageal echocardiogram would be indicated if a less invasive work-up did not reveal any abnormalities. Angiography may be necessary at a later time but would be done as a confirmatory rather than screening tool of the neck vessels and not brain. While relatively simple and noninvasive, a lipid profile may or may not show any abnormalities. A patient who has been on statin therapy and reached appropriate levels may have built atherosclerotic plaques for years before starting therapy.

32.2 **D.** This patient's blood glucose is below 50, which is one of the major contraindications for tPA administration. These also include head trauma within the last 3 months, history of intracranial hypertension or subarachnoid hemorrhage, a brain tumor, arterial puncture of any kind, platelets less than 100,000, heparin use with an elevated PTT, INR greater than 1.7, oral direct thrombin inhibitors or Factor Xa inhibitors, systolic blood pressures greater than 185 mm Hg or diastolic blood pressures greater than 100 mm Hg, and severe hypo- or hyperglycemia. Until this patient's blood glucose is increased, she cannot have tPA.

CLINICAL PEARLS

▶ The use of intravenous rTPA is currently restricted to a 3-hour time window (up to 4.5 by European guidelines) after the onset of symptoms, with potential benefit when used up to 6 hours after the onset of a stroke.

▶ NIHSS is a useful and rapid tool in the assessment of severity of stroke and can be used in determining treatment options.

▶ The use of UNFH, LMWH, heparinoids, thrombin inhibitors, or oral anticoagulants in the acute phase of stroke improves functional outcomes.

REFERENCES

Foster C, Mistry N, Peddi PF, Sharma S. *The Washington Manual of Medical Therapeutics.* 33th ed. Philadelphia, PA: Lippincott Williams & Wilkins; 2010.

Fugate JE, Rabinstein AA. Absolute and relative contraindications to IV rtPA for acute ischemic stroke. Demaerschalk BM, ed. *The Neurohospitalist.* 2015;5(3):110-121.

Van der Worp HB, Acute ischemic stroke. *N Engl J Med.* 2007;357:2203-2204.

A 63-year-old man underwent sigmoid colectomy and colostomy formation for peritonitis and sigmoid volvulus. At the time of the operation, he was noted to have necrosis and perforation of the sigmoid colon with extensive fecal contamination. On postoperative day 8, the patient remains on the ventilator with $PaO_2/FiO_2 = 260$. Over the past 48 hours, he has developed worsening oliguria with urine output of less than 300 mL over the 18 hours. The patient is becoming visibly jaundiced. A CT scan of the abdomen reveals no intrahepatic ductal dilatation, moderate amount of postoperative inflammatory changes throughout the peritoneal cavity, and no signs of active intra-abdominal infections.

▸ What are the likely causes of the patient's current condition?
▸ How would you monitor and quantify the patient's organ dysfunction?
▸ What are your therapeutic strategies and goals for this patient?

ANSWERS TO CASE 33:
Multiorgan Dysfunction

Summary: This is a 63-year-old man who had an operation for sigmoid volvulus, and his course was complicated by colonic perforation and fecal peritonitis. The patient is now developing organ dysfunction despite probable adequate source control. He is showing signs of pulmonary dysfunction with compromised oxygenation (P/F ratio = 260); in addition, he has new onset compromised renal and hepatic functions as seen by his decreased urine output and visible jaundice. All of these organs are now working well, despite there being no evidence of continued intra-abdominal pathology.

- **Likely causes of the patient's current condition:** The patient's initial peritonitis and subsequent inflammatory response has led to organ dysfunction in multiple systems.

- **Monitoring and quantifying the organ dysfunction:** Continuous monitoring of his organ functions is mandatory, and the level of dysfunction is quantified using the multiple organ dysfunction scale.

- **Therapeutic strategies and goals for this patient:** The therapy for multiple organ dysfunction is mainly supportive. Mechanical support may be necessary, such as ventilator support for pulmonary failure and hemodialysis for renal failure.

ANALYSIS

Objectives

1. Learn to identify, quantify, and manage multiple organ dysfunction associated with critical illnesses.

2. Learn the factors that may contribute to the development of multiple organ dysfunction syndrome (MODS).

3. Learn the supportive care for patients with MODS.

Considerations

This patient presented with a single identifiable cause for his illness: sigmoid perforation with fecal peritonitis. His illness has not resolved with the removal of his diseased colon, irrigation of the peritoneal cavity, and antibiotic administration. Instead, despite appropriate treatment of his peritonitis, his overall status is continuing to deteriorate. His pulmonary function has declined with a P/F ratio that is indicative of acute lung injury. Likewise, he has acute kidney injury demonstrated by his progressive oliguria. His hepatic function has also deteriorated as evidenced by his visible jaundice. The organ dysfunction that occurs days following the inciting event and continues despite there solution of his initial illness is indicative of secondary multiple organ dysfunction syndrome (MODS). Continued supportive care with aggressive investigation to identify new or untreated infectious and/or inflammatory sources is the mainstay of care for this patient.

APPROACH TO:
Multiple Organ Dysfunction Syndrome

DEFINITIONS

MULTIPLE ORGAN DYSFUNCTION SYNDROME: The continued dysfunction of two or more organ systems that occurs as a result of disruption in homeostasis. The organ dysfunction may continue despite the resolution of the initial event.

SYSTEMIC INFLAMMATORY RESPONSE SYNDROME (SIRS): Occurs when two of the following are present:

1. Body temperature less than 36°C or greater than 38°C

2. Heart rate greater than 90 beats/min

3. Respiratory rate greater than 20 breaths/min

4. White blood cell count less than 4000 cells/mm^3 or greater than 12,000 cells/mm^3 **or** the presence of greater than 10% immature neutrophils (bandforms)

ACUTE KIDNEY INJURY (AKI): AKI was formerly referred to as acute renal failure (ARF). AKI is defined by a rapid decline in renal function (less than 48 h). The decrease in renal function is determined using urine output and/or serum creatinine levels. An absolute increase in serum creatinine of ≥0.3 mg/dL **or** a percentage increase in serum creatinine of ≥50% is indicative of AKI. Also, a reduction in urine output, defined as <0.5 mL/kg/h for more than 6 hours, is AKI.

ACUTE LUNG INJURY/ACUTE RESPIRATORY DISTRESS SYNDROME: Hypoxemic respiratory failure, of which the most severe form is acute respiratory distress syndrome (ARDS). Acute lung injury (ALI) is defined as a P/F ratio of less than 300. ARDS is hypoxemic failure with a P/F ratio of <200, bilateral fluffy infiltrates on chest x-ray, and no evidence of congestive heart failure.

CLINICAL APPROACH

Multiple organ dysfunction syndrome (MODS) is a clinical syndrome that has its origins in the ICU. MODS did not exist prior to the ability to keep patients alive who would have otherwise died from their disease processes. Once ICU care began to evolve and became successful at sustaining patients after life-threatening illnesses, we began to see patients develop remote organ dysfunction despite resolution of their initial insults. Patients who develop MODS have increased length of ICU stays and a 20-fold increase in mortality rate when compared to patients without MODS.

Pathophysiology

There are multiple factors that may contribute to the development of MODS. Originally, it was thought that MODS only occurred in patients who had severe sepsis.

Although sepsis is responsible for almost three-fourths of MODS cases, any clinical scenario that leads to significant inflammation or host injury responses can cascade into MODS. The beginning of MODS starts with the normal, appropriate physiologic response to a single inciting event, such as pneumonia, pancreatitis, or a gunshot wound to the abdomen. This initial insult activates macrophages, which in turn release pro-inflammatory mediators as well as activate coagulation factors. The pro-inflammatory mediators interact with white blood cells, resulting in their recruitment and activation. The inflammatory mediators also can cause microvascular thromboses, apoptosis derangements, and increased capillary permeability. The procoagulant effects act in conjunction with the previously activated coagulation system. This combined with the activation of the coagulation factors serves to act as a local protective mechanism against injury.

Once the original injury is treated, the inflammatory mediators and coagulation factors return to normal when healing has been achieved. However, occasionally, despite the resolution of the inciting event, the normal physiologic response acts as a positive feedback loop, leading to over-amplification of the immune response. The activation of the white blood cells can also release pro-inflammatory mediators with further activation of monocytes/macrophages and release of additional pro-inflammatory mediators. This continued inflammation and coagulation causes cellular damage, which in turn activates more inflammatory mediators; subsequently, further cellular damages occur with subsequent organ failure. Once this organ system fails, inflammatory mediators are continued to be released, acting on other organ systems until there is multiorgan dysfunction.

Once patients have been treated for their original injury and continue to have clinical deterioration, MODS should be considered as the diagnosis. Although the pulmonary system is often noted to be the first organ system to fail, there is no standard progression of organ failure. The degree of organ dysfunction is often graded by the Multiple Organ Dysfunction Syndrome Score (Table 33–1). There is no single therapy for MODS, and the treatment is largely supportive. The goal of therapy is to decrease the continued cellular injury in each organ so that the positive feedback loop can be interrupted with an aim toward return of normal homeostasis.

Table 33–1 • MULTIPLE ORGAN DYSFUNCTION SCORE (MODS)					
	SCORE				
Organ System	0	1	2	3	4
Respiratory (P/F)	>300	226-300	151-225	76-150	<75
Renal (serum Cr) (μmol/L)	<100	101-200	201-350	351-500	>500
Hepatic (serum bilirubin) (μmol/L)	<20	21-60	61-120	121-240	>240
Cardiovascular (PAR*)	<10	10.1-15	15.1-20	20.1-30	>30
Hematologic (platelet count/mm³)	>120,000	81-120,000	51-80,000	21-50,000	<20,000
Neurologic (GCS)	15	13-14	10-12	7-9	<6

*PAR = pulse adjusted rate = (HR × CVP)/MAP

The best treatment of MODS is to identify which patients are at increased risk for developing MODS and begin preemptive therapy to limit the progression to MODS. This is best accomplished by optimizing cardiac and pulmonary performance early in the disease process, providing early and adequate nutritional support, utilizing antibiotics appropriately to decrease the risk of resistant "super" infections, and minimizing the use of blood transfusions.

The identification of organ failure in patients with MODS necessitates continuous monitoring and supportive therapy for that organ. Increased vigilance should also be used to monitor and detect for new organ dysfunction during treatment. The increase in number, duration, and severity of organ dysfunction identification, the worse the short-term and long-term prognosis associated with the process.

The pulmonary system is often the earliest organ system to demonstrate dysfunction. Patients who develop MODS are often already intubated, but despite treatment of their original illnesses, the patients are unable to wean from ventilator support. Acute lung injury (ALI) is an umbrella term for hypoxemic respiratory failure. The most severe form of ALI is acute respiratory distress syndrome (ARDS). In acute lung injury, there is a failure of normal gas exchange. The inflammation that occurs affects oxygen uptake more than carbon dioxide elimination. This occurs early because of atelectasis and intravascular thrombosis. As it progresses, an increase in capillary permeability leads to an increase in alveolar fluid, which increases the distance for oxygen diffusion to occur. Identification of a P/F ratio of less than 300 indicates that the patient has acute lung injury. A P/F ratio of less than 200 is suggestive of ARDS. A P/F ratio less than 200 with bilateral fluffy infiltrates and no evidence of congestive heart failure is the definition of ARDS. Once acute lung injury or ARDS is diagnosed, lung protective ventilation should be initiated. The goal for treatment of these patients is to continue to provide adequate oxygenation without further damaging to the alveoli. This is best accomplished with low tidal volumes (5-7 mL/kg), increased positive end-expiratory pressure (PEEP), and limiting peak/plateau pressures. These lung protective ventilation strategies decrease the incidence of volutrauma and barotraumas and result in decreased levels of inflammatory mediators released by the injured lungs.

The biggest risk factor for developing MODS is circulatory failure within the first 24 hours of admission. This is why early management of resuscitation is extremely important in critically ill patients. The cause of circulatory failure during MODS is multifactorial. During the initial phase of inflammation, TNF and reactive oxygen species inhibit cardiac contractility. Additionally, the early cytokines released result in increased vascular permeability and vasodilation. This combination results in loss of effective preload, contractility, and afterload. The initial treatment for circulatory failure is intravascular volume repletion. However, this treatment may contribute to the worsening of the system, as the fluids administered may not stay intravascular because of the increased vascular permeability. Even though volume repletion is necessary, excess fluid administration can contribute to the increase in organ failure and the cascade of multiple organ dysfunction. The use of vasopressors is advocated only once it is determined that the intravascular volume has been repleted. Likewise, the use of blood and blood products can be used to increase intravascular volume but are associated with complications. The injudicious use of vasopressors and blood transfusions is known to increase morbidity and mortality. The use of $ScVO_2$, lactate, and base excess can help guide the initial resuscitation.

AKI, formerly referred to as acute renal failure (ARF), is a decline in renal function as determined by either a rise in serum creatinine levels or a decrease in urine output. Serum creatinine levels that increase by 0.3 mg/dL or by 50% from baseline is AKI. Urine output that is less than or equal to 0.5 mL/kg/h for more than 6 hours is also AKI. In MODS, the causes of AKI are both intrinsic and pre-renal. Early in the course of MODS, hypotension can lead to early AKI, while late causes can sometimes be attributed to nephrotoxic drugs and contrast-induced nephropathy. Hypoxemia can lead to cellular destruction and altered renal function. Renal replacement therapy may be necessary to support a patient with MODS and AKI.

Patients with MODS can develop hepatic dysfunction as identified by cholestasis and jaundice. Bilirubin levels are used to determine the severity of dysfunction on the MODS scoring system. The elevation of bilirubin is most likely a result of bile leakage from hepatic canalicula that have been damaged by cytotoxins and inflammatory mediators. The elevation of acute phase reactants, such as C-reactive protein and α_1 anti-trypsin, is common during the inflammatory stages of MODS. The hepatic dysfunction identified in MODS is usually not life-threatening. There is no specific supportive therapy aimed directly at the liver, so continued support of the other systems is all that is necessary. Implementation of enteral nutritional support rather than parenteral nutritional support can help minimized the cholestasis produced by gut inactivity.

CASE CORRELATION

- See also Case 8 (Respiratory Failure), Case 22 (Acute Liver Failure), and Case 23 (Acute Kidney Injury).

COMPREHENSION QUESTIONS

33.1 A 63-year-old, otherwise healthy man is admitted to the ICU with sepsis and right lower lobe pneumonia. He is started on broad-spectrum antibiotics and is being mechanically ventilated. The ventilator settings are Assist Control ventilation, tidal volume of 9 mL/kg, oxygen concentration of 60%, and a PEEP of 8. Two days later, his chest x-ray shows bilateral fluffy infiltrates and a PaO_2/FIO_2 ratio of 195. His oxygen saturation is 85%. The best treatment for this patient is:

    A. Increase the tidal volume on the ventilator

    B. Decrease the amount of PEEP

    C. Add additional antibiotic coverage

    D. Increase the PEEP and decrease the tidal volume

    E. Perform bronchoscopy to rule-out atypical pneumonia

33.2 A man with history of chronic alcohol abuse is admitted with severe pancreatitis that does not appear to be necrotic on CT scan. He is admitted to the ICU with respiratory failure and low urine output. His bilirubin is 3.8 mg/dL, but he has no history of cholelithiasis and ultrasound shows normal ductal anatomy. The most likely cause of his multiorgan failure is:

A. Pancreatic enzymes traveling in vasculature to degrade proteins

B. Infection of the pancreas

C. Blockage of the biliary system

D. Malnutrition from chronic alcoholism

E. Release of inflammatory cytokines from monocytes

33.3 A 21-year-old man sustained a gunshot wound to the abdomen. He had multiple small bowel enterotomies repaired, and a short segment of bowel was resected. After 36 hours, he remains intubated and develops an increasing white blood cell count, tachycardia, and fever. The *least* likely cause of his fever and white count is:

A. Intra-abdominal abscess

B. MODS

C. Pneumonia

D. Missed bowel injury

E. Deep venous thrombosis

33.4 The best treatment for MODS is:

A. Preventative

B. Large volume resuscitation

C. Dialysis

D. Lung protective ventilation

E. Enteral nutritional

ANSWERS

33.1 **D.** This patient is hypoxic and has a diagnosis of acute respiratory distress syndrome (ARDS). The essentials of treating ARDS revolve around decreasing the incidence of both volutrauma and barotrauma. The goal is to decrease the tidal volume, increase the PEEP, and maintain adequate oxygenation. Permissive hypercapnia is allowed as long as the pH does not fall below 7.2. The low oxygen saturations in this patient should be treated by decreasing his tidal volume and increasing the PEEP using the ARDS net protocol strategy (national guidelines based on low tidal volumes) for lung protective ventilation. A typical pneumonia is mostly encountered in immune-compromised hosts and is therefore not a likely diagnosis in this otherwise healthy man.

33.2 **E.** While the other mechanisms may be the instituting and contributing factors, the systemic inflammatory response is secondary to the release of cytokines from monocytes that have been activated. Under normal circumstances, the cytokine release decreases as the patient's inciting pathology improves. Occasionally, the inflammatory cascade does not subside and becomes a positive feedback loop. This is the beginning of MODS.

33.3 **B.** Increasing WBC, fever, and tachycardia in this patient can represent a number of possible complications. Given the circumstances of his injury, missed intra-abdominal injury and intra-abdominal infections are distinct possibilities. Similarly, this patient who is a trauma victim and who recently underwent emergency laparotomy for intra-abdominal injuries is at risk for the development of pneumonia. The timing of these symptoms does not fit the typical picture of MODS, which generally occurs more days to weeks following the initial insult. ADVT is possible in this patient since he is ill and immobilized.

33.4 **A.** The best treatment for MODS is supportive and prevention. Resuscitation, dialysis, enteral nutrition, and lung protective ventilation are all treatment or supportive modalities used when treating a patient with MODS. However, identifying which patients are at risk for developing MODS and instituting early and appropriate care before MODS starts is the best treatment. Once MODS occurs, supportive care through the above modalities is often necessary.

CLINICAL PEARLS

► The best treatment for MODS is supportive and prevention.

► The pulmonary system is often the earliest organ system to demonstrate dysfunction.

► The biggest risk factor for developing MODS is circulatory failure within the first 24 hours of admission.

REFERENCES

Barie PS, Hydo LJ, Pieracci FM, Shou J, Eachempati SR. Multiple organ dysfunction syndrome in critical surgical illness. *Surg Infect (Larchmt)*. 2009 Oct;10(5):369-377.

Mosenthal AC. Multiple organ dysfunction and failure. In: Cameron JL, Cameron AM, eds. *Current Surgical Therapy*. 11th ed. Philadelphia, PA: Elsevier Saunders; 2014:1267-1271.

Mizock BA. The multiple organ dysfunction syndrome. *Dis Mon*. 2009 Aug;55(8):476-526.

A 69-year-old man was admitted to the hospital 10 days ago for a colonic volvulus complicated by colonic perforation and fecal peritonitis. He underwent surgery and was placed on IV antibiotics and mechanical ventilation. Yesterday, he was extubated from mechanical ventilation and was doing well up to this morning. This morning, the patient has had persistent pulse rates ranging from 100 to 110 beats/min, and he is noted to be somnolent and does not interact with his family. The patient's visiting family members are concerned because they feel that he is "not the same person as usual." A CT scan of the brain is performed and demonstrates no abnormalities.

▶ What are the potential causes of this patient's condition?
▶ What are common endocrine disorders associated with critical illnesses?

ANSWERS TO CASE 34:
Endocrinopathies in the ICU Patient

Summary: A 69-year-old man is recovering from sepsis due to peritonitis from a GI process; the patient is now noted to have altered mental status and tachycardia. A normal CT scan of the brain suggests that anatomic causes are unlikely to be responsible for his current condition.

- **Potential causes of the patient's current picture:** The cardiovascular and neurological abnormalities observed in critically ill patients can have a variety of possible causes, including hypoxia from pulmonary pathology, analgesics and sedation medication-related changes, and critical illness-induced endocrinopathies.

- **Common endocrine disorders associated with critical illnesses:** Endocrine-related changes following critical illnesses may include *behavioral changes* (psychomotor, cognitive, and sleep disorders), *cardiovascular changes* (vasodilatory shock, multiple organ dysfunction syndrome), *metabolic changes* (defects in glucose metabolism, protein wasting), and *immunologic changes* (increased susceptibility to infections caused by increased immune suppression related to the shift of TH_1/TH_2 balances toward an excess of TH_2 cells).

ANALYSIS
Objectives

1. To learn the cardiovascular, metabolic, behavioral, and immune disorders that may be produced by endocrine changes associated with critical illnesses.
2. To learn to recognize the manifestations of endocrinopathies in the ICU.
3. To learn the medications that may contribute to endocrinopathies.

Considerations

This patient has been critically ill in the ICU and has had a prolonged ICU course following intra-abdominal infection and sepsis. Even though he has taken steps toward improvement, his persistent tachycardia and mental status change now require further investigation for the causes. At this point, complete blood count, chemistries, arterial blood gas, chest x-ray, electrocardiogram, and cardiac enzymes may be useful in identifying cardiopulmonary causes. Potential new sources of infections may be evaluated with a thorough physical examination, appropriate cultures, and imaging studies. In addition, anatomic causes should be evaluated with a brain CT.

The possibility of endocrinopathies should also be entertained when a patient with critical illness develops cardiovascular, metabolic, and neuropsychiatric derangements, as critical illness can affect the homeostatic processes in several organ systems. A severe septic insult can initially overwhelm the body's innate stress responses primarily regulated by the sympathetic nervous system and hypothalamus-pituitary-adrenal (HPA) axis, leading to early hemodynamic instability that is often associated with mental status changes. Subsequent to these initial responses, critically ill individuals may enter into a state of hypercatabolism, which could be produced by thyroid dysfunction and manifest clinically as tachycardia, atrial fibrillation, or agitation. In older individuals, hyperthyroidism may also manifest as lethargy. Elevated metabolic activity secondary to hyperthyroidism can be evaluated by thyroid function studies. Delirium and cognitive impairment occur quite frequently among individuals following recovery from acute respiratory distress syndrome (ARDS), in which significant cognitive dysfunction, anxiety, and depression are often reported. The exact causes of these neuropsychiatric changes have not been determined; however, it has been theorized that intense inflammatory mediator and cytokine responses may alter neurohormonal homeostasis and lead to neuropsychiatric dysfunctions.

APPROACH TO:

Endocrinopathies in the ICU Patient

CLINICAL APPROACH

Sepsis in the Critically Ill Patient

A systematic guideline as delineated by the Surviving Sepsis campaign provides a multidisciplinary approach to optimize treatment of septic patients. In the initial management, fluid resuscitation begins with isotonic crystalloid for the goals of mean arterial pressure (MAP) >65 mm Hg, central venous pressure 8 to 12, urine output >0.5 mL/kg/h, and superior vena cava oxygen saturation ($Scvo_2$) >70% or mixed venous oxygen saturation (Svo_2) >65%. Vasoactive agents, such as norepinephrine or dopamine, are started when patients are unable to maintain MAP >65 mm Hg despite adequate fluid administration. Transfusion of packed red blood cells may also be initiated for a general hemoglobin goal of 7 to 9 g/dL; however, for patients with lactic acidosis, hemorrhage, or coronary ischemia, the hemoglobin goal should be 10 g/dL. Source control with broad-spectrum antibiotics should be started immediately, with subsequent narrowing of coverage as soon as culture results are available. In managing critical illness, physicians should remain vigilant in considering endocrine derangements, such as adrenal insufficiency, hyper- or hypoglycemia, vasopressin deficiency, and thyroid dysfunction.

Endocrine Response to Critical Illness

Two physiologic pathways are activated during periods of acute stress: the sympathetic nervous system and the endocrine system. The sympathetic nervous system is activated via secretion of catecholamines from the adrenal medulla, leading to changes in the cardiovascular, metabolic, immunologic, and endocrine systems. **In the acute phase of illness, the endocrine system is responsible for an adaptive response to maintain organ perfusion, decrease anabolism, and up-regulate the immune response.**

In the chronic phase of illness, the endocrine system may play a role in the development of persistent hypercatabolism and contribute to organ dysfunction.

Sympathetic Nervous System and Arginine Vasopressin

The "fight or flight" response from the sympathomimetic system is produced by norepinephrine, epinephrine, and dopamine release from the adrenal medulla. These hormones produce complex adaptive responses throughout the body, leading to increased alertness, skin vasoconstriction, vasodilation of skeletal and coronary arteries, bronchodilatation, tachycardia, tachypnea, pupillary dilatation, and glycogenolysis. Catecholamines are also released from mesenteric organs during stress and contribute to a significant percentage of total levels in the body. Catecholamine release from a typical systemic inflammatory response syndrome (SIRS) reaction typically decreases within 3 to 5 days, which may be inadequate in periods of severe stress such as in septic shock. **Three major pathways are theorized to contribute to development of vasodilatory shock: (1) overproduction of nitric oxide (NO), (2) hyperpolarization of vascular smooth muscle membranes, and (3) relative deficiency of vasopressin.**

Some patients with sepsis have insufficient host catecholamine responses and therefore may benefit from exogenous administration of vasoactive medication to maintain end-organ perfusion. Dopamine or norepinephrine is often given as a first-line agent when septic shock patients are refractory to appropriate fluid management. Arginine vasopressin is a neurohypophyseal hormone that acts on V_1 vascular smooth muscle cell receptors and V_2 renal tubular cell receptors to cause hemostasis, arterial vasoconstriction, and antidiuresis. With sepsis, some patients may develop relative vasopressin deficiency with downregulation of V_1 receptors and may benefit from low-dose exogenous vasopressin. Thus, patients with septic shock refractory to fluid management and high-dose conventional vasopressors may be candidates for vasopressin.

Hypothalamic-Pituitary-Adrenal Axis

Acute stress also activates the hypothalamic-pituitary-adrenal (HPA) axis, which is essential for survival. Initiation of this pathway begins with the increased secretion of corticotrophin-releasing hormone from the paraventricular nucleus of the hypothalamus, which in turn stimulates the anterior pituitary to produce ACTH. ACTH then signals for the adrenal cortex to produce cortisol. Cortisol has several important physiologic actions on metabolism, including stimulatory effects on the cardiovascular and immune system. During stress, cortisol increases blood glucose concentration by activating hepatic gluconeogenesis and inhibiting glucose uptake by peripheral tissues. Cortisol also activates lipolysis in adipose tissue to increase free fatty acid release. Cortisol increases blood pressure by sensitizing vascular smooth muscle to catecholamines. Immunologically, cortisol produces anti-inflammatory effects by reducing the number and function of T and B lymphocytes, monocytes, neutrophils, and eosinophils at the site of inflammation.

Approximately 10% to 20% of critically ill patients may exhibit some adrenal insufficiency, with the incidence reported as high as 60% among patients with septic shock. Glucocorticoid resistance is a phenomenon described in septic patients.

Observations suggest that mediators released in patients with critical illness, and sepsis in particular, may either stimulate or impair the synthesis and activation of cortisol via actions on the HPA axis and the glucocorticoid receptor signaling system.

Three laboratory assays are commonly used to diagnose adrenal insufficiency. The first is serum **cortisol** level, which reflects total hormone concentration. The disadvantage of analyzing serum cortisol level is that free cortisol, rather than the protein-bound fraction, is actually responsible for the physiologic activities of the hormone. In most critically ill patients, corticosteroid-binding globulin levels are decreased. Furthermore, with acute stimulation of the adrenal gland, free cortisol increase is substantially more pronounced than the increase of total cortisol concentrations. Consequently, the total serum cortisol level may not accurately reflect free cortisol levels and adrenal functions in critically ill patients. The second test is the Free cortisol level measurement, which is preferable in ICU patients; however, this assay is not widely available. **The third test is the cosyntropin stimulation test, which is a measurement of change (increase) in serum cortisol following the administration of 250 μg dose of synthetic ACTH. An increase <9 μg/dL within 60 minutes is indicative of an inability for the adrenal glands to appropriately respond to ACTH stimulation.** However, this test has its limitations, as it does not assess the integrity of the HPA axis, the response of the HPA axis to other stresses such as hypotension or hypoglycemia, or the adequacy of stress cortisol levels.

In a multicenter, randomized controlled trial, Annane and colleagues reported improved survival in catecholamine-dependent patients with septic shock that was unresponsive to cosyntropin who were given a 7-day course of steroids. In another randomized control trial reported in 2008 (The Corticus Trial), no difference in mortality was found with steroid administration in septic patients with or without appropriate responses to cosyntropin stimulation. This study did find a shorter duration for shock reversal in the steroid-treated patients when compared to patients receiving placebos. These apparently conflicting results may be explained by the sicker patients in the Annane study. In 2008, based on a meta-analysis of six randomized control trials, the American College of Critical Care Medicine issued a consensus statement that **hydrocortisone may be considered in the management of some patients with septic shock, particularly those patients who have responded poorly to fluid resuscitation and vasopressor agents; however, this should not be standard protocol for all septic patients.** The decision to treat septic patients with corticosteroids should be based on clinical criteria and not on results of cosyntropin stimulation tests or other adrenal function testing.

Insulin

Critical illness and sepsis frequently cause hyperglycemia in patients with or without a history of diabetes mellitus. The causes of critical illness–induced hyperglycemia include catecholamine-mediated inhibition of insulin release, as well as glucocorticoid and proinflammatory cytokine-induced glucose synthesis and release. In addition, pancreatic β-cell dysfunction, hepatic glucose production dysfunction, and peripheral insulin resistance are other factors that contribute to the hyperglycemia. In critically ill patients, hyperglycemia contributes to increased morbidity and mortality through a variety of mechanisms, including augmentation of oxidative burden, activation of stress-signaling pathways, and impairment of neutrophil function. Furthermore, hyperglycemia is associated with the increased risk for myocardial infarction, impairment of wound healing, and increased mortality in patients following surgery, trauma, or neurotrauma.

Intensive insulin therapy was found to have reduced mortality benefits in a randomized control trial involving mechanically ventilated cardiac surgical patients. These benefits were observed in patients with and without known diabetes, and the benefits appeared to be most significant among patients with sepsis-induced multiple-organ failure and an ICU stay of >5 days. Target glucose values of 80 to 110 mg/dL were originally suggested as being most beneficial for ICU patients based on the above-mentioned study; however, **more recent evidence suggests that target values of 140 to 180 mg/ dL are more appropriate and produce fewer hypoglycemia-related complications when compared to target glucose values of 80 to 110 mg/dL.**

Hypothalamic-Pituitary-Thyroid Axis

Thyroid hormones produced by the thyroid gland are regulated by thyrotropin-releasing hormone (TRH) and thyroid-stimulating hormone (TSH) released by the hypothalamus and anterior pituitary, respectively. Thyroid hormones act to increase the basal metabolic rate, affect protein synthesis, and increase the sensitivity of tissues to catecholamines. Thyroxine (T_4) is the principal hormone produced by the thyroid and can be subsequently deiodinated to the active form, triiodothyronine (T_3) in extrathyroidal tissues. Approximately 99% of all T_3 and T_4 is bound to thyroxine-binding globulins and other plasma proteins; the physiologically active form of thyroid hormone is unbound, and its level can be measured via laboratory testing.

Euthyroid sick syndrome, also known as low T_3 to T_4 syndrome or nonthyroidal illness syndrome, is commonly identified in critically ill patients. This is characterized by an acute decrease in T_3 followed by a decrease in T_4 within 24 to 48 hours. This is caused by inhibition in T_4 to T_3 conversion, leading to an increase in reverse-T_3 (rT_3). TSH often increases briefly at onset but usually remains within the low to normal range without a circadian rhythm. Although this may reflect an adaptive mechanism aimed at reducing hypercatabolism, this disease process is associated with an increased mortality despite a lack of overt hyper- or hypothyroid symptoms. A small randomized control trial found no mortality benefit in exogenous administration of T_4 versus placebo in critically ill patients with this disorder. Another nonrandomized cohort study showed no clinical outcome difference in patients undergoing continuous TRH infusion. Current recommendations call for no intervention to correct the thyroid hormone levels in euthyroid sick syndrome.

Somatotropic Axis

Growth hormone (GH) is secreted by the anterior pituitary in a pulsatile fashion and has anabolic effects in the body, increasing lipolysis and protein synthesis and reducing glucose uptake in hepatocytes. Its activity is mediated by insulin-like growth factor 1 (IGF-1), which is bound by IGF-binding proteins (IGFBP), thereby reducing its bioavailability but prolonging its half-life. The acute phase of critical illness is characterized by a reduced pulsatile release of GH, high basal GH levels, and low levels of IGF-1 and IGFBP. Cytokine release during stress causes a widespread GH resistance with the down-regulation of GH receptors, causing reduced anabolic activity and providing metabolic energy while wasting muscle protein. This has deleterious effects in critically ill patients, including delaying wound healing, depressing immune function, and contributing to respiratory muscle dysfunction. Two large clinical trials investigating whether exogenous GH would reverse hypercatabolism found no benefit, and in fact, they found an increased risk of infection and death. Currently, there is no evidence to show that pharmacologic agents acting on the somatotropic axis have any benefit on clinical outcome in critically ill patients.

Hypothalamic-Pituitary-Gonadal Axis

Gonadal hormones, which interact with androgen and estrogen receptors, are mediated by luteinizing hormone (LH) and follicle-stimulating hormone (FSH) released by the anterior pituitary; LH and FSH in turn are regulated by gonadotropin-releasing hormone secreted by the hypothalamus. In males, a low level of testosterone is associated with acute and chronic critical illness and is directly associated with mortality. Female patients may experience the "hypothalamic amenorrhea of stress." Although estrogen supplementation has been shown to be beneficial in critically ill patients, current recommendations do not endorse routine use of sex hormone replacement. Furthermore, estrogen use can increase the risk of venous thromboembolism.

Sleep Disturbances in the ICU

Sleep disturbances in the ICU are common, and these disturbances may include decreased nocturnal sleep, reduced or absence of deep sleep, and disrupted circadian patterns. In addition, ICU patients commonly report anxiety, fear, and nightmares associated with sleep during and after their ICU stays. The normal sleep–wake cycle is controlled by complex interactions between neurotransmitters such as catecholamines, glutamate, histamine, melatonin, and acetylcholine. Melatonin production by the pineal gland follows a diurnal variation pattern and is responsible in promoting nocturnal sleep. Septic patients have been found to have a continuous, non-fluctuating secretion of melatonin. Altered melatonin production is believed to be beneficial during sepsis, as it possesses antioxidant properties. ICU patients may also have sleep disruption due to disturbances in the HPA axis activity, which modulates cortisol release following stress. Cortisol is known to inhibit sleep. Because of these endogenous changes as well as the external stimuli, 60% of all ICU patients report sleep disturbances.

Drug-Induced Endocrine Disorders

Drug-induced pituitary-adrenal axis dysfunction Etomidate is often used for rapid-sequence induction during intubation. Continuous infusion of etomidate was utilized during the 1980s, but this practice was discontinued when it was found to be associated with increased mortality due to adrenal dysfunction. Single-dose etomidate has been reported to contribute to adrenal dysfunction; however, its uncommon occurrence suggests that the risk is minimal. Single-dose etomidate may produce clinically significant adrenal insufficiency in septic patients in whom any level of adrenal dysfunction could contribute to worse clinical outcomes; therefore, the current recommendations suggest that ketamine may be a more appropriate agent for rapid-sequence induction in the septic patient population. The etomidate effect on adrenal dysfunction is believed to be due to a dose-dependent blockade of the enzyme involved in the final conversion of cholesterol to cortisol.

Chronic glucocorticoid therapy is common in ICU patients. Patients with a history of chronic glucocorticoid therapy are at risk for the development of adrenal insufficiency during stress states; however, the dose and duration of prior steroid use do not predict the likelihood of insufficiency. It is recommended that patients in shock and with history of chronic steroid use receive steroid repletion, and patients without shock should be closely monitored for signs of insufficiency rather than receiving empiric replacement.

Drugs causing up-regulation of cytochrome P-450 (CYP-450) activity may increase cortisol metabolism (breakdown) and contribute to adrenal insufficiency. Examples of this class of agents are rifampin, phenobarbital, and phenytoin. The medication effects can be observed within 7 days of therapy initiation and require close monitoring of clinical effects.

Antifungal agents causing CYP-450 inhibition may produce adrenal insufficiency by suppressing CYP-450-dependent steroidogenesis. Ketoconazole is the most well-documented antifungal agent associated with adrenal insufficiency. Fluconazole and itraconazole are agents that produce adrenal insufficiency much less frequently in comparison to ketoconazole. Due to the potential of causing clinically significant adrenal insufficiency, patients receiving antifungal therapy should be closely monitored.

Thyroid dysfunction can be induced by a dopamine infusion, which is associated with the occurrence of **nonthyroidal illness syndrome.** This effect is related to the reduction of TSH concentration and reduction in thyroxine production. Dopamine effects on thyroid functions can be observed within 24 hours after the initiation of dopamine infusion, and these effects are completely reversed within 24 hours following termination of dopamine infusion.

Lithium is concentrated in the thyroid and may cause a **decrease in thyroxine release.** Hypothyroidism and goiter formation may occur in individuals with prolonged lithium intake; hypothyroidism is reported in approximately 20% of individuals taking lithium for 10 years or longer.

Amiodarone is frequently prescribed for the management of atrial or ventricular arrhythmias. By weight, **37% of amiodarone is made up of iodine,** and this medication is structurally similar to thyroxine. Long-term and short-term administration of amiodarone have the potential of producing **thyrotoxicosis.** Amiodarone-induced thyrotoxicosis 1 (AIT-I) describes the amiodarone-induced thyrotoxicosis that occurs in individuals with preexisting thyroid diseases. This problem is treated with antithyroid medications such as methimazole or propylthiouracil. ATI-II is an amiodarone-induced thyroiditis causing destruction of the gland and release of thyroid hormone; this condition is best treated with glucocorticoids. Due to the long half-life of amiodarone (50-100 days), ATI diseases may occur long after discontinuation of the medication.

Interestingly, **amiodarone can also cause hypothyroidism**; however, the mechanisms that cause amiodarone-induced hypothyroidism are undetermined at this time. Women and those with a history of Hashimoto thyroiditis are at increased risk for amiodarone-induced hypothyroidism. Most cases of hypothyroidism are mild and can be managed with thyroxine replacement or the discontinuation of amiodarone.

CLINICAL CASE CORRELATION

- See also Case 15 (Cardiac Arrhythmias), Case 19 (Sepsis), and Case 33 (Multiorgan Dysfunction).

COMPREHENSION QUESTIONS

34.1 A 44-year-old man is hospitalized for septic shock due to pneumonia, and he has received crystalloid resuscitation to achieve a CVP of 18 mm Hg. Thereafter, a norepinephrine drip was initiated. Despite these measures, his mean arterial pressures remained below 65 mm Hg. Vasopressin drip at 0.03 U/min was initiated without improvement. He is believed to be on the appropriate antimicrobial regimen for his infection. Which of the following is the most appropriate management in this patient?

   A. Proceed with a cosyntropin stimulation test and give hydrocortisone if the patient is demonstrated to have insufficient adrenal response

   B. Give 100 μg of thyroxine

   C. Measure plasma vasopressin level

   D. Administer cortisol 100 mg intravenously

   E. Transfuse 2 U of packed red blood cells

34.2 A 55-year-old woman with a history of goiter develops fever, tachycardia, and anxiety 12 hours following the initiation of amiodarone drip for ventricular arrhythmias. Her serum TSH is noted to be <0.01. Which of the following statement best describes her current condition?

   A. This patient is experiencing amiodarone-induced hypothyroidism.

   B. This condition is best treated by corticosteroid administration.

   C. This patient is experiencing amiodarone-induced thyroiditis.

   D. This patient's condition is best treated with propylthiouracil.

   E. This condition is best treated with iodine administration.

34.3 Which of the following statements best describes the current recommended approach to glycemic control in the ICU?

A. Strict glucose control targeting glucose levels of 80 to 110 mg/dL is strongly recommended for postoperative patients.

B. Glucose control targeting glucose levels of 140 to 180 mg/dL is associated with lower morbidity and mortality than glucose target levels of 80 to 110 mg/dL.

C. Glycemic control in the ICU has not been shown to provide clinical benefits.

D. Hyperglycemia is generally not a problem unless individuals are receiving total parenteral nutrition.

E. Serum glucose levels >180 mg/dL is associated with improved neurological outcomes following head injury.

ANSWERS

34.1 **D.** This patient has persistent septic shock despite sufficient fluid resuscitation to restore intravascular volume. He remains refractory to norepinephrine and low-dose vasopressin infusions. Based on the meta-analysis findings of six randomized control trial and the American College of Critical Care Medicine consensus recommendations, hydrocortisone should be considered in this individual. Thyroxine replacement and blood transfusions do not play a role in the treatment of vasopressor-refractory septic shock. Measurement of serum vasopressin levels does not play a significant role in clinical decision-making in this setting.

34.2 **D.** This patient has clinical and biochemical evidence of hyperthyroidism. The condition may or may not be the result of amiodarone-induced hyperthyroidism. In either case, the appropriate treatment is antithyroid medications such as propylthiouracil. Amiodarone can also produce hyperthyroidism by causing an autoimmune thyroiditis; however, this process generally takes more than 12 hours to appear.

34.3 **B.** Current evidence suggests that glycemic control targeting glucose levels of 140 to 180 mg/dL rather than 80 to 110 mg/dL is associated with fewer occurrences of hypoglycemia-associated complications.

CLINICAL PEARLS

▶ Dopamine and norepinephrine are first-line agents to maintain end-organ perfusion in septic shock after patients have been adequately volume resuscitated.

▶ Arginine vasopressin may be indicated in critically ill patients who are refractory to high-dose vasopressors and are suspected to have relative vasopressin deficiency.

▶ Hydrocortisone should be considered in septic shock when hypotension is refractory to fluid and vasopressor agents and the patient has clinical evidence of adrenal insufficiency.

▶ Treatment of septic patients with corticosteroids should be a clinical decision and should not be determined on the basis of adrenal function testing results.

▶ Insulin therapy with target glucose levels of 140 to 180 mg/dL is beneficial in critically ill patients.

▶ Nonthyroidal illness syndrome may occur in critically ill patients; however, no intervention is currently recommended to restore normal thyroid levels.

▶ Gonadal steroids have a linear relationship with mortality in critically ill patients; however, current literature does not support exogenous replacement.

REFERENCES

Annane D. Effect of treatment with low doses of hydrocortisone and fludrocortisones on mortality in patients with septic shock. *JAMA.* 2002;288:862.

Bello G, Paliani MG, Pontecorvi A, Antonelli M. Treating nonthyroidal illness syndrome in the critically ill patients: still a matter of controversy. *Curr Drug Targets.* 2009;10:778-787.

Gabrielli A, Layon AJ, Yu M, eds. *Civetta, Taylor, and Kirby's Manual of Critical Care.* Philadelphia, PA: Lippincott Williams & Wilkins; 2012:848-856.

Marik PE, Pastore SM, Annane D, et al. Recommendations for the diagnosis and management of corticosteroid insufficiency in critically ill adult patients: consensus statements from an international task force by the American College of Critical Care Medicine. *Crit Care Med.* 2008;36:1937-1949.

Sprung CL, Annane D, Keh D, et al. Hydrocortisone therapy for patients with septic shock. *N Engl J Med.* 2008;358:111-124.

The NICE-SUGAR Study Investigators. Intensive versus conventional glucose control in critically ill patients. *N Engl J Med.* 2009:360:1283-1297.

Thomas Z, Bandali F, McCowen K, Malhotra A. Drug-induced endocrine disorders in the intensive care unit. *Crit Care Med.* 2010;38(6):S219-S230.

A 19-year-old G1P0 woman at 29 weeks' gestation arrives to the hospital because of severe dyspnea of 6 hours' duration. Her prenatal course has been unremarkable, and she denies any medical problems. Her blood pressure is 160/114 mm Hg, HR 105 beats/min, RR 40 breaths/min and labored, and oxygen saturation 90%. The fetal heart tones are in the 140 beats/min range. The patient denies prior history of elevated blood pressure. A urine protein to creatinine ratio is 0.6. The serum ALT is 84 IU/L (normal <35), and AST is 90 IU/L (normal <35). The prenatal records show the following normal BP previously, and normal urine protein.

▶ What is the most likely diagnosis?
▶ What is your immediate next step?
▶ What are your priority laboratory tests?
▶ What is your management plan?

ANSWERS TO CASE 16:
Preeclampsia With Severe Features

Summary: A 19-year-old G1P0 woman at 29 weeks' gestation has acute onset of severe dyspnea, RR of 40 breaths/min and labored, new onset severely elevated BP of 160/114, elevated protein/creatinine ratio, and elevated liver function tests. The prenatal records show normal BPs in the pregnancy with a borderline elevated BP and 1+ proteinuria at the last visit (26 weeks).

- **Most likely diagnosis:** Preeclampsia with severe features (pulmonary edema).

- **Immediate next step:** The highest priority must be to improve oxygenation. Sufficient oxygen must be provided to raise the O_2 saturation above 94%, and if the patient is tiring, then ventilator support may be required. The second priority is to lower the BP with an IV antihypertensive agent. If pulmonary edema is confirmed, IV diuresis such as furosemide should be given.

- **Priority laboratory tests:** CBC with platelet count, and renal function test (creatinine).

- **Management:** Stabilize maternal status (optimize oxygenation, lower BP to safe level below 160/110 mm Hg), stabilize fetal status, administer corticosteroids for fetal lung maturity, start magnesium sulfate for seizure prophylaxis, and move toward delivery.

ANALYSIS

Objectives

1. Know the clinical presentation and diagnostic criteria for four categories of hypertensive disorders of pregnancy.

2. Know the serious sequelae of severe features of preeclampsia, including pulmonary edema.

3. Understand the management of preeclampsia with severe features at the preterm and term gestations.

Considerations

The patient is nulliparous, which is a risk factor for preeclampsia. She has preeclampsia based on new onset BP exceeding 140/90 mm Hg with proteinuria (urine protein/creatinine ratio exceeding 0.3). The patient has a record of normal BPs in her first 24 weeks of pregnancy (with borderline BP and 1+ proteinuria at 26 weeks), which is evidence that she does not have chronic hypertension. She has **preeclampsia with severe features** based on any one of three criteria: elevated **blood pressure, elevated liver function tests, and likely pulmonary edema.** An O_2 sat of 90% correlates to a Po_2 level of 60 mm Hg. Thus, the most immediate next step would be improving oxygenation. The patient should be given 100% oxygen by face mask, and if lung auscultation confirm pulmonary edema, then IV furosemide should be given. Concurrently, the BP needs to be lowered from the severe level ($\geq 160/110$ mm Hg) to prevent stroke. The physical examination and an urgent portable chest x-ray can help to assess for cardiomyopathy, pulmonary embolism, or asthma. Stabilization of maternal status has priority over fetal status; however, there should not be undue delay to evaluate the fetal status: fetal heart rate pattern and ultrasound for fetal weight, and amniotic fluid measurement. **Deciding whether to deliver a preeclamptic patient with severe features depends on the risk to maternal/fetal well being, the stability of the patient, and the gestational age.** In the face of pulmonary edema, delivery must be enacted, since the pregnant woman's life is in immediate jeopardy. In the face of marked prematurity, some severe features such as mildly elevated but stable liver function tests may be observed carefully without delivery. The **key laboratories to draw are the CBC with platelet count, liver function tests (LFTs), and serum creatinine.** The **management of this patient includes magnesium sulfate for seizure prophylaxis and delivery.** Because of the preterm gestation, antenatal **corticosteroid administration** is important to promote lung maturity, as is **GBS prophylaxis** such as with IV Penicillin.

APPROACH TO:
Hypertensive Disease in Pregnancy

DEFINITIONS

CHRONIC HYPERTENSION: Blood pressure of 140/90 mm Hg before pregnancy or at less than 20 weeks' gestation, or persisting more than 12 weeks postpartum

GESTATIONAL HYPERTENSION: Hypertension without proteinuria (or other features of preeclampsia) at greater than 20 weeks' gestation persistent for at least 4 hours

PREECLAMPSIA: Hypertension (140 systolic or 90 diastolic) over 6 hours with the new onset of proteinuria (>300 mg over 24 hours, or a urine protein to creatinine ratio >0.3) usually at a gestational age greater than 20 weeks. In the absence of proteinuria, hypertension and one of the following findings may suffice: thrombocytopenia, impaired LFT, renal insufficiency, pulmonary edema, cerebral disturbances, or visual impairment

ECLAMPSIA: Seizure disorder associated with preeclampsia

HELLP SYNDROME: Hemolysis, elevated liver function tests, low platelets, possibly a subset of severe preeclampsia, associated with significant fetal/maternal morbidity and mortality.

POSTERIOR REVERSIBLE ENCEPHALOPATHY SYNDROME (PRES): A clinico- neuroradiological syndrome with headache, encephalopathy, seizures, and cortical visual disturbances, usually diagnosed with clinical features and MRI (showing enhancement in the posterior parietal areas). Prompt recognition and treatment of PRES with antihypertensives, anti-epileptics, and ICU monitoring is important to prevent long-term neurological sequelae.

SEVERE FEATURE OF PREECLAMPSIA: Vasospasm associated with preeclampsia of such extent that maternal end organs are threatened, usually necessitating delivery of the baby regardless of gestational age.

SUPERIMPOSED PREECLAMPSIA: Development of preeclampsia in a patient with chronic hypertension, often diagnosed by an increased blood pressure and/or new onset proteinuria, which can be with or without severe features.

SUPERIMPOSED PREECLAMPSIA WITH SEVEVE FEATURES: Development of preeclampsia in a patient with chronic hypertension with severe hypertension despite maximum therapy, cerebral/visual symptoms, pulmonary edema, low platelets, elevated LFT, or new onset renal insufficiency (Cr ≥ 1.1 mg/dL).

CLINICAL APPROACH

Hypertensive disorders complicate 3% to 4% of pregnancies and can be organized into several categories:

- Gestational hypertension
- Preeclampsia with or without severe features
- Chronic hypertension
- Superimposed preeclampsia with or without severe features
- Eclampsia

Gestational hypertensive patients have only increased blood pressures without proteinuria or other features of preeclampsia. Up to one-third of those who are thought to have gestational hypertension are later found to have preeclampsia.

Preeclampsia is characterized by hypertension and proteinuria; less commonly, there is absence of proteinuria but evidence of vasospastic disease via other end-organ manifestations (Table 35–1). Although not a criterion, nondependent edema is also usually present. An elevated blood pressure is diagnosed with a systolic blood pressure at or higher than 140 mm Hg or diastolic blood pressure at or higher than 90 mm Hg. Two elevated BPs, measured 6 hours apart (BP taken in the seated position), are needed for the formal diagnosis of preeclampsia, although at term, presumptive diagnoses with persistent hypertension over a shorter interval often

Table 35–1 • DIAGNOSIS OF PREECLAMPSIA
New onset hypertension (140 mm Hg systolic or 90 mm Hg diastolic) twice over 6 hours with any of the following: • Proteinuria (≥300 mg/24 h, or Protein/Cr ≥0.3, or dipstick ≥1+) • Thrombocytopenia (plt <100,000/µL) • Impaired LFT (2 × normal) • Renal insufficiency (Cr ≥1.1 mg/dL) • Pulmonary edema • New onset cerebral disturbance or visual impairment

Table 35–2 • SEVERE FEATURES OF PREECLAMPSIA ANY ONE OF THE FOLLOWING:
• Systolic BP ≥160 mm Hg or diastolic BP ≥110 mm Hg on two occasions 4 h apart • Platelet <100,000/μL • Impaired LFT (2 × normal) or severe persistent epigastric or RUQ pain • Progressive renal insufficiency (Cr ≥ 1.1 mg/dL) • Pulmonary edema • New onset cerebral or visual disturbance

guides management. Proteinuria is usually based on timed urine collection, defined as equal to or greater than 300 mg of protein in 24 hours, although a P/Cr ratio ≥0.3 is accurate.

Preeclampsia is further categorized as **with or without severe features.** See Table 35–2. With severe vasospasm to the brain, headache or visual disturbances can occur. Capillary leakage can lead to pulmonary edema. Right upper quadrant or epigastric pain or elevated LFTs result from hepatic injury.

Chronic hypertension includes preexisting hypertension or hypertension that develops prior to 20 weeks' gestation. These patients are at risk for intrauterine growth restriction (IUGR), fetal demise, or placental abruption. A patient with chronic hypertension is at risk for developing preeclampsia and, if this develops, her diagnosis is labeled as **superimposed preeclampsia**; this diagnosis is made on the basis of new onset of severe and uncontrollable hypertension, or new onset proteinuria, or a severe feature (Table 35–2). **Eclampsia** occurs when the patient with preeclampsia develops convulsions or seizures, but it can occur without elevated blood pressure or proteinuria.

Pathophysiology

The underlying pathophysiology of preeclampsia is vasospasm and "leaky vessels," but its origin is unclear. It is cured only by termination of the pregnancy, and the disease process almost always resolves after delivery. Vasospasm and endothelial damage result in leakage of serum between the endothelial cells and cause local hypoxemia of tissue. Hypoxemia leads to hemolysis, necrosis, and other end-organ damage. The **vasospasm leads to increased systemic vascular resistance (hypertension), decreased intravascular volume, and decreased oncotic pressure**; these changes make a patient more susceptible to pulmonary edema and sensitive to fluid shifts (fluid overload with IV fluids, and hypotension with blood loss).

Clinical Evaluation

Patients are usually unaware of the hypertension and proteinuria, and typically the presence of symptoms indicates severe disease. Hence, one of the important roles of prenatal care is to identify patients with hypertension and proteinuria prior to severe disease. Complications of preeclampsia include placental abruption, eclampsia (with possible intracerebral hemorrhage), coagulopathies, renal failure, hepatic subcapsular hematoma, hepatic rupture, and uteroplacental insufficiency. Fetal growth restriction, poor Apgar scores, and fetal acidosis are also more often seen.

Risk factors for preeclampsia include nulliparity, extremes of age, African-American race, personal history of severe preeclampsia, family history of preeclampsia, chronic hypertension, chronic renal disease, obesity, antiphospholipid syndrome, diabetes, and multifetal gestation. The history and physical examination is focused on end-organ disease.

It is important to review and evaluate the blood pressures prior to 20 weeks' gestation (to assess for chronic hypertension). Patients with chronic hypertension may sometimes already have mild proteinuria; thus, it is important to establish a baseline to later document superimposed preeclampsia (substantial increase in proteinuria). Also, one should document any sudden increase in weight (indicating possible edema). On physical examination, serial blood pressures should be checked along with a urinalysis.

Laboratory tests should include a complete blood count (CBC; check platelet count and hemoconcentration), urinalysis and 24-hour urine protein collection or protein/creatinine ratio (check for proteinuria), liver function tests, LDH (elevated with hemolysis), and creatinine. Fetal testing (such as biophysical profile) is also usually performed to evaluate uteroplacental insufficiency.

Management

After the diagnosis of preeclampsia is made, the management will depend on the gestational age of the fetus and the severity of the disease (see Figure 35–1 for one management scheme). **Gestational hypertensive or preeclamptic patients without severe features** can be observed and delivered at term (**37 weeks**), and magnesium sulfate use is individualized. **Chronic hypertensive patients who are well controlled and uncomplicated can be observed and delivered at 38 to 39 weeks.** When severe features complicate preeclampsia or superimposed preeclampsia, the risks of the preeclampsia must be weighed against the risk of prematurity.

When the fetus is premature, the following issues are considered:

1. What are the immediate threats to maternal status, how stable is the patient, and can these threats be ameliorated?

2. What are the immediate threats to fetal status, how stable is the fetus, and can these threats be ameliorated?

3. What is the gestational age? If less than 34 weeks' gestation, can delivery be safely delayed for 48 hours to allow corticosteroids to have maximum efficacy?

4. What is the natural history of the severe feature, and does it seem to be worsening rapidly?

Observation of a patient with severe features should be performed in a tertiary center, since the risks to both the woman and the fetus are substantial. **With an unstable patient, delivery is always warranted regardless of gestational age. NSAIDs may elevate the BP in postpartum preeclamptic patients and should be avoided.**

Acute Management of Severe Hypertension

The acute-onset of severe hypertension (160 mm Hg systolic or 110 mm Hg diastolic, NOTE "or") that persists more than 15 minutes is considered a hypertensive emergency. **Therapy should be initiated quickly to avoid stroke.** Systolic hypertension is

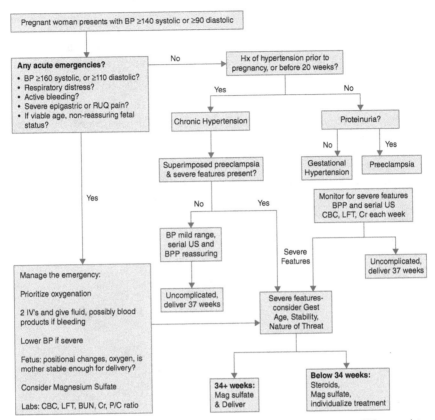

Figure 35-1. Suggested Algorithm for Management of Hypertension in Pregnancy. CBC = complete blood count; LFT = liver function tests; BUN = blood urea nitrogen; Cr = creatinine; P/C ratio = protein to creatinine ratio.

as important or even more important as a predictor of cerebral injury. **First-line agents include IV labetolol, IV hydralazine, or oral nifedipine;** typically after an initial dose, the BP is retaken 20 minutes later and further higher dose therapy is given if the BP is still in the severe range.

Eclampsia

Eclampsia is one of the most feared complications of preeclampsia, and the greatest risk for occurrence is just prior to delivery, during labor (intrapartum), and within the first 24 hours postpartum. During labor, the preeclamptic patient should be started on the anticonvulsant magnesium sulfate. Since magnesium is excreted by the kidneys, it is important to monitor urine output, respiratory depression, dyspnea (side effect of magnesium sulfate is pulmonary edema), and abolition of the deep tendon reflexes (first sign of toxic effects is hyporeflexia). Hypertension is not affected by the magnesium. Severe hypertension needs to be controlled with antihypertensive medications such as hydralazine or labetalol. After delivery, magnesium sulfate is discontinued approximately 24 hours postpartum. The hypertension and proteinuria frequently will resolve. Occasionally, the patient's blood pressure remains high and an antihypertensive medication is needed after delivery. After discharge, the patient usually follows up in 1 to 2 weeks to check blood pressures and proteinuria.

Collaboration Between Obstetricians and Intensivists

Over the past 15 years, the maternal mortality rate in the United States has climbed to be double and in some states three-fold higher than in 1990. There are many reasons for this increase, including higher cesarean rate, patients with more co-morbidities getting pregnant, delayed childbirth, and higher rate of obesity. Pregnant or postpartum women who develop critical illnesses should be co-managed by intensivists and obstetricians/maternal fetal medicine specialists. Good communication, coordination of care, and team work is important in this setting.

CLINICAL CASE CORRELATION

- See also Case 36 (ICU patients with obstetrical issues).

COMPREHENSION QUESTIONS

35.1 A 29-year-old G1P0 woman at 28 weeks' gestation is admitted to the hospital for preeclampsia. Her blood pressure (BP) is 150/100 mm Hg, and her protein excretion is 500 mg in 24 hours. On hospital day 7, she is diagnosed with severe features of preeclampsia and the decision is made to administer magnesium sulfate and deliver the baby. Which of the following findings is most likely present in this patient to necessitate delivery?

A. Elevated uric acid levels

B. 5 g of proteinuria excreted in a 24-hour period

C. 4+ pedal edema

D. Platelet count of 115,000/μL

E. PT INR of 1.9 and PTT of 50 s

35.2 Which of the following is the best management of an 18-year-old G1P0 woman at 28 weeks' gestation with a blood pressure of 160/110 mm Hg, elevated liver function tests, and a platelet count of 60,000/μL?

A. Oral antihypertensive therapy

B. Platelet transfusion

C. Magnesium sulfate therapy and induction of labor

D. Intravenous immunoglobulin therapy

35.3 A 19-year-old G1P0 woman at 39 weeks' gestation is diagnosed with pre-eclampsia based on blood pressures in the range of 150/90 mm Hg and 2+ proteinuria on urine dipstick. She complains of a severe headache. The patient is placed on magnesium sulfate and develops flushing and fatigue. She asks about the need for the magnesium sulfate. You explain that it is to prevent the seizures that may complicate preeclampsia and may even cause death. The patient asks how seizures associated with preeclampsia can cause mortality. Which of the following is the most common mechanism?

    A. Intracerebral hemorrhage

    B. Myocardial infarction

    C. Electrolyte abnormalities

    D. Aspiration

35.4 A 33-year-old woman at 29 weeks' gestation is noted to have blood pressures of 150/90 mm Hg and a protein/creatinine ratio of 0.6. The platelet count, liver function tests, and creatinine are normal. Which of the following is the best management for this patient?

    A. Induction of labor

    B. Cesarean section

    C. Antihypertensive therapy

    D. Expectant management

35.5 A 25-year-old G1P0 woman at 28 weeks is diagnosed with severe preeclampsia based on BP of 160/100 mm Hg and a platelet count of 98,000/mm^3. The patient is treated with hydralazine for the hypertension. Which of the following is the most appropriate reason for delivery?

    A. Blood pressures persist in the range of 150/95 mm Hg

    B. Urine protein increases to 5 g over 24 hours

    C. The patient reaches 32 weeks gestation

    D. The patient develops pulmonary edema

    E. Repeat platelet count is 95,000/mm^3

35.6 On postpartum day 1, a 28-year-old G1P1 woman reports some headache and problems with her vision bilaterally. Her BP is 150/95 mm Hg and P/C ratio is 0.5. Her neurological examination is normal, but her vision is impaired in both eyes. Which of the following is the best next step?

    A. Antihypertensive agent

    B. IV mannitol

    C. MRI of the brain

    D. CT imaging of the brain

    E. Ophthalmic eye drops to both eyes

Choose the best management plan (A-E) for each of the clinical scenarios (35.7-35.10):

    A. Corticosteroids

    B. Antihypertensive agent

    C. Biophysical profile

    D. Magnesium sulfate and delivery

    E. Continued observation

35.7   A 32-year-old G2 P1 woman is at 35 weeks with chronic hypertension. The BP is in the 140/95 mm Hg range.

35.8   A 28-year-old G1P0 woman is at 30 weeks' gestation with superimposed preeclampsia. The BP is 150/100. The platelet count is 95,000/μL and LFT is two times normal. BPP is 10/10.

35.9   A 30-year-old G2P1 woman is at 31 weeks with chronic hypertension, using oral labetolol. Her BP in the office is 160/95 and 162/90. The urine protein is negative.

35.10   A 24-year-old G3P2 woman at 34 weeks' gestation is noted to have preeclampsia. The BP is 150/90 and P/C ratio is 0.5. A fetal ultrasound shows the estimated fetal weight is at the eighth percentile.

ANSWERS

35.1 **E.** A severe feature of preeclampsia (Table 35–2) may or may not necessitate immediate delivery. In this case, disseminated intravascular coagulation (DIC) is the most concerning condition and requires delivery at any gestational age. Pedal edema is not pathologic; nondependent edema, such as of the face and hands, may be consistent with preeclampsia but does not indicate severity of disease. Low platelets are associated with HELLP syndrome, a form of hemolytic anemia in pregnancy, and are very worrisome. Uric acid levels are known to be elevated with preeclampsia; however, it is not a criterion for severe preeclampsia. In general, the criteria for severe preeclampsia indicate end-organ threat and generally require delivery for gestational age at or greater than 34 weeks, and depending on the nature of the threat and the stability of the patient, perhaps delivery at gestational age.

35.2 **C.** Although the pregnancy is only 28 weeks, in light of the severe features of preeclampsia with marked thrombocytopenia, the best treatment is magnesium sulfate and delivery. When preeclampsia with severe features is diagnosed, delivery depends on the nature of the threat, the stability of the patient/fetus, and the gestational age. If the platelet count were higher (90,000/μL), expectant management may be entertained at a tertiary center. Oral antihypertensive therapy, such as labetalol, may be given to the patient to control blood pressure; however, it should not be used as the "treatment" for severe preeclampsia. The platelet levels are not low enough to require transfusion; although intravenous immunoglobulin (IVIG) is used for various autoimmune diseases, it is not indicated in this patient.

35.3 **A.** The most common cause of maternal death due to eclampsia is intracerebral hemorrhage. Eclampsia is one of the most feared complications of preeclampsia, and the greatest risk for occurrence is just prior to delivery, during labor (intrapartum), and within the first 24 hours postpartum. Patients with gestational hypertension or preeclampsia without severe features do not necessarily require magnesium sulfate for seizure prophylaxis. This patient has a severe headache, which is a severe feature. Magnesium sulfate has been proven to be superior to other anticonvulsants such as valium, Dilantin, or phenobarbital. One dictum that is useful in the emergency room or obstetrical unit is that "a pregnant patient greater than 20 weeks' gestation without a history of epilepsy who presents with seizures has eclampsia until otherwise proven."

35.4 **D.** In the preterm patient with mild preeclampsia, expectant management is generally employed until severe features are noted or the pregnancy reaches 37 weeks. In other words, the risks of prematurity usually outweigh the risks of the preeclampsia until end-organ threat is manifest. Had this patient been at term, the best step in management would be to induce labor; this is because at term, the risks of prematurity are minimal. Severe, but not mild hypertension associated with preeclampsia, should be controlled with hypertensive medication. Antihypertensive agents are useful in chronic hypertension but not preeclampsia unless the BP is in the severe range; lowering these BPs can help avoid stroke. For the patient in this scenario, neither induction nor cesarean section is indicated since she is not yet at term. It is not a requirement for a preeclamptic patient to deliver by cesarean. This patient can be followed as an outpatient with twice weekly BP checks and once a week platelet count, Cr and LFTs.

35.5 **D.** Pulmonary edema is an indication for delivery at a preterm gestation. Proteinuria of 5 g over 24 hours is no longer criteria of a severe feature of preeclampsia and does not correspond to maternal or fetal outcome. Mild thrombocytopenia (80,000-100,000/mm3) that is stable may be judiciously observed in this patient (in a tertiary care center). A DIC panel should be performed to ensure there is not a coagulopathy, since that would be an indication for immediate delivery.

35.6 **C.** This patient is postpartum and likely has preeclampsia based on the elevated BP and the proteinuria. The symptoms may be due to PRES syndrome, which needs to be quickly diagnosed by MR imaging, since aggressive therapy must be enacted to prevent long-term brain dysfunction. An antihypertensive agent does not generally need to be used unless the BP is severe (160 mm Hg systolic or 110 mm Hg diastolic). CT imaging can discern an intracranial bleed and is useful if the patient had an eclamptic episode. Eye drops would be indicated in conjunctivitis.

35.7   **C.** A biophysical profile should be performed. A patient with chronic hypertension that is well controlled should be monitored carefully for superimposed preeclampsia, complications such as abruption, serial ultrasound examinations to assess for IUGR, and fetal testing such as BPP weekly. The patient should be delivered at 38 to 39 weeks.

35.8   **A.** Corticosteroid therapy is the single most important intervention to impact the neonatal outcome in a pregnancy less than 34 weeks when delivery is expected imminently (within 7 days). Magnesium sulfate is often given during this time of carefully monitoring the platelet count and liver function tests, but not necessarily delivering. This change in carefully observing patients with stable mild thrombocytopenia and stable elevated LFTs is based on the knowledge of antenatal corticosteroid impact on neonatal outcome.

35.9   **B.** This patient has severely elevated BP and must receive an antihypertensive agent ASAP to reduce the risk of stroke. This may be IV labetolol, IV hydralazine, or oral nifedipine. Although corticosteroids and BPP are viable answer choices, the highest priority is to lower the BP.

35.10 **C.** This patient likely has IUGR. The next step would be to evaluate possible fetal compromise with BPP and umbilical artery Doppler studies. At 34 weeks, corticosteroid therapy is not effective. Magnesium sulfate and delivery is an option, but more information such as assessment of fetal status would give a more complete picture. The BPs are in the mild range, so an antihypertensive agent is not needed.

CLINICAL PEARLS

▶ In general, the treatment of gestational hypertension or preeclampsia without severe features at or beyond 37 weeks' gestation is delivery. Use of magnesium sulfate is individualized.

▶ The management of preeclampsia without severe features in a preterm pregnancy is observation until severe features are noted or term gestation is reached.

▶ Severe features complicating preeclampsia or superimposed preeclampsia at a gestational age of 34 weeks or higher should be given magnesium sulfate and delivered. Those below 34 weeks may be judiciously observed in specialized facilities.

▶ The most common cause of significant proteinuria in pregnancy is preeclampsia.

▶ Magnesium sulfate is the best anticonvulsant to prevent eclampsia.

▶ The first sign of magnesium toxicity is loss of deep tendon reflexes.

▶ Chronic hypertension is diagnosed when a pregnant woman has hypertension prior to 20 weeks' gestation, or if the hypertension persists beyond 12 weeks postpartum.

▶ Gestational hypertension is when a pregnant woman has hypertension after 20 weeks of gestation without proteinuria or other evidence of preeclampsia.

▶ Acute onset severe hypertension (160 mm Hg systolic or 110 mm Hg diastolic) persisting more than 15 minutes is considered a hypertensive emergency. IV labetolol, IV hydralazine, or oral nifedipine are first-line agents.

REFERENCES

American College of Obstetricians and Gynecologists. Diagnosis and management of preeclampsia and eclampsia. *ACOG Practice Bulletin*. Washington, DC: 2012.

Castro LC. Hypertensive disorders of pregnancy. In: Hacker NF, Gambone JC, Hobel CJ, eds. *Essentials of Obstetrics and Gynecology*. 5th ed. Philadelphia, PA: Saunders; 2009:173-182.

Cunningham FG, Leveno KJ, Bloom SL, et al. Pregnancy hypertension. *Williams Obstetrics*. 24th ed. New York, NY: McGraw-Hill; 2014:706-756.

Task Force on Hypertension in Pregnancy. Hypertension in pregnancy. ACOG. 2013.

A 25-year-old G1P0 woman at 11 weeks' gestation is noted to be lethargic by her husband. The patient was noted to have numerous episodes of nausea and vomiting over the past 1 1/2 months, which has persisted despite antiemetic therapy and adjustments in her diet. The patient had been discharged from the hospital 2 weeks ago due to emesis. She was brought in by EMS when her husband arrived after work to find her unarousable. On examination, the patient is lethargic but will respond to painful stimuli and open her eyes. Her blood pressure is 92/44 mm Hg, heart rate 130 beats/min, and respiratory rate is 14 breaths/min. O_2 saturation is 99% on room air. The patient's mucous membranes are dry. She otherwise has a normal examination. The fetal heart tones are 150 beats/min. The urinalysis shows a dipstick of specific gravity 1.027 and 3+ ketones.

▶ What is the most likely diagnosis?
▶ What is your next step in management?
▶ What is the differential diagnosis?

ANSWERS TO CASE 36:

Hyperemesis Gravidarum and Obstetric Emergencies Less than 26 Weeks' Gestation

Summary: A 25-year-old G1P0 woman at 11 weeks' gestation has a 6-week history of persistent emesis. She is found to be lethargic and noted to be hypovolemic with blood pressure of 92/44 mm Hg and heart rate of 130 beats/min. Her respiratory rate is 14 breaths/min. The fetal heart tones are 150 beats/min. The urinalysis shows a dipstick of specific gravity 1.027 and 3+ ketones.

- **Most likely diagnosis:** Hyperemesis gravidarum, severe

- **Next step in management:** Immediate isotonic fluid replacement, and also assess for electrolyte abnormalities and correction of these problems

- **Differential diagnosis:** Acute pancreatitis, molar pregnancy or twin pregnancy, peptic ulcer disease, hyperthyroidism, and cholelithiasis

ANALYSIS

Objectives

1. Know the common complications in pregnant women less than 26 weeks' gestation.

2. Understand the diagnostic strategy and management of those complications.

3. Know the physiologic changes in pregnancy and their impact on common diseases in pregnancy.

Considerations

The patient described in this scenario is significantly ill and needs aggressive fluid replacement, electrolyte replacement, and correction of metabolic abnormalities. Replacement with 2 L of normal saline quickly is warranted. Assessment of comprehensive metabolic panel, electrolytes, amylase, lipase, urinalysis for leukocytes, calcium, magnesium, and CBC with differential should be performed. She has complicated hyperemesis gravidarum and needs a diagnostic workup such as pelvic ultrasound if not previously performed, right upper quadrant ultrasound, and thyroid function tests. The patient should be admitted to the hospital. Antiemetic therapy, fluid replacement and nothing by mouth should be initiated. The patient should be followed carefully once discharged to ensure that she does not become so volume depleted again.

APPROACH TO:
Medical Complications in Pregnancies Before 26 Weeks

INTRODUCTION

There are numerous emergencies or urgencies that bring a pregnant woman into the emergency department. For this chapter, the discussion will be focused on hyperemesis gravidarum, spontaneous abortion, asthma exacerbation, hyperthyroidism/thyroid storm, preterm premature rupture of membranes, and pyelonephritis.

Hyperemesis Gravidarum

Nausea and vomiting in pregnancy is very common, affecting up to 75% of pregnant women. However, hyperemesis gravidarum, which is defined as intractable emesis with volume depletion and metabolic/electrolyte alterations, is less common, with prevalence of about 2% of pregnancies. Typically, it occurs in women in the first trimester. The emergency physician should not be lulled into complacency because nausea and vomiting is so common in pregnant women. The evaluation should include addressing the degree of volume depletion and exploring the possibility of metabolic issues such as electrolyte abnormalities, renal or liver function abnormalities, and the possibility of other etiologies. A urinalysis should also be performed. Hyperemesis gravidarum is a diagnosis of exclusion.

Pregnant women are typically young and healthy and can have significant hypovolemia with compensation without appearing ill. A careful history should be taken regarding the amount of oral intake, medications taken if any, and the presence of other possible causes of emesis. The differential diagnosis includes pancreatitis, gallstones, peptic ulcer disease, appendicitis, ovarian torsion, pyelonephritis, and gastroenteritis. Additionally, a high hCG level as associated with molar pregnancies or multiple gestation is seen with hyperemesis. Thus, an ultrasound should be performed to assess for adnexal masses and to define the type of pregnancy.

Treatment depends on the severity of the patient's condition. Patients with mild volume depletion can be given IV hydration or a trial of oral fluids and prescribed antiemetic medications. Pyridoxine (vitamin B_6) has efficacy as a first-line agent. Ondansetron (Zofran), while pregnancy Class B, has become the most common parenteral and oral antiemetic used in US emergency departments due to its efficacy, and it has become the first choice in hyperemesis in the last several years. As an adjunctive agent, corticosteroids have also been used. Patients who have failed outpatient therapy or who have moderate to severe volume depletion should be hospitalized for more intensive therapy and monitoring. Rarely, patients will be so severely affected that total parenteral nutrition is required.

Spontaneous Abortion

Patients who present with vaginal bleeding during pregnancy are said to have a threatened abortion. In this circumstance, approximately 10% of cases will involve ectopic pregnancy (see Case 26), 40% will result in a spontaneous abortion and 50% will result in a normal pregnancy carried to term. When the patient presents to the emergency department, a careful history and physical examination should be performed, including assessing for cramping, passage of tissue, risk factors for ectopic pregnancy, and hemodynamic alterations. The physical examination should be focused on assessing volume status, abdominal tenderness, pelvic examination for the state of the cervix, and the presence of adnexal masses or tenderness. The hCG level and transvaginal ultrasound usually help to determine the type of pregnancy. For instance, if the hCG level is above the threshold of 1500 mIU/mL and nothing is seen in the uterus indicating an intrauterine pregnancy, in the absence of history indicative of tissue passing, the presentation is consistent with an ectopic pregnancy. Women with threatened abortion should be instructed to bring in any passed tissue for histologic analysis.

An inevitable abortion must be differentiated from an incompetent cervix. With an inevitable abortion, the uterine contractions (cramping) lead to the cervical dilation. With an incompetent cervix, the cervix opens spontaneously without uterine contractions and, therefore, affected women present with painless cervical dilation. This disorder is treated with a surgical ligature at the level of the internal cervical os (cerclage). Hence, one of the main features used to distinguish between an incompetent cervix and an inevitable abortion is the presence or absence of uterine contractions.

The treatment of an **incomplete abortion**, characterized by the **passage of tissue and an open cervical os**, is dilatation and curettage of the uterus. The primary complications of persistently retained tissue are bleeding and infection. A completed abortion is suspected by the history of having passed tissue and experiencing cramping abdominal pain, now resolved. The cervix is closed. Serum hCG levels are still followed to confirm that no further chorionic villi are contained in the uterus.

Asthma Exacerbation

Asthma is one of the most common medical conditions complicating pregnancy, with an incidence of 4% to 9%. The clinical course of asthma in pregnancy is relatively unpredictable; however, there is evidence to suggest that worsening of asthma may be related to baseline asthma severity. Approximately one-third of pregnant asthmatics experience worsening of symptoms, while one-third improve and one-third remain the same. Exacerbations are more common in the second and third trimester and are less frequent in the last 4 weeks of pregnancy. Asthma typically follows a similar clinical course with successive pregnancies. As such, this patient would be expected to do relatively well given that her asthma symptoms were well controlled prior to this pregnancy and in previous pregnancies.

Asthma symptoms correlate poorly with objective measures of pulmonary function. Therefore, the next step in the evaluation of this patient is to perform an objective measure of airway obstruction. The single best measure is the **forced expiratory volume (FEV$_1$)**, which is the volume of gas exhaled in 1 second by a forced exhalation after a full inspiration. This value, however, can only be obtained by spirometry, thus limiting its clinical use. The **peak expiratory flow rate (PEFR)** correlates well with FEV$_1$ and can be measured with inexpensive, disposable portable peak flow meters. Both the FEV$_1$ and PEFR remain unchanged throughout pregnancy and may be used as measures of asthma control and severity.

Treatment of an acute exacerbation during pregnancy is **similar** to that of non-pregnant asthmatics. In other words, a rule of thumb is that pregnant women should be treated similarly to nonpregnant asthmatics. Patients should be taught how to recognize the signs and symptoms of early exacerbations so that they may begin treatment at home promptly. **Initial treatment consists of a short-acting inhaled β_2-agonist** (albuterol), up to three treatments of two to four puffs by MDI (metered-dose inhaler) at 20 minute intervals for up to three treatments, or a single nebulizer treatment for up to 1 hour. A good response is characterized by PEFR greater than 80% of personal best and resolution of symptoms sustained for 4 hours. Patients may be continued on β_2-agonists every 3 to 4 hours for 24 to 48 hours. Inhaled corticosteroids (ICS) should be initiated, or if already taking ICS, the dose should be doubled. A follow-up appointment with their physician should be made as soon as possible. Inadequate response to initial therapy (PEFR <80%) or decreased fetal activity warrants immediate medical attention.

Prevention of hypoxia is the ultimate goal for the pregnant woman who presents to the hospital during an acute asthma attack. Initial assessment should include a brief history and physical examination to assess the severity of asthma and possible trigger factors such as a respiratory infection. Patients with imminent respiratory arrest include those who are drowsy or confused, have paradoxical thoracoabdominal movement, bradycardia, pulsus paradoxus, and decreased air movement (no wheezing). Intubation and mechanical ventilation with 100% oxygen should be performed in these circumstances, and the patient should be admitted to the intensive care unit. Because of the changes in the respiratory physiology in pregnancy (ie, a respiratory alkalosis with partial metabolic compensation), different thresholds for action exist (Table 36–1). A $Paco_2$ greater than 35 mm Hg, with a pH less than 7.35 in the presence of a falling Pao_2, is a sign of impending respiratory failure in a pregnant asthmatic. Intubation is warranted when the $Paco_2$ is 45 mm Hg or more and rising.

Premature Rupture of Membranes

Premature rupture of membranes (PROM) is defined as the ROM prior to the onset of labor. Preterm PROM (PPROM) is the ROM that occurs prior to 37 completed weeks. Approximately 3% of all pregnancies are complicated by PPROM, and it is the underlying etiology of one-third of preterm births. Normal fetal membranes are biologically very strong in preterm pregnancies. The weakening mechanism is likely multifactorial. Studies have shown PPROM to be associated with

Table 36–1 • ARTERIAL BLOOD GAS FINDINGS IN PREGNANCY			
Parameter	Nonpregnant	Pregnancy	Mechanism
pH	7.40	7.45	Respiratory alkalosis
Po_2	80-100 mm Hg	90-110 mm Hg	Increased minute ventilation
Pco_2	40 mm Hg	28 mm Hg	Respiratory alkalosis
Hco_3	24 mEq/L	18 mEq/L	Partial metabolic acidosis compensation

intrinsic (intrauterine stretch/strain from polyhydramnios and multifetal pregnancies, cervical incompetence) and extrinsic factors (ascending bacterial infections). There is evidence demonstrating an association between ascending infection from the lower genital tract and PPROM. This section will be restricted to gestational age less than 26 weeks.

PPROM is associated with significant maternal and fetal morbidity and mortality. The time from rupture of membranes to delivery is known as "latency." The latency period is inversely proportional to the gestational age at PPROM. A latency period of 1 week or less is present in 50% to 60% of PPROM patients. During this period amnionitis occurs in 13% to 60%, and abruptio placentae occurs in 4% to 12%. Multiple complications have been associated with PPROM; however, both maternal and fetal complications decrease with increasing gestational age at the time of PPROM.

The primary maternal morbidity is chorioamnionitis. Incidence varies with population and gestational age at PPROM, with reported frequency from 15% to 40%. Chorioamnionitis typically precedes fetal infection, but this is not always the case, and therefore close clinical monitoring is required. Fetal morbidity and mortality varies with gestational age and complications, particularly infection. The most common complication is respiratory distress syndrome (RDS). Other serious fetal complications include necrotizing enterocolitis, intraventricular hemorrhage, and sepsis. The three causes of neonatal death associated with PPROM are prematurity, sepsis, and pulmonary hypoplasia. Preterm infants born with sepsis have a mortality rate four times higher than those without sepsis.

Management of PPROM starts with initial evaluation and diagnosis of rupture of membranes. The primary patient complaint is experiencing a "gush" of fluid, but some patients will report persistent leakage of fluid. Patient history of rupture of membranes is accurate in 90% of cases. Diagnosis is established on sterile speculum evaluation. Confirmatory findings include pooling of amniotic fluid in posterior fornix and/or leakage of fluid on Valsalva; positive nitrazine test of fluid (vaginal pH 4.5-6.0, amniotic fluid pH 7.1-7.3, nitrazine turns dark blue above 6.0-6.5); and amniotic fluid *ferning* on microscopy. Should the initial tests be ambiguous or negative in the face of continued clinical suspicion, other diagnostic modalities can be utilized. The ultrasound finding of oligohydramnios is usually confirmatory.

At the time of the initial evaluation, the patient's cervical os should be **visually** assessed for dilatation and possible prolapse of umbilical cord or fetal limb. In general, a digital examination of the cervix should be avoided since bacteria may be theoretically inoculated with an examination. Ultrasound evaluation of the gestational age, fetal weight, fetal presentation, placental location, and assessment of amniotic fluid index (AFI) are vital for treatment planning. A low AFI (<5.0 cm) and low maximum vertical fluid pocket (<2.0 cm) at the time of initial assessment is associated with shorter latency, increased RDS, and increased composite morbidity.

Management

Patients diagnosed with PPROM would benefit from an admission to the hospital in all likelihood until delivery. Once PPROM is verified, the treatment plan must balance the maternal, fetal, neonatal risks/benefits of prolonged pregnancy or expeditious delivery and possible inclusion of medical intervention. For those gestations that are previable, observation in the hospital or careful follow-up with an obstetrician is advisable.

In the absence of clinical signs of labor, abruption, or maternal or fetal signs of infection, most patients in this gestational age will benefit from an expectant management with daily assessment of the maternal and fetal well-being.

Maternal and Fetal Assessment

1. **Maternal:** The criteria for the diagnosis of clinical chorioamnionitis include maternal pyrexia, tachycardia, leukocytosis, uterine tenderness, malodorous vaginal discharge, and fetal tachycardia. During inpatient observation, the woman should be regularly examined for such signs of intrauterine infection, and an abnormal parameter (such as fever, fetal or maternal tachycardia) may indicate intrauterine infection. The frequency of maternal and fetal assessments (temperature, pulse, and fetal heart rate auscultation) should be between 4 and 8 hours.

2. **Fetal:** Electronic fetal heart rate tracing is useful when the gestation is considered viable because fetal tachycardia may represent a sign of fetal infection and is frequently used in the clinical definition of chorioamnionitis in some studies. Fetal tachycardia is often the earliest sign of infection. However, checking intermittent fetal heart activity for previable gestation is preferable.

Use of Steroids: A meta-analysis of 15 randomized controlled trials involving more than 1400 women with preterm rupture of the membranes demonstrated that antenatal corticosteroids reduced the risks of respiratory distress syndrome. This is generally administered from 24 to 34 weeks' gestation to enhance fetal lung maturity in the absence of infection.

Use of Antibiotics: The use of antibiotics following PPROM was associated with a statistically significant reduction in chorioamnionitis. There was a significant reduction in the numbers of babies born within 48 hours and 7 days. Neonatal infection was significantly reduced in the babies whose mothers received antibiotics.

PPROM Under 23 Weeks: There are insufficient data to make recommendations in the setting of PPROM under 23 to 24 weeks including the possibility of home, day care, and outpatient monitoring. It would be considered reasonable to maintain the woman in hospital for at least 48 hours before a decision is made to allow her to go home. The management of these cases should be individualized and outpatient monitoring restricted to certain groups of women after careful consideration of other risk factors and access to the hospital.

Hyperthyroidism

Hyperthyroidism in pregnancy is more difficult to recognize due to the hyperdynamic physiologic changes in pregnancy. However, unintended weight loss, nervousness, palpitations, tachycardia, or tremor are clinical manifestations that warrant evaluation. The diagnosis is made based on clinical suspicion and thyroid function tests, such as thyroid-stimulating hormone (TSH) and free T4 levels. The immediate treatment includes β-blocking agents and thioamides.

The patient who presents acutely to the emergency department should be started on β-blockers urgently to relieve the adrenergic symptoms of tachycardia, tremor, anxiety, and heat sensitivity by decreasing the maternal heart rate, cardiac output, and myocardial oxygen consumption. Longer-acting agents, such as atenolol and metoprolol 50 to 200 mg/d, are recommended. β-Blockers are contraindicated in patients with asthma and congestive heart failure and should not be used at the time of delivery due to possible neonatal bradycardia and hypoglycemia.

Thioamides inhibit thyroid hormone synthesis by reduction of iodine organification and iodotyrosine coupling. Both propylthiouracil (PTU) and methimazole have been used during pregnancy, but PTU is preferred during the first trimester. After the first trimester, physicians should consider switching to methimazole because the risk of liver failure associated with PTU use becomes greater than the risk of teratogenicity. Teratogenic patterns associated with methimazole include aplasia cutis and choanal/esophageal atresia; however, these anomalies do not occur at a higher rate in women on thioamides compared to the general population.

Side effects of thioamides include transient leukopenia (10%), agranulocytosis (0.1%-0.4%), thrombocytopenia, hepatitis, and vasculitis (<1%) as well as rash, nausea, arthritis, anorexia, fever, and loss of taste or smell (5%). Agranulocytosis usually presents with a fever and sore throat. If a CBC indicates agranulocytosis, the medication should be discontinued. Treatment with another thioamide carries a significant risk of cross-reaction as well.

Initiation of thioamides in a patient with a new diagnosis during pregnancy requires a dose of PTU 100 to 150 mg three times daily or methimazole 10 to 20 mg twice daily. Free T_4 levels are used to monitor response to therapy in hyperthyroid patients and should be checked in 4 to 6 weeks. The PTU or methimazole can be adjusted in 50 mg or 10 mg increments, respectively, with a therapeutic range for free T_4 of 1.2 to 1.8 ng/dL. The goal of treatment is to maintain the free T_4 in the upper normal range using the lowest possible dose in order to protect the fetus from hypothyroidism. The required dose of thioamide during pregnancy can increase up to 50% for patients with a history of hyperthyroidism prior to conception. The patient's TSH should be checked at the initial prenatal visit and every trimester. Medication adjustments, testing intervals, and therapeutic goals for the free T_4 are the same as for patients with new-onset disease.

The most common cause of hyperthyroidism is Graves disease, which occurs in 95% of all cases at all ages. The diagnosis of Graves disease is usually made by the presence of elevated free T_4 level or free thyroid index with a suppressed TSH in the absence of a nodular goiter or thyroid mass. The differential diagnosis of hyperthyroidism, in the order of decreasing frequency, includes subacute thyroiditis, painless (silent or postpartum) thyroiditis, toxic multinodular goiter, toxic adenoma (solitary autonomous hot nodule), iodine-induced (iodinated contrast or amiodarone), iatrogenic overreplacement of thyroid hormone, factitious thyrotoxicosis, *strumaovarii* (ovarian teratoma), and gestational trophoblastic disease. The general symptoms of hyperthyroidism include palpitations, weight loss with increased appetite, nervousness, heat intolerance, oligomenorrhea, eye irritation or edema, and frequent stools. The general signs include diffuse goiter, tachycardia, tremor, warm, moist skin, and new-onset atrial fibrillation. Diagnosis during pregnancy is even more difficult because the signs and symptoms of hyperthyroidism may overlap with the hypermetabolic symptoms of pregnancy. Discrete findings with Graves disease include a diffuse, toxic goiter (common in most young women), ophthalmopathy (periorbital edema, proptosis, and lid retraction in only 30%), dermopathy (pretibial myxedema in <1%), and acropachy (digital clubbing).

The pathogenesis of Graves disease is characterized by an autoimmune process with production of thyroid-stimulating immunoglobulins (TSIs) and TSH-binding inhibitory immunoglobulins (TBIIs) that act on the TSH receptor on the thyroid gland to mediate thyroid stimulation or inhibition, respectively. These antibodies, in effect, act as TSH agonists or antagonists to stimulate or inhibit thyroid growth, iodine trapping, and T_4/T_3 synthesis. Maternal Graves disease complicates one out of every 500 to 1000 pregnancies. The frequency of poor outcomes depends on the severity of maternal thyrotoxicosis, with a risk of preterm delivery of 88%, stillbirth of 50%, and risk of congestive heart failure of over 60% in untreated mothers.

Thyroid Storm

Maternal thyroid storm is a medical emergency characterized by a hypermetabolic state in a woman with uncontrolled hyperthyroidism. Thyroid storm occurs in less than 1% of pregnancies but has a high risk of maternal heart failure. Usually there is an inciting event, such as infection, cesarean delivery, or labor, which leads to acute onset of fever, tachycardia, altered mental status (restlessness, nervousness, confusion), seizures, nausea, vomiting, diarrhea, and cardiac arrhythmias. Shock, stupor, and coma can ensue without prompt intervention, which includes OB-ICU admission, supportive measures, and acute medical management. Therapy includes a standard series of drugs, each of which has a specific role in suppression of thyroid function: PTU or methimazole blocks additional synthesis of thyroid hormone, and PTU also blocks peripheral conversion of T_4 to T_3. Saturated solutions of potassium iodide or sodium iodide block the release of T_4 and T_3 from the gland. Dexamethasone decreases thyroid hormone release and peripheral conversion of T_4 to T_3. Propranolol inhibits the adrenergic effects of excessive thyroid hormone. Phenobarbital can reduce extreme agitation or restlessness and may increase catabolism of thyroid hormone. Fetal surveillance is performed throughout, but intervention for fetal indications should not occur until the mother is stabilized.

Pyelonephritis

A pregnant woman is at greater risk for pyelonephritis and its complications such as sepsis and acute respiratory distress syndrome (ARDS). Most cases of pyelonephritis in pregnancy are caused by infection with gram-negative aerobic bacteria, but an increasing number are due to group B *Streptococcus*. Approximately 7% of affected women will develop pulmonary insufficiency due to ARDS (Figure 36–1), presumably related to release of endotoxin. For these reasons, a pregnant patient with pyelonephritis should be admitted to the hospital. The diagnosis is established with the classic triad of fever, costovertebral angle (CVA) tenderness, and pyuria.

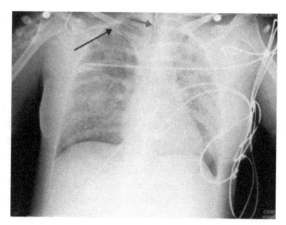

Figure 36–1. CXR showing diffuse bilateral alveolar opacities consistent with ARDS. (Reproduced, with permission, from Kasper D, Fauci A, Hauser S, et al. *Harrison's Principles of Internal Medicine.* 19th ed. New York, NY: McGraw-Hill Education; 2015. Figure 308E–30).

The patient should be placed on IV hydration and antibiotics aimed at the most common etiology, *Escherichia Coli*, and monitored for complications. Bacteria and/ or their component toxins can produce a sepsis syndrome that, unchecked, will develop into septic shock. The cornerstone of management is early diagnosis, but often that is not easy. A program of early goal-directed therapy has been shown to reduce mortality from septic shock. However, not all patients with septic shock require the same treatment interventions. The woman in our case scenario, for example, requires aggressive fluid resuscitation and transfer to an intensive care unit. Per hour, 1 to 2 L (not the 125 cc/h she was receiving) would be appropriate. The total volume needed should be determined by monitoring central venous pressure. An arterial catheter should be placed to monitor blood pressure and obtain timely pH and blood gas measurements. If adequate fluid resuscitation has not elevated the mean arterial pressure above 65 mm Hg, then vasopressors would be indicated. Adequate oxygenation should be maintained, with endotracheal intubation and mechanical ventilation, if necessary. The ceftriaxone she was receiving likely does not need to be changed, but some authorities prefer ampicillin and gentamicin for the treatment of pyelonephritis in pregnancy. Surgical intervention is seldom necessary for septic shock secondary to pyelonephritis, but prolonged hypotension and ischemia can lead to gangrene of the extremities and amputation in severe cases. When septic shock results from necrotizing fasciitis, extensive debridement of necrotic tissue is an essential component of management. Antibiotic therapy should include vancomycin for methicillin-resistant *Staphylococcus* and clindamycin for *Streptococcus*; there is evidence that clindamycin may directly inhibit the synthesis of group A streptococcal toxins.

COMPREHENSION QUESTIONS

36.1 A 35-year-old woman G2P1 at 24 weeks' gestation comes into the emergency department with fever of 102°F, dysuria, and costovertebral angle tenderness. The urinalysis shows numerous bacteria and leukocytes. The patient asks whether she can be treated as an outpatient. Which of the following is the best response?

A. Outpatient therapy with oral cephalexin is acceptable.

B. Outpatient therapy with an initial dose of ceftriaxone IM and then oral nitrofurantoin is acceptable.

C. Outpatient therapy is acceptable if this is the patient's first episode of pyelonephritis.

D. Inpatient therapy is preferred in this patient.

36.2 The patient in Question 27.1 is treated with antibiotic therapy for 2 days and develops acute shortness of breath and is noted to have an O_2 sat of 89% on room air. Which of the following is the most likely cause of her hypoxemia?

A. Pulmonary embolism

B. Pneumonia

C. ARDS

D. Aspiration

36.3 A 28-year-old G1P0 woman is noted to be at 7 weeks' gestation by dates. She comes into the ED with vaginal bleeding. The physical examination is otherwise unremarkable. There are no adnexal masses or tenderness and the uterus is nontender and the cervix is closed. The hCG level is 2000 mIU/mL, and the transvaginal ultrasound shows no intrauterine gestation, no adnexal masses, and no free fluid. Which of the following is the most likely diagnosis?

A. Ectopic pregnancy

B. Completed abortion

C. Incomplete abortion

D. Molar pregnancy

36.4 A 31-year-old woman G3P2 woman at 19 weeks' gestation complains of jitteriness, weight loss, and palpitations. She has a history of Graves disease and had been taking PTU and propranolol until she stopped 2 weeks ago due to concern about the medications' effect on her pregnancy. The patient is noted to have a temp of 102°F, BP 160/100 mm Hg, heart rate 130, and she is confused and disoriented. Which of the following is the most likely diagnosis?

A. Acute β-blocker withdrawal syndrome

B. Sepsis due to PTU-induced neutropenia

C. Thyroid storm

D. Hyperparathyroidism

36.5 A 27-year-old G1P0 woman at 18 weeks' gestation complains of significant nausea and vomiting throughout her pregnancy and has not been able to keep any foods or liquids down. She has been admitted to the hospital numerous times. Her BP is 100/60 mm Hg and heart rate 110 beats/min, and urinalysis shows negative nitrates, negative leukoesterase, and ketones 2+/4. Which of the following statements is most accurate about this patient?

A. The presence of ketones in the urine is consistent with significant volume depletion.

B. The patient's gestational age of 18 weeks is expected for hyperemesis gravidarum.

C. Vitamin B_1 is useful for this patient's condition.

D. The patient may be expected to have hyperkalemia.

36.6 A 31-year-old G2P1 woman is noted to be at 20 weeks' gestation. She presents to the ED with a history of leakage of fluid per vagina earlier in the day. On speculum examination, there is no fluid in the vagina. The fern and nitrazine tests are negative. Which of the following is the best next step for this patient?

A. Inform the patient that she does not have rupture of membranes.

B. Hospitalize the patient and assume that she has rupture of membranes.

C. Treat with an oral antibiotic for presumed UTI.

D. Perform an ultrasound examination.

ANSWERS

36.1 **D.** Pregnant women with pyelonephritis should be admitted to the hospital in general because of the complications such as sepsis, preterm labor, miscarriage, or ARDS. Endotoxin-induced pulmonary injury is a well-documented complication of pyelophritis and occurs more commonly in pregnant women.

36.2 **C.** A patient who develops acute shortness of breath and hypoxemia after treatment for pyelonephritis should be assumed to have endotoxin-mediated pulmonary injury, or ARDS. A chest x-ray will usually reveal patchy bilateral infiltrates in the lung fields. The treatment is supplemental oxygen and supportive therapy.

36.3 **A.** When the hCG level exceeds the threshold of 1500 mIU/mL and no gestational sac is seen on TV ultrasound, the likelihood of an ectopic pregnancy is high (in the range of 85%). These patients usually go to laparoscopy to confirm the diagnosis. When the hCG level is below the threshold, then the next step is generally to repeat the hCG level in 48 hours to assess for a normal rise (>66% rise), which would indicate a normal intrauterine pregnancy, versus an abnormal rise (<66%), which would be either an ectopic pregnancy or a miscarriage.

36.4 **C.** Thyroid storm is present with hyperthyroidism in conjunction with CNS dysfunction (seizures, confusion, lethargy), and/or autonomic instability (fever). Thyroid storm carries a worse prognosis and usually requires immediate admission to the ICU and aggressive therapy consisting of PTU, β-blockers, and steroids. A common precursor to thyroid storm is a patient who has stopped taking medications and a stressor such as infection or surgery.

36.5 **A.** With hyperemesis gravidarum, the presence of moderate to significant ketones is associated with significant volume depletion. The patient is typically hypokalemic. The usual gestational age for hyperemesis is the first trimester, although less commonly, women can persist later and even rarer, throughout the pregnancy. Vitamin B_6 is a useful adjunctive treatment.

36.6 **D.** When the history suggests PROM but the speculum examination is negative, ultrasound to assess for amniotic fluid volume is helpful. If oligohydramnios is diagnosed, the patient is assumed to have ROM and should be admitted to the hospital.

CLINICAL PEARLS

▶ Nausea and vomiting in pregnancy is common and usually self-limited after the first trimester, and it is not associated with significant volume or metabolic derangements.

▶ Hyperemesis, which is associated with significant volume and/or metabolic derangement, is a diagnosis of exclusion.

▶ The physiologic changes of pregnancy should be considered when interpreting arterial blood gases (ABGs). For instance, when the P_{CO_2} exceeds 40 mm Hg in a pregnant asthmatic, severe hypercarbia is present and intubation should be considered.

▶ Dyspnea and hypoxemia after treatment for pyelonephritis is usually caused by endotoxin-related pulmonary injury, ARDS.

▶ Hyperthyroidism is typically treated with methimazole or PTU, and a β-blocker.

▶ When the hCG level exceeds the threshold of 1200 to 1500 mIU/mL and no gestational sac is seen in the uterus on transvaginal ultrasound, then an ectopic pregnancy is highly likely.

▶ The history for a gush of fluid followed by constant leakage is 90% accurate for rupture of membranes.

▶ In there is strong clinical suspicion, and the speculum examination is negative for ROM, an ultrasound assessment for amniotic fluid volume is helpful.

REFERENCES

American College of Obstetricians and Gynecologists. Diagnosis and treatment of gestational trophoblastic disease. *ACOG Practice Bulletin 53.* Washington, DC: 2004.

American College of Obstetricians and Gynecologists. Medical management of abortion. *ACOG Practice Bulletin 67.* Washington, DC: 2005.

American College of Obstetricians and Gynecologists. Premature rupture of membranes. *ACOG Practice Bulletin 160.* Washington, DC: 2016.

Andrews JI, Shamshirsaz AA, Diekema DJ. Nonmenstrual toxic shock syndrome due to methicillin-resistant *staphylococcus aureus. Obstet Gynecol.* 2008;112:933-938.

Carney LA, Quinlan JD, West JM. Thyroid disease in pregnancy. *Am Fam Physician.* 2014;89(4): 273-278.

Katz VL. Spontaneous and recurrent abortion: etiology, diagnosis, treatment. In: Katz VL, Lentz GM, Lobo RA, Gersenson DM, eds. *Comprehensive Gynecology.* 6th ed. Philadelphia, PA: Mosby; 2012;(16):335-359.

Lu MC, Hobel CJ. Antepartum care: preconception and prenatal care, genetic evaluation and teratology, and antenatal fetal assessment. In: Hacker NF, Gambone JC, eds. *Essentials of Obstetrics and Gynecology.* 6th ed. Philadelphia, PA: Saunders; 2016:76-95.

Martin SR, Foley MR. Intensive care in obstetrics: an evidence-based review. *Am J Obstet Gynecol.* 2006;195:673-689.

Neal DM, Cootauco AC, Burrow G. Thyroid disease in pregnancy. *Clin Perinatol.* 2007;34:543-557.

Parillo JE. Septic shock—vasopressin, norepinephrine, and urgency. *N Engl J Med.* 2008;358:954-956.

A 46-year-old man was brought to the hospital because family members found him lethargic and complaining of abdominal pain. The patient has a history of chronic low back pain and has been under the care of a physician for the past several weeks. He has been prescribed acetaminophen/hydrocodone (Vicodin) and has been supplementing this medication with extra-strength acetaminophen (500 mg tablets) purchased from the drug store. His family members reported that they found several empty medication bottles at home. His laboratory studies from the emergency department revealed normal white blood cell count, hemoglobin, hematocrit, and platelet counts. His serum aspartate aminotransferase (AST) and alanine aminotransferase (ALT) are 1,300 IU/L and 1,700 IU/L, respectively.

▶ What is the most likely cause of the patient's current condition?
▶ What is the best next step in management?
▶ How is this disease process staged?

ANSWERS TO CASE 37:
Poisoning

Summary: This patient is a 46-year-old man with lethargy and abdominal pain, found to have elevated transaminase enzymes in the setting of possible excess acetaminophen ingestion. His presentation to the emergency department is consistent with hepatotoxicity secondary to acetaminophen overdose.

- **Likely cause of current condition:** Acetaminophen overdose.

- **Next step in management:** Gastric lavage may be helpful following massive ingestions, as this maneuver may be effective in retrieving undigested pills or pill fragments 30 to 60 minutes after the ingestion. Activated charcoal will absorb most toxins (due to its large surface area) and should be administered only to awake patients or comatose patients after appropriate airway protection. The dose is 1 g/kg orally or via gastric tube, with the goal of a 10:1 (charcoal:toxin) ratio.

- **Disease stages:** There are four distinct stages of acetaminophen-induced hepatotoxicity: (1) preclinical toxic effects (no laboratory abnormalities); (2) hepatic injury (elevated transaminase enzymes); (3) hepatic failure; (4) recovery. Each stage has a different prognosis and management strategy. This patient would appear to be stage 2 based on his initial evaluation.

ANALYSIS

Objectives

- Learn the clinical manifestations, management, and outcome of acetaminophen, salicylate, tricyclic antidepressants, alcohol, oral hypoglycemics, cyanide, and propofol overdoses.

- Learn when activated charcoal is indicated in the management of substance ingestion/overdose.

- Recognize the importance of airway, breathing, and circulation management in patients with substance ingestion/overdose.

Considerations

This patient was given a prescription for Vicodin (acetaminophen/hydrocodone) and was supplementing this medication with extra-strength acetaminophen to treat his back pain. The additional over-the-counter acetaminophen is sufficient to exceed the liver's ability to safely metabolize acetaminophen. Significant hepatic injury is evident by the patient's elevated transaminase enzymes. Due to the potential for decreased GI motility from opiates, such as hydrocodone, the acetaminophen toxicity could be potentiated because the compound would remain in the patient's system over a prolonged period of time. Early intubation may be important, as the patient's current condition is not entirely known, and intubation may help facilitate gastric lavage. It would be extremely helpful to examine all the empty pill bottles found at the patient's home to determine the types and possibly the quantity of the medications ingested. Early treatment should include gastric decontamination with activated charcoal administration.

APPROACH TO:
Poisoning

CLINICAL APPROACH

Priorities

Assess the patient's airway, with careful attention to the patient's airway-protective reflexes. The most common factor contributing to increased morbidity related to drug overdose is airway compromise caused by a flaccid tongue, aspiration of gastric content, or apnea from respiratory depression. Securing the patient's airway with endotracheal intubation is necessary if the patient's level of consciousness is compromised. Cardiac monitoring and assessment of respiratory rate and function may give clues to other potential co-ingestants. Continued monitoring of the patient's level of alertness and assessment of serum glucose are important, as the patient may have also ingested other substances in addition to those mentioned by the family. After stabilization of the patient's airway, breathing and circulation, the acetaminophen level and time of ingestion will be used in concert with the liver enzyme levels and coagulation studies to determine the course of treatment and the extent of hepatic injury. Additional tests to evaluate for concomitant ingestion of other substances include salicylate level, alcohol level, serum electrolytes, serum osmolality, urine toxicology screens (to screen for drug abuse), lactate, serum ketones, and an ECG.

Additional History

Approach all poisoned patients as if they have potentially life-threatening polysubstance intoxication (ingestion of multiple substances). Additional history is always helpful to determine which other substances the patient could have accessed. Family members, emergency medical personnel (paramedics, fire department), and the patient's primary doctor are often helpful in providing additional insight. The timing of ingestion and dosage of medication are also of extreme importance and will help guide treatments. In some situations, it is helpful to have all the patient's pill bottles brought from home. It is always helpful to consult your local Poison Control Center for assistance with patient management once all the suspected or confirmed ingested toxic substances are identified.

Decontamination

The technique for decontamination will largely depend on the timing, amount, and type of substance ingested. Gastrointestinal decontamination may involve gastric lavage, activated charcoal administration, or whole bowel irrigation given the circumstance. Gastric lavage has little clinical evidence to support its use but is currently used for massive ingestions of extremely toxic substances, with the aim of retrieving undigested pills or pill fragments, usually within 30 to 60 minutes after the ingestion. **Activated charcoal is a highly effective absorbent which functions to absorb most toxins (due to its large surface area), and it should be administered to awake patients or to comatose patients with secured airways. The dose is 1 g/kg orally or via gastric tube, with the goal of a 10:1 (charcoal:toxin) ratio.** Repeat doses of charcoal may enhance elimination of substances. Iron, lithium, and heavy metals are poorly absorbed by activated charcoal. Whole bowel irrigation utilizes nonabsorbable surgical bowel cleansing solutions at high flow rates to force intestinal contents out by way of large volume force. This technique is indicated with ingestion of: (1) substances not absorbed by charcoal, (2) drug-filled condoms or packets, (3) sustained-release tablets. Hemodialysis and antidotes may also hasten elimination for specific substances.

Psychiatric Evaluation

All poisoned patients must be assessed for suicidal ideation, risk factors for depression, prior history of suicide attempts, and prior psychiatric illnesses. This information can be obtained by the patient, if possible, and corroborated by the family. Although the potential for accidental overdose exists, these are more likely in the pediatric, elderly, and disabled populations. Therefore, the need for further evaluation by a psychiatrist should be considered after medical stabilization.

MANAGEMENT OF ACETAMINOPHEN TOXICITY

The American Association of Poison Control Centers estimated that acetaminophen was responsible for over 70,000 visits to healthcare facilities and 300 deaths in 2005. Acetaminophen poisoning can be due to ingestion of a single overdose (typically with suicide attempts) or ingestion of excessive repetitive doses or too-frequent dosages with therapeutic intent.

Pathophysiology of Acetaminophen Toxicity

Acetaminophen toxicity can occur with daily intake of greater than 4 g/d, and most acute hepatic failure from ingestion occurs with ingestion in excess of 10 g/d. Acetaminophen is normally metabolized by the liver, primarily via glucuronidation and sulfation into nontoxic metabolites. However, approximately 5% of acetaminophen is metabolized via cytochrome P450 2E1 to N-acetyl-p-benzoquinone imine (NAPQI), which is extremely toxic to the liver. When acetaminophen is taken in therapeutic doses, NAPQI is rapidly detoxified by glutathione to form nontoxic metabolites (cysteine and mercapturic conjugates). However, in an acetaminophen overdose NAPQI depletes glutathione reserves, and this toxic metabolite interacts with hepatic macromolecules to cause the liver injury.

There are four distinct stages of acetaminophen-induced hepatotoxicity: (1) preclinical toxic effects (no laboratory abnormalities); (2) hepatic injury (elevated transaminase enzymes); (3) hepatic failure; and (4) recovery. Each stage has a different prognosis and management strategy. Patients with frank hepatic failure have a mortality rate of 20% to 40%.

Clinical Assessment

The initial assessment of any patient with a potential overdose should focus on evaluating airway, breathing, circulation, disability and decontamination. Early in acute acetaminophen ingestions, the majority of patients remains asymptomatic or will complain of nausea, vomiting, and anorexia. However, 24 to 48 hours postingestion, patients begin to show signs of liver injury and liver failure.

After stabilization of the airway, breathing, and circulation, the **acetaminophen level and time of ingestion** will be used in concert with the liver enzyme levels and coagulation studies to determine the extent of injury and course of treatment. Additional history to pinpoint the time of ingestion is key in guiding therapy. Activated charcoal administration should be considered. Perhaps one of the greatest contributions to the management of patients with acetaminophen overdose is the **Rumack-Matthew Nomogram** (Figure 37–1). The nomogram was first published in 1975 and was developed from the acetaminophen levels of untreated patients. It describes the mathematic relationship between acetaminophen level, time of ingestion, and potential for hepatic injury. The upper line of the nomogram defines the toxic level likely to be associated with acute overdose, and is also known as **the "200 line,"** as any level of 200 or greater within 4 hours of ingestion requires antidote treatment. The lower line ("150 line") on the nomogram defines serum levels 25% below those expected to cause hepatotoxicity and was instituted by the FDA to improve clinical outcomes with antidote treatment.

The nomogram helps the clinician interpret the acetaminophen level. Any acetaminophen level obtained prior to 4 hours postingestion is unable to predict the likelihood of hepatotoxicity but is able to confirm acetaminophen ingestion. Acetaminophen levels obtained 4 to 24 hours after ingestion can be plotted on the nomogram to determine probability of hepatic injury. If levels plot above the lower line on the nomogram, antidote treatment should be initiated. Any elevated acetaminophen level detected 24 hours after ingestion should be considered toxic and warrants antidote treatment. The majority of poisoned patients present after polypharmacy ingestions. In cases in which patients have taken co-ingestants that may delay GI absorption (ie, extended-release acetaminophen preparations, opiates, or anticholinergics), it has been recommended that an 8-hour level follow a non-toxic 4-hour acetaminophen level and that treatment be guided by the nomogram (Figure 37–1). **The nomogram is not valid in cases of chronic ingestions.**

N-acetylcysteine (NAC) is the FDA-approved antidote for acetaminophen toxic-ity and functions to aid in glutathione repletion. Glutathione is synthesized from amino acids glutamate, glycine, and cysteine (cysteine availability is the rate-limiting step in production). NAC is readily absorbed and hydrolyzed to cysteine, which provides the substrate for glutathione synthesis. Glutathione functions to convert NAPQI to a nontoxic metabolite that is easily eliminated from the body via renal clearance. NAPQI is capable of causing liver injury by two separate mechanisms. First, NAPQI can bind covalently to intracellular proteins and cause hepatocellular necrosis. Second, a high rate of NAPQI formation can cause depletion of intrahe-patic glutathione stores and cause increased liver toxicity. NAC is of maximal benefit if given within 8 to 10 hours of ingestion, as this is usually prior to NAPQI accumu-lation. Although the benefit of NAC diminishes after 12 hours, treatment should

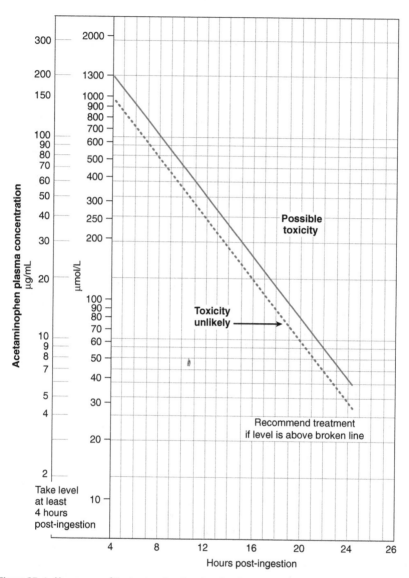

Figure 37–1. Nomogram of Acetaminophen Level vs. Time Post Ingestion. (Reproduced, with permission, from Tintinalli JE, Stapczynski JS, Ma OJ, et al. *Tintinalli's Emergency Medicine: A Comprehensive Study Guide.* 7th ed. New York: McGraw-Hill Education, 2011. Figure 184–2).

not be withheld despite a delay of 24 hours or more. Mortality reduction with NAC treatment has been shown in cases where hepatic failure has already developed.

NAC can be given orally, with a loading dose of 140 mg/kg, followed by a maintenance dose of 70 mg/kg every 4 hours. Uncomplicated cases with no evidence of hepatic injury may be treated for 20 hours, or five maintenance doses. However, if there is evidence of hepatic injury, NAC treatment should be continued until liver function tests have improved. Intravenous NAC is indicated if the patient is unable to tolerate the oral formulation or has decreased level of consciousness, vomiting or ileus. NAC can be given intravenously with a loading dose of 150 mg/kg over 15 minutes, followed by 50 mg/kg over 4 hours, then 100 mg/kg over 16 hours. Liver enzymes, as well as coagulation studies, are monitored until 36 hours after ingestion. If evidence of liver injury develops, then intravenous NAC treatment is continued until liver improvement in function tests occurs.

OTHER COMMON TOXIC INGESTIONS

Management of Salicylate Toxicity

Salicylates are commonly used for their anti-inflammatory and analgesic properties and can be found in aspirin, Pepto-Bismol, over-the-counter cold medications, and topical muscle and joint preparations (Aspercreme, Bayer Joint Cream, Icy Hot Cream). The daily therapeutic dose ranges from 40 to 60 mg/kg/d. Mild toxicity can be seen with doses of 150 to 200 mg/kg/d with marked toxicity at 300 to 500 mg/kg/d.

Toxicity from salicylate occurs via **two main mechanisms.** First, salicylate may directly stimulate the central respiratory centers, causing hyperventilation, respiratory alkalosis, and a compensatory metabolic acidosis. This metabolic acidosis is further exacerbated by the interruption of glucose and fatty acid metabolism, leading to increased carbon dioxide production. Mild salicylate toxicity may result in respiratory alkalosis (hyperventilation) with compensatory metabolic acidosis as bicarbonate is excreted in the urine. However, with moderate to severe toxicity the respiratory alkalosis is accompanied by a high anion-gap metabolic acidosis, as the kidneys deplete sodium bicarbonate and potassium.

Patients typically present with nausea, vomiting, tinnitus, tachypnea, and lethargy. Pulmonary edema, coma, and cardiovascular collapse can occur with severe toxicity. Management is aimed at supporting the patient's airway, breathing, and circulation with close attention to ensure adequate ventilation to allow the compensatory mechanisms to maintain a suitable arterial pH. Activated charcoal administration should be considered. Laboratory tests of significance include a salicylate level, electrolytes (to calculate the anion gap), arterial blood gas, and ECG (evidence of hypokalemia). Treatment is aimed at enhancing the elimination of salicylates by the kidneys, which is dependent on hydrogen ion gradients. Therefore, the treatment of choice remains sodium bicarbonate, which functions to treat the metabolic acidosis and enhance renal clearance. Sodium bicarbonate is given as a continuous infusion with a goal urine pH of 7.5-8.0. Potassium supplementation should be added to IV fluids, as potassium is rapidly depleted in salicylate toxicity. **Hemodialysis** should be considered in acute intoxication with serum salicylate levels of 100 mg/dL in association with **severe acidosis.**

Management of Tricyclic Antidepressant Toxicity

Tricyclic antidepressants (TCAs) were traditionally used to treat depression but are now more commonly used to treat chronic pain syndromes and for migraine prophylaxis in adult patients. TCAs are commonly prescribed to pediatric patients to treat enuresis, attention deficit disorder, and obsessive compulsive disorder.

Tricyclic antidepressants have a narrow therapeutic window. **TCAs have anticholinergic properties** that may delay GI absorption. TCAs also have α-adrenergic blockade effects and can cause hypotension and contribute to acidemia along with respiratory depression from CNS effects. However, the most serious complications from TCAs are related to cardiovascular and CNS effects. Cardiac conduction defects can develop as the result of the membrane-depressant qualities due to myocardial fast sodium channel blockade, leading to prolonged PR, QRS, and QT intervals. Hypotension may occur from α-adrenergic blockade. Anticholinergic properties may cause tachycardia. CNS effects mainly manifest as lethargy and coma (due to the anticholinergic properties), in addition to seizures (attributed to central CNS activity).

Supportive care should be immediately initiated to stabilize the airway and support breathing. Intravenous fluids and cardiac monitoring should be instituted for circulatory support. Decontamination with activated charcoal should be considered. Sodium bicarbonate should be administered for patients with QRS prolongation or hypotension. Sodium bicarbonate is believed to reverse the sodium blockade and subsequent myocardial suppressant effects of TCAs. Sodium bicarbonate may also be utilized for serum alkalinization, with a goal of achieving serum pH of 7.45 to 7.55, which has been shown to elevate blood pressure and shorten the QRS interval.

Management of Alcohol Toxicity

A variety of alcohols can be found commercially available in liquor, cold medicines, mouthwash, food extracts, colognes, after-shave solutions, antifreeze, and rubbing alcohol. Up to 15% of the U.S. population is considered to be at risk for alcohol dependence.

Alcohol dehydrogenase is the primary enzyme that metabolizes ethanol, isopropyl alcohol, methanol, and ethylene glycol. The genetic polymorphisms of alcohol dehydrogenase will determine the rate of alcohol metabolism. Patients with alcohol toxicity are typically grossly inebriated, with evidence of slurred speech, ataxia, impaired judgment, and lack of coordination. Severe toxicity may present with progressive CNS depression and coma. Methanol toxicities typically cause changes in vision in addition to inebriation. Isopropyl alcohol and ethylene glycol typically present gross intoxication similar to that associated with ethanol toxicity.

Ethanol toxicity typically causes CNS depression, which is additive when in combination with benzodiazipines, barbituates, or opiods. Hypoglycemia occurs commonly due to impaired gluconeogenesis along with poor nutrition in patients with history of chronic alcohol abuse. Occult head injury, hypoxemia, aspiration, and underlying metabolic disturbance must also be considered in all intoxicated patients. Treatment is mainly supportive with intravenous fluids, glucose and thiamine. In cases of **alcoholic ketoacidosis** (defined by anion-gap metabolic acidosis and elevated β-hydroxybutyrate), supplemental glucose and volume replacement are essential. There is no specific antidote for ethanol or isopropyl alcohol intoxication. However, methanol and ethylene glycol toxicity should be treated with fomepizole or ethanol to saturate the alcohol dehydrogenase enzyme and prevent further production of toxic metabolites. Methanol may also be eliminated by hemodialysis in cases of severe toxicity.

Management of Hypoglycemic Agent Toxicity

There are several oral agents used to lower serum glucose in the treatment of type 2 diabetes mellitus. Typically, these medications are divided into two categories, hypoglycemics and antihyperglycemics. Agents referred to as antihyperglycemics work to reduce glucose levels but rarely cause hypoglycemia, even when used in excess. These agents include metformin (glucophage), alpha-glucosidase inhibitors, and glitazones. The aforementioned agents work by reducing hepatic glucose production (metformin and glitazones), as well as decreasing intestinal glucose absorption (metformin and α-glucosidase inhibitors). In contrast, the hypoglycemics, namely sulfonylureas, typically cause hypoglycemia in cases of overdose or decreased elimination. Sulfonylurea lowers blood glucose by increasing insulin release from the pancreas and enhancing peripheral sensitivity to insulin.

Patients with **sulfonylurea toxicity** may present with signs of hypoglycemia such as diaphoresis, delirium, progressive decreased level of consciousness, syncope, or coma. The method of toxicity may be an intentional or unintentional overdose, as well as decreased elimination secondary to renal insufficiency. The duration of action for many sulfonylureas exceeds 24 hours. Therefore, patients are typically admitted to the hospital and treated with dextrose-containing intravenous fluids in addition to close glucose monitoring. Patients may require intravenous octreotide when they are unresponsive to intravenous dextrose. Octreotide is a synthetic somatostatin analog, which suppresses pancreatic insulin release. Adjunctive therapy for patients with sulfonylurea overdose includes alkalinization of the urine to increase renal elimination of sulfonylureas.

Although antihyperglycemics rarely cause hypoglycemia at toxic levels, these agents do exhibit toxicity through other mechanisms. For instance, metformin is known to cause lactic acidosis with overdose and with renal insufficiency. Severe cases of acidosis may warrant hemodialysis.

Management of Cyanide Toxicity

Cyanide toxicity is most commonly encountered in victims of smoke inhalation from industrial or residential fires and is due to the formation of gaseous hydrogen cyanide from burning plastics. Cyanide toxicity can also occur in the ICU as a result of **high-dose or prolonged nitroprusside infusions.** Nitroprusside releases cyanide during metabolism, which is normally converted to a nontoxic metabolite in the liver. However, cyanide may accumulate with prolonged use and/or high dosages. A rare cause of cyanide toxicity in the United States is the over-ingestion of cyanide-containing foods, such as cassava, apricot seeds, apple seeds, and spinach.

Cyanide causes cellular metabolism to switch from aerobic to anaerobic by the uncoupling of oxidative phosphorylation, which produces lactic acidosis. Patients typically present with malaise, headache, confusion, and generalized weakness. Cardiovascular collapse, syncope and coma may occur with severe toxicity.

The safest antidote for cyanide toxicity is intravenous hydroxocobalamin, which combines with cyanide to form cyanocobalamin (Vitamin B12), which is subsequently excreted by the kidneys. The cyanide antidote kit should be used if hydroxocobalamin is not accessible. The cyanide antidote kit consists of amyl nitrites, sodium nitrites, and sodium thiosulfate. Amyl nitrite pearls and intravenous sodium nitrite are capable of inducing methemoglobinemia in cells to help bind cyanide. However, nitrites should be avoided in cases of smoke inhalation, where carboxyhemoglobinemia may coexist. Instead, if hydroxocobalamin is not available, sodium thiosulfate should be administered intravenously, which enhances the conversion of cyanide to thiocyanate that is also excreted by the kidneys.

Management of Propofol Toxicity

Propofol is a lipid-soluble, sedative-hypnotic agent commonly used in surgical and critical care units. It is **metabolized by the liver** via oxidation by CYP-450 2B6 and is excreted by the kidneys. Its primary site of action is at the GABA-A receptors. Due to its rapid onset of action and quick metabolism (mean duration of action is 3-5 minutes for a single bolus), propofol is used with increasing frequency in the ICU for patients receiving mechanical ventilation. It is contraindicated in patients with egg or soybean allergies because of the additives in the formulation of the emulsion in which it is administered. Standard dosing of propofol for sedation is 25 to 75 μg/kg/min (or 1.5-3 mg/kg/h).

Adverse effects with use of propofol range from pain at the site of injection to death. Patients may experience hypotension, arrhythmias (both bradycardia and supraventricular tachyarhythmias have been described), acute pancreatitis secondary to hypertriglyceridemia, and/or bronchospasm as a result of propofol administration. **Propofol infusion syndrome includes rhabdomyolysis, acute renal failure, lactic acidosis, and hemodynamic instability as a result of prolonged (>48 hours) and/or high-dose infusion (>5 mg/kg/h) of propofol.**

There is no specific antidote for propofol toxicity. The treatment is immediate discontinuation of the propofol infusion followed by supportive care. Supportive care may include administration of IV fluids, vasopressors and antiarrhythmic agents.

CASE CORRELATION

- See also Case 22 (Acute Liver Failure).

COMPREHENSION QUESTIONS

37.1 A 25-year-old woman is admitted to the ICU for altered level of consciousness after a polypharmacy ingestion. An acetaminophen level of 80 μg/dL
is obtained 12 hours after the ingestion. After stabilization of the patient's
airway, breathing, and circulation, the ICU team discussed antidote treatment
with liver function tests pending. Which statement is most accurate regarding
the next step of management for this patient?

  A. Sodium bicarbonate infusion should be initiated with a goal serum
pH 7.45-7.55.

  B. N-acetylcysteine treatment should not be considered until the liver
function tests are available.

  C. Octreotide can be considered if the patient does not respond to IV
dextrose administration.

  D. N-acetylcysteine treatment should be started, and serial liver function
tests should be monitored during treatment.

  E. Initiate NG lavage of gastric contents.

37.2 A 54-year-old man is admitted to the burn ICU with confusion and decreased
level of consciousness, along with several third-degree burns throughout his
body from an industrial fire. The patient was intubated for airway protection after soot in the posterior pharynx and airway edema were noted upon
arrival. Cyanide toxicity is suspected. What is the best treatment method for
cyanide toxicity in this patient?

  A. Sodium bicarbonate infusion should be initiated with a goal serum
pH 7.45-7.55.

  B. Amyl nitrite pearls and intravenous sodium nitrite should be administered.

  C. Hydroxocobalamin should be administered intravenously.

  D. Methemoglobinemia should be the goal of treatment.

  E. Nitroprusside should be administered.

37.3 A 33-year-old man was admitted to the ICU after having been found comatose
in his home with a suicide note and an empty bottle of aspirin (30 count). His
salicylate level returns at 111 mg/dL, and his serum pH is 7.01. What is the
best treatment plan for this patient?

  A. Octreotide can be considered if the patient does not respond to IV
dextrose administration.

  B. Sodium bicarbonate infusion should be initiated with a goal serum
pH 7.45-7.55.

  C. Hemodialysis should be initiated to enhance elimination and correct the
acidosis.

  D. N-acetylcysteine treatment should be started and serial liver function
tests should be monitored during treatment.

  E. Potassium supplementation in intravenous fluid should be administered.

37.4 A 40-year-old woman with diabetes on a sulfonylurea was admitted from the emergency department for acute kidney injury with Cr 3.2 mg/dL in the setting of hypoglycemia (glucose initially noted to be 30 mg/dL). Which of the following therapies is the first-line treatment?

A. Intravenous dextrose infusion with close glucose monitoring

B. Fomepizole therapy, initiated immediately

C. Intravenous octreotide, administered immediately

D. Sodium bicarbonate infusion with a goal urine pH 7.5-8.0

E. Calcium chloride administration

ANSWERS

37.1 **D.** The patient's alcohol level is clearly past the line indicating probable hepatic toxicity when plotted on the nomogram for 12 hours after ingestion. Therefore, NAC therapy is warranted. Remember that **the nomogram functions to assist the medical team with the decision on whether or not to initiate NAC therapy.** Serial liver function tests are followed while the patient is receiving NAC therapy to help determine the length of therapy. Gastric lavage may be of value when initiated within 30 to 60 minutes following ingestion to help evacuate pill fragments. Sodium bicarbonate and octreotide are not indicated for the treatment of acetaminophen toxicity.

37.2 **C.** Hydroxocobalamin is the preferred treatment for cyanide toxicity, especially in the setting of smoke inhalation. Amyl nitrites and sodium nitrite should be avoided with smoke inhalation exposures, as carbon monoxide toxicity is also common with these types of exposures. Since amyl nitrite and sodium nitrite function by inducing methemoglobinemia, this may be detrimental to the patient's oxygen carrying capacity with concomitant carboxyhemoglobinemia. If hodroxocobalamin is unavailable in these situations, treating with thiosulfate is the next best option for cyanide toxicity from smoke inhalation exposures. Sodium bicarbonate is not indicated in the treatment of cyanide toxicity. Nitroprusside administration in high doses or prolonged fashion can contribute to cyanide toxicity, and its administration has no role in treatment of inhalation-related cyanide toxicity.

37.3 **C.** Hemodialysis is indicated in salicylate toxicity with a serum level above 100 mg/dL with profound acidosis. Sodium bicarbonate is the mainstay of treatment with salicylate toxicity; however, the goal of treatment is to alkalinize the urine to enhance salicylate elimination. Therefore, the goal of sodium bicarbonate therapy is to maintain a urinary pH of 7.5 to 8.0. Octreotide and N-acetylcysteine are not indicated in salicylate toxicity. Potassium supplementation is helpful during treatment of salicylate toxicity as depletion often occurs; however, replacement of potassium does not actually address the salicylate toxicity.

37.4   **A.** The mainstay of treatment for sulfonylurea-induced hypoglycemia is the administration of dextrose-containing IV fluids and close monitoring for greater than 24 hours. Octreotide is warranted only after patients display that they are unresponsive to dextrose containing IV fluids. Fomepizole is used for ethylene glycol poisoning. Sodium bicarbonate can be applied as an adjunctive measure to facilitate the elimination of sulfonylurea in the treatment of sulfonylurea toxicity if the patient's renal function is adequate. In this patient with a serum creatinine of 3.2 mg/dL and acute kidney injury, alkalinization most likely will not work. Calcium chloride does not have any therapeutic benefits in a patient with sulfonylurea poisoning.

CLINICAL PEARLS

▶ NAC is the FDA-approved medication for patients with acetaminophen toxicity, and it is of maximal benefit when administered within 8-10 hours after ingestion. Benefits may be seen even when administered after 24 hours post-ingestion.

▶ Acute ethanol ingestion may serve a protective role against acetaminophen toxicity by occupying the cytochrome P450 2E1 system and decreasing the metabolism of acetaminophen to NAPQI.

▶ Chronic ethanol ingestion up-regulates the cytochrome P450 2E1 system and increases the conversion of acetaminophen to the toxic metabolite NAPQI.

▶ Propofol infusion syndrome includes rhabdomyolysis, acute renal failure, lactic acidosis, and hemodynamic instability. This syndrome may be the result of prolonged (>48 hours) high-dose infusion (>5 mg/kg/h) of propofol.

REFERENCES

Heard K. Acetylcysteine for acetaminophen poisoning. *N Eng J Med.* 2008;359:258-292.

Lank PM, Corbridge T, Murray PT. In: Hall JB, Schmidt GA, Kress JP, eds. *Principles of Critical Care.* 4th ed. New York, NY: McGraw-Hill Education; 2015:1192-1223.

Stolbach A, Goldfrank LR. Toxicology. In: Gabrielli A, Layon AJ, Yu M, eds. *Civetta, Taylor, & Kirby's Critical Care.* Philadelphia, PA: Lippincott Williams & Wilkins; 2009:987-1014.

A 66-year-old man fell down a flight of stairs. He sustained several rib fractures and a small right frontal-parietal cerebral contusion. While in the emergency center he developed progressive dyspnea, which led to intubation and mechanical ventilation. Shortly after arrival to the ICU, his nurse notifies you that the patient appears anxious and agitated despite having received 8 mg of morphine sulfate intravenously over the past 1 hour. His heart rate is 110, BP is 146/90, respiratory rate is 28, Glasgow coma scale (GCS) is 10T (E4, M5, V1), and O_2 saturation is 100%. He appears uncomfortable and is making attempts to remove his monitoring leads and urinary catheter.

▶ What are the appropriate next steps in assessment?
▶ What are appropriate interventions at this time?

ANSWERS TO CASE 38:
Pain Control

Summary: A 66-year-old man with rib fractures and small right frontal-parietal cerebral contusion following a fall is intubated secondary to progressive dyspnea. He now appears agitated, uncomfortable, and in danger of self harm.

- **Appropriate next steps in the assessment:** Identify potential reasons for pain and agitation in this patient using validated scales and establish treatment goals.

- **Appropriate interventions at this time:** Administer a combination of sedative and analgesic medications. An appropriate combination for this patient is propofol for sedation, titrated to the Richmond Agitation Sedation Scale (RASS) of 2, and fentanyl for pain control.

ANALYSIS

Objectives

1. Learn the principles and strategies for monitoring pain and anxiety in the ICU.

2. Learn the various medication treatment strategies available for pain and sedation management in the ICU.

3. Learn management considerations for mechanically ventilated patients.

4. Learn management considerations for patients who are at risk for developing alcohol, benzodiazepine, and opioid withdrawal.

Considerations

This patient is clearly agitated and has progressed to become a danger to himself, as evidenced by his attempt to remove his catheter and lines. In order to avoid further harm to the patient, we must address his agitation and pain immediately. Prior to the next step in management, however, we must consider the patient's comorbid conditions, current injuries, and goals of care. The patient has experienced head trauma; subsequently, a fast onset/offset agent that will allow easily performed neurologic checks would be ideal. The ICU team must evaluate how long they anticipate the patient to require mechanical ventilation based on the severity of his respiratory failure and his overall condition. This initial assessment must occur quickly and will guide the ICU care practitioner toward particular agents and techniques of sedation and pain management. In this situation, a bolus of short-acting sedative agent with rapid onset, such as propofol, is a very reasonable choice.

APPROACH TO PAIN CONTROL

Background and Pain Monitoring

The ICU care practitioner is responsible for maintaining a patient's comfort while in the ICU. Mechanically ventilated patients in the ICU can exhibit even further stress superimposed on their acute medical problems, and examples of these additional stresses include anxiety related to unfamiliar surroundings and distress with potential and experienced pain from invasive and frequent ICU care. Agitation, anxiety, and pain can bring about many adverse side effects, including increased endogenous catecholamine activity, myocardial ischemia, hypercoagulability, hypermetabolic states, sleep deprivation and delirium, possibly resulting in self-injury via removal of life-sustaining devices. Although such adverse effects should be actively avoided, the care providers must be mindful of the potential detrimental effects associated with pharmacological treatment of pain and agitation. A fine balance must be established to maximize the benefits while minimizing the risks of drug accumulation in tissue stores, which may prolong clinical effects and ICU stay.

When developing sedation and pain management strategies, it is important to consider the anticipated duration of treatment and the anticipated duration of mechanical ventilation. Addressing the target of intervention will help determine the most practical medication strategies. Very often, a combination of opioids and benzodiazepines are used for analgesia and sedation. Alternatively, other agents may be selected, depending on the patient's clinical status (Table 38–1). Benzodiazepines (midazolam, lorazepam, and diazepam) have been the cornerstone of anxiolytic, amnestic, and sedative therapy for the ICU patient, while opioids have a long history of efficacy and safety for adequate analgesia in the ICU patient.

Generally speaking, **elderly patients usually have increased sensitivity to centrally acting sedation medications such as benzodiazepines and opioids**, both in a therapeutic sense and a propensity to develop adverse side effects. The ability to handle medications changes with age-related changes in body composition together with alterations in renal and liver function. Thus nonopioids such as intravenous acetaminophen can be effective in elderly patients.

Multiple modalities of pain regimens exist, such as epidural infusions, nerve blocks, and paravertebral blocks, which are particularly relevant for the elderly patient with rib fractures described at the beginning of the case. Epidural analgesia is a method whereby narcotics, anesthetic agents or combinations thereof are introduced into the spinal epidural space at the thoracic or lumbar level to provide regional anesthesia; agents can be delivered by either a bolus or continuous infusion. The major advantage of epidural analgesia is its apparent effectiveness in the absence of sedation; epidurals have been shown to increase functional residual capacity, lung compliance and vital capacity and decrease airway resistance. Epidurals can be technically demanding to insert, can cause hypotension and can pose the risk of an epidural hematoma, a serious injury where spinal paralysis can occur. Multi-modality pain regimens can be very effective in critically ill patients.

Pain is common, and the majority of management algorithms incorporate testing for pain, with patient self-report being the most accurate means of assessment if the patient is able to communicate. Self reporting for pain is facilitated using a numerical rating scale (NRS) or visual aid (Figure 38–1). A number of other tools for pain observation, such as the behavioral pain scale (BPS) and critical pain observation tool (CPOT), have been validated (Table 38–2). These tools utilize facial expression, body movement, muscle tension, and ventilator synchrony to help assess a patient's pain. The validity of these scales declines with increased depth of sedation.

Table 38–1 • PAIN MEDICATIONS

Class of Medication	Mechanism of Action	Uses	Adverse Effects	Examples
Opioids	Mu-1 receptors for analgesia in CNS and peripheral tissue Mu-2 receptors mediate respiratory depression, nausea, vomiting, constipation	Mainstay drug for analgesia therapy in ICU	Depress respiratory drive, decrease GI motility—ileus, little cardiovascular effects in euvolemic patients but can result in significant hypotension in hypovolemic patients, dependence and withdrawal effects with prolonged infusion	Morphine Fentanyl Remifentanyl Methadone Hydromorphone
Benzodiazepines	Potentiate effects of gamma-aminobutyric acid (GABA) via benzodiazepine receptor—suppress CNS activity	Mainstay for sedation in ICU—do not have analgesic properties	Respiratory depression	Lorazepam (Ativan) Midazolam (Versed)
Propofol	Potentiates effects of GABA receptor (different receptor than benzodiazepines), very lipophilic—crosses blood brain barrier rapidly	Rapid onset and offset action for sedation, used for short term sedation, used to treat status epilepticus and is a common anesthesia induction agent	Highly lipophilic compound – can cause hypertriglyceridemia Pain at injection site Propofol infusion syndrome: rare, seen with high infusion rates >48 h, characterized by arrhythmias, heart failure, metabolic acidosis, hyperkalemia, rhabdomyolysis	

α₂ receptor agonists	Binds to α₂ receptors releasing norepinephrine and decreasing sympathetic activity—net effect sedation, analgesia and amnesia, sedative properties facilitated through locus coeruleus site in CNS and analgesic effects accentuate opioid receptors	Commonly used following cardiac and neurosurgical procedures, not associated with respiratory depression	Biphasic cardiovascular effect: initial bolus may cause vasoconstriction causing bradycardia and hypertension; continuous infusion associated with hypotension secondary to vasodilation	Dexmedetomidine Clonidine
Neuromuscular blocking agents (NMBA)	Block neuromuscular transmission at neuromuscular junction, causing paralysis of affected skeletal muscles; clinically relevant drugs acts postsynaptically at acetylcholine receptors of motor nerve end-plate	Indicated for patients on modes of mechanical ventilation that produce agitation interfering with ventilation/oxygenation, closed head injury with increased ICP, tetanus and decreased venous O_2 in hypermetabolic, agitated states	Most feared complication is accidental extubation. Considered a causative factor for critical illness myopathy—causing prolonged weakness after use, especially in those patients using steroids	Rocuronium Vecuronium Atracurium Cistracurium

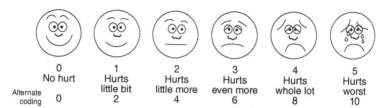

Figure 38–1. Visual-Analog Scale of Pain. (Reproduced, with permission, from Hockenberry MJ, Wilson D: *Wong's essentials of pediatric nursing*, ed 8, St. Louis, 2009, Mosby. Used with permission. Copyright Mosby).

Sedation scales, the most common being Ramsay Sedation Scale (RSS), RASS, and Sedation Agitation Scale (SAS) are used to direct the management of agitation, establish a target level of sedation for medication titration, and detect when oversedation is present (Table 38–3 and Table 38–4). The Ramsay score of 2 or 3 is optimal. In the absence of organic or natural causes of obtundation (ie, central nervous system pathology), a Ramsay score of 5 or 6 represents oversedation.

Once a patient is started on sedative and analgesic medications, the goal should be to minimize the risk of continued infusion of these agents. A focused downward titration of sedative drugs over time can be accomplished with daily interruption of sedative infusions (DIS). Retrospective, controlled studies conducted in mechanically ventilated patients receiving continuous IV sedation demonstrated that a daily interruption in the sedation until the patient was awake decreased the duration of mechanical ventilation and ICU length of stay. DIS minimizes drug accumulation and shortens the duration of mechanical ventilation. Both sedative and analgesic agents should be interrupted once daily unless there is evidence for ongoing patient distress. Once drugs are interrupted, the ICU team must be vigilant for evidence of patient distress—overt physical agitation, hemodynamic lability (HTN or tachycardia) or ventilator asynchrony. A bolus should be given to de-escalate symptoms, and both sedative and analgesic drugs should be restarted at half the previous infusion doses with subsequent titration. Performing DIS in every patient may not be appropriate, as there is some concern that DIS could provoke brief episodes of intense withdrawal from drugs or alcohol in those individuals. For example, in traumatic head injury patients, DIS may lead to significant increases in intracranial

Table 38–2 • BEHAVIORAL PAIN SCALE			
Score	Facial Expression	Verbalization	Body Position
0	Neutral/positive facial expression, calm	Normal conversation, laugh	Inactive, laying relaxed with all extremities or sitting, walking
1	Negative facial expression, concerned	Completely quiet or sobbing and/or complaining but not because of pain	Restless movements, shifting fashion and/or touching wound or wound area
2	Negative facial expression, grimace, distorted face	Crying, screaming and/or complains about pain	Lying rigid and/or drawn up with arms and legs to the body

Table 38–3 • RICHMOND AGITATION SEDATION SCALE (RASS)		
Score	Term	Description
+4	Combative	Overtly combative or violent and an immediate danger to staff
+3	Very agitated	Pulls on or removes tubes/catheters or has aggressive behavior to staff
+2	Agitated	Frequent nonpurposeful movement or patient ventilator dyssynchrony
+1	Restless	Anxious or apprehensive but movements not aggressive or vigorous
0	Alert and calm	
−1	Drowsy	Not fully alert but has sustained (>10 seconds) awakenings with eye contact to voice
−2	Light sedation	Briefly (<10 seconds) awakens with eye contact to voice
−3	Moderate sedation	Any movements (but no eye contact) to voice
−4	Deep sedation	No response to voice, but any movement to physical stimuli
−5	Unarousable	No response to voice or physical stimulation

pressure (ICP) and decreased cerebral perfusion pressures. Abrupt sedation interruptions have been shown to increase circulating levels of stress hormones, such as cortisol and catecholamines; such increases have been associated with a slight but significant increase in ICPs. In such patients, sedation should not be stopped abruptly but withdrawn progressively with titration of the sedation doses to ICP targets. Further research is needed to clarify the most optimal approach to selecting patients for DIS. Currently, the optimal way to approach DIS at the bedside is to consider and discuss the risks and benefits of DIS for each patient daily.

THERAPEUTIC APPROACH

In agitated and anxious patients, the clinician can first attempt nonpharmacologic interventions such as comfortable positioning, verbal reassurance, and encouraging the presence of family and friends, though such interventions are often inadequate

Table 38–4 • THE RAMSAY SEDATION SCORING SYSTEM	
Score	Response
1	Anxious and agitated or restless; or both
2	Cooperative, oriented and tranquil
3	Responding to commands only
4	Brisk response to a light glabellar tap
5	Sluggish response to a light glabellar tap
6	No response to a light glabellar tap

alone and patients may ultimately require medical intervention. In the case study at the beginning of the chapter, initial assessment of the patient's agitation places him at a RASS +3, as he is removing his catheters and is clearly agitated. Because the patient is awake, we can ask him directly about pain, instructing him to quantify his pain numerically if he is able to do so.

Prior to initiating a sedation and pain regimen in an ICU patient, the patient's injuries, comorbidities, and goals of care must always be addressed. The patient with head trauma may require frequent neurologic examinations in the immediate observation period. In this situation, propofol may be the best choice given its rapid onset and offset. Midazolam (Versed) can also be used as a sedative, though its offset is longer than propofol and frequent neurologic examinations would not be as easy to administer. When initiating a sedative agent, a level of sedation should always be identified, using the RASS sedation scale as a guideline. An appropriate level of sedation would allow the patient to be easily awakened and comfortable, consistent with RASS −1 or −2. Sedation and analgesia in the ICU are multidisciplinary, as the bedside nurses will be the crucial component of evaluating the patient's sedation level. As such, it is important to communicate the sedation goals with the entire healthcare team.

Opioids are the mainstay of analgesic care in the ICU. These drugs are also very good at palliating coughing and the subjective sense of dyspnea, which is particularly important for patients who are mechanically ventilated. Amongst the opioids, fentanyl has a rapid onset of action (1 min) and rapidly redistributes into peripheral tissues, resulting in a short half-life (0.5-1 h) after a single dose. As a continuous infusion, fentanyl can be titrated to the patient's comfort as identified by a pain scale described earlier. If the patient is easily awakened, we can address pain by simply asking the patient to quantify the pain. If the patient is not easily awakened, tools such as facial expression, body movement and ventilator synchrony can be utilized, again with the bedside nurse being the most important person in this assessment.

After initiation of sedation and analgesia, it is important to continuously clinically re-evaluate the patient. If the patient appears to be improving from a respiratory standpoint and is clinically prepared to undergo spontaneous breathing trials in preparation for extubation, the patient's sedation should be titrated downwards and the patient slowly awoken, as sedation can hinder one's respiratory status. The ICU clinician must be vigilant in this aspect—always reassessing the patient's clinical status and de-escalating medications (or escalating medications if needed) in order to minimize the risks of medical sedation and analgesia.

Prevention and Treatment of Agitation Related to Substance Ingestion or Substance Administration

Alcohol abuse contributes to a number of health problems; consequently, it is not uncommon to encounter patients with chronic alcohol ingestion history in the ICU. Chronic excessive alcohol consumption causes depression of the central α and β receptors and an increase in the inhibitory neurotransmitter GABA. At the same time, chronic alcohol use causes an increase in NMDA receptors, which are responsible for central excitatory activities. When alcohol consumption stops in an individual with a chronic consumption history, the combination of excess excitatory activities and the withdrawal of inhibitory activities can lead to symptoms of withdrawal, which include a number of neuropsychiatric and hemodynamic manifestations. Alcohol withdrawal symptoms may include **tremulousness** (onset within hours, peak 10-30 h, subsides at approximately 40 h), **seizures** (onset 6-48 h, peak 13-24 h), **hallucination** (onset 8-48 h, may persist 1-6 d), and **delirium tremens** (onset 48-96 h). Recognition of patients at risk for alcohol withdrawal is important and can be determined based on social history and history of prior withdrawal episodes. The treatments are supportive care and benzodiazepine administration, and in some cases of delirium tremens, the addition of propofol and neuroleptics may be considered.

Chronic ingestion and the administration of exogenous opioids can lead to diminished endogenous opioid peptides; with the discontinuation of exogenous opioids, patients may develop withdrawal symptoms. Early symptoms of opioid withdrawal may include yawning, rhinorrhea, and sneezing. Later manifestation of withdrawal may include restlessness, irritability, tachycardia, tremor, hyperthermia, vomiting, and muscle spasm. Withdrawal symptoms may begin within 6 to 12 hours after the last dose of short-acting opioid or after 36 to 48 hours of the last dose of long-acting opioids, such as methadone. It is important to remember that opioid withdrawal can occur when long-term administration of opioids is discontinued or tapered too rapidly. A course of tapering over days to weeks may be implemented to avoid this problem.

Benzodiazepine withdrawal can occur in the ICU setting when infusions are decreased or interrupted. Patients receiving higher doses of the medications for prolonged periods of time (>7 days) have increased susceptibility for developing withdrawal. Close monitoring and slow tapering schedules may be needed when considering benzodiazepine discontinuation in ICU patients.

CLINICAL CASE CORRELATION

- See also Case 8 (Airway Management/Respiratory Failure), Case 9 (Ventilator Management), and Case 30 (Altered Mental Status).

COMPREHENSION QUESTIONS

38.1 A 45-year-old man with multiple abdominal gunshot wounds is intubated in the ICU and has been receiving continuous infusion of propofol and fentanyl for 3 days. His morning labs reveal a potassium of 6.3 mEq/L and bicarbonate of 16 mEq/L, and the patient had three episodes of unsustained ventricular tachycardia overnight. What is your next step in management?

A. Administer calcium gluconate, insulin and β blockers for his hyperkalemia

B. Cardioversion

C. Discontinue propofol

D. Resuscitate with fluids to increase bicarbonate

E. Hemodialysis

38.2 A 37-year-old woman is admitted to the ICU for severe pancreatitis complicated by acute respiratory distress syndrome (ARDS) requiring mechanical ventilation. She continues to have difficulty ventilating and agitation on increasing doses of fentanyl and Versed IV infusions, and it is becoming increasingly difficult to ventilate her. What is the most appropriate next step?

A. Continue to increase Versed as tolerated

B. Change sedative agent from Versed to Propofol

C. Administer a neuromuscular blocking agent in addition to current regimen

D. Administer a second analgesic, as her difficulty ventilating and agitation are secondary to poorly controlled pain

E. Provide a trial of pressure support ventilation

38.3 A 67-year-old woman with end-stage renal disease and coronary artery disease is admitted to the ICU for respiratory failure secondary to pneumonia. Which analgesic agent is most appropriate for this patient?

A. Ketorolac

B. Fentanyl

C. Morphine

D. Meperidine

ANSWERS

38.1 **C.** Propofol infusion syndrome is a rare but serious and potentially fatal adverse effect, typically seen with infusion rates >83 µg/kg/min for more than 48 hours and carrying with it a mortality rate of up to 85%. This syndrome is characterized by dysrhythmias, heart failure, metabolic acidosis, hyperkalemia, and rhabdomyolysis. High-risk patients include those receiving high doses of the drug, those with history of hypertriglyceridemia, and those concurrently receiving parenteral lipids for nutrition. Treatment consists of immediate cessation of propofol infusion and then correction of hemodynamic and metabolic abnormalities.

38.2 **C.** Some patients may remain delirious, agitated and have difficulty maintaining ventilation, regardless of whether they are on an effective dose of anxiolytic drugs. If the patient is tracheally intubated, mechanically ventilated, and receiving adequate sedation, using a neuromuscular blockade to paralyze the patient is a therapeutic option. In patients with ARDS who are difficult to ventilate and often agitated, neuromuscular blockades may be a reasonable alternative to help improve ventilation and gas exchange.

38.3 **B.** Fentanyl is metabolized by the liver, creating inactive metabolites which are renally excreted. This makes fentanyl a good choice for patients with renal insufficiency. Morphine is conjugated by the liver to metabolites that include morphine-6-glucuronide, a potent metabolite. Both morphine and morphine-6-glucuronide are eliminated by the kidney; thus, patients with renal dysfunction may suffer from prolonged drug effects. Like morphine, meperidine is renally excreted. A metabolite of meperidine, normeperidine, is a potent CNS stimulate that can potentiate seizures, especially in patients with renal dysfunction. Ketorolac is an NSAID that reversibly inhibits cyclo-oxygenase-1 and 2 enzymes and is contraindicated in patients with advanced renal impairment, as NSAID use may compromise existing renal function.

CLINICAL PEARLS

▶ Prior to initiating a sedation and pain regimen in an ICU patient, the patient's injuries, comorbidities and goals of care must always be addressed.

▶ Opioids are the mainstay of analgesic care in the ICU.

▶ Sedation scales, the most common being RSS, RASS, and SAS are used to direct the management of agitation, establish a target level of sedation for medication titration, and detect when oversedation is present.

▶ Once a patient is started on sedative and analgesic medications, the goal should be to minimize the risk of continued infusion of these agents.

▶ Daily interruption of sedative infusions (DIS) minimizes drug accumulation and shortens the duration of mechanical ventilation.

REFERENCES

Devlin JW, Roberts RJ. Pharmacology of commonly used analgesics and sedatives in the ICU Benzodiazepines, propofol, and opioids. *Crit Care Clin.* 2009;25:431-449.

Murray MJ, Bloomfield EL. Sedation and neuromuscular blockade. In Gabrielli A, Layon AJ, Yu M, eds. *Civetta, Taylor, & Kirby's Critical Care.* 4th ed. Philadelphia, PA Lippincott, Williams, & Wilkins; 2009:961-971.

Rajaram SS, Zimmerman JL. Substance abuse and withdrawal alcohol, cocaine, opioids, and other drugs. In Gabrielli A, Layon AJ, Yu M, eds. *Civetta, Taylor, & Kirby's Critical Care.* 4th ed. Philadelphia, PA Lippincott, Williams, & Wilkins; 2009:1015-1027.

Skoglund K, Enblad P, Hillered L, Marklund N. The neurological wake-up test increases stress hormone levels in patients with severe traumatic brain injury. *Crit Care Med.* 2012;40:216-222.

Sokol S, Patel BK, Lat I, Kress JP. Pain control, sedation, and use of muscle relaxants. In Hall JB, Schmidt GA, Kress JP, eds. *Principles of Critical Care.* 4th ed. New York, NY McGraw-Hill; 2015: 145-155.

Zapanis A, Leung S. Tolerance and withdrawal issues with sedation. *Crit Care Nurs Clin N Am.* 2005;17:211-223.

A 56-year-old man was at a mall, where he had a witnessed sudden cardiac arrest. He received immediate cardiopulmonary resuscitation (CPR) from bystanders. When the paramedics arrived, they noticed that the patient was in ventricular fibrillation and initiated cardioversion and continued CPR. After several rounds of cardioversion and medications, the patient's rhythm returned to sinus tachycardia with a rate of 120 beats/min and a blood pressure of 96/40 mm Hg. In the emergency center, he was noted to have sinus tachycardia with a rate of 115 beats/min, BP of 98/60 mm Hg, and Glasgow coma score (GCS) of 7T. You are called to see the patient to prepare his admission to the ICU.

▶ What are your priorities in this patient's management?
▶ What are post-resuscitation treatment strategies that have been shown to improve outcome?

ANSWERS TO CASE 39:
Post-Resuscitation Management in the ICU

Summary: A 56-year-old man with witnessed ventricular fibrillation-induced cardiac arrest has been successfully resuscitated following CPR, cardioversion, and pharmacological interventions. He is now intubated and admitted to the ICU for further care.

- **Priorities in this patient's management:** Minimize post-cardiac arrest brain injury, address his post-cardiac arrest myocardial dysfunction, minimize his systemic ischemia/reperfusion responses, address the problems that caused his cardiac arrest in the first place, and lastly prognosticate outcome.

- **Post-resuscitation strategies that improve outcome:** Coronary reperfusion with either percutaneous intervention and/or thrombolytic therapy has been shown to improve survival in cardiac arrest survivors if acute change in coronary plaque morphology is the underlying cause for the cardiac arrest. Other strategies that have been shown to improve neurological outcome in post-cardiac arrest patients include controlled reoxygenation, therapeutic hypothermia, and glucose management.

ANALYSIS

Objectives

1. To learn the post-cardiac arrest syndrome and strategies directed toward its management, including optimization of neurological outcome, optimization of myocardial function, glucose management, and controlled reoxygenation.

2. To be able to describe the use of therapeutic hypothermia to reduce neurological injury after resuscitation.

Considerations

This 56-year-old man is admitted to the ICU after successful resuscitation from an apparent ventricular fibrillation (VF)-induced cardiac arrest. Neurological and cardiac dysfunction are common problems in the post-cardiac arrest resuscitation setting. Therapeutic hypothermia (TH), which is defined as lowering the core body temperature to 32°C to 34°C, can help post-resuscitation neurological and myocardial dysfunction. Maintaining oxygenation saturation in the 94% to 96% range will help decrease re-perfusion hyperoxic injuries. Finally, hyperglycemia is common following resuscitation. While prior interventions attempted to maintain tighter glycemic control in this setting, more recent evidence has found that moderate hyperglycemia correlates to better outcome. Thus, targeting the patient's glucose levels to the 144 to 180 mg/dL range is the current treatment recommendation.

APPROACH TO:
The Post-Resuscitation Patient

DEFINITIONS

POST-CARDIAC ARREST SYNDROME: This syndrome includes post-cardiac arrest brain injury, post-cardiac arrest myocardial dysfunction, ischemia/reperfusion injuries, and the underlying disease process that contributed to the event.

THERAPEUTIC HYPOTHERMIA (TH): Therapeutic maneuvers to improve neurologic outcomes by rapid reduction of core body temperature to 32°C to 34°C following cardiac arrest, with hypothermia maintained for 24 to 48 hours after induction.

POST-CARDIAC ARREST MYOCARDIAL DYSFUNCTION: This is a biventricular dysfunction due to multiple factors that occurs transiently following resuscitation from cardiac arrest.

POST-CARDIAC ARREST ENCEPHALOPATHY: Ischemic brain injury in which the two main manifestations are depressed level of consciousness and seizures.

CLINICAL APPROACH

Introduction

Survival after in-hospital and out-of-hospital cardiac arrest is poor. For the subset of patients with return of spontaneous circulation following resuscitation, the probability of survival is significantly better. Approximately one-third of patients admitted to the ICU following cardiac arrest survive to discharge from the hospital. Post-cardiac arrest syndrome describes a number of complex pathophysiologic processes which are grouped into four major categories: post-resuscitation brain injury, ischemia/reperfusion injuries, myocardial dysfunction, and persistence of the precipitation of the cardiac arrest. Neuronal susceptibility to ischemia is not uniform within the brain. These differential responses may be related to the different brain regions' cellular energy requirements and adaptive heat-shock responses. The hallmark of anoxic encephalopathy is disorder of consciousness and arousal. In addition to depressed level of arousal, 10% to 40% of post-cardiac arrest patients develop seizure activities that have to monitored and treated.

Most of the treatment strategies and rationale are based on recent post-arrest resuscitation literature and include TH and early cardiac intervention. Several organizations now recommend bundling of post-resuscitation care to include therapeutic hypothermia, early coronary angiography and PCI (percutaneous coronary intervention), hemodynamic support with inotropes or vasopressors, and rapid extubation.

Therapeutic Hypothermia (TH)

Rapid reduction of the patients' temperatures to 32°C to 34°C has been shown in several randomized controlled trials to improve neurological recovery in patients following VF-induced cardiac arrest. TH should be instituted as quickly as possible following successful resuscitation, and this can be accomplished in most patients with the application of surface cooling using cooling blankets and ice packs. This approach has been definitvely shown to improve neurologic outcomes in patients suffering from out-of-hospital VF arrest. Some experts have proposed applying the cooling strategy more broadly to include patients with cardiac arrest from other causes; however, the beneficial effects of TH in these other patients have not been as clearly supported by clinical evidence. TH has now been incorporated into the International Consensus Guidelines for Resuscitative Care since 2005. During TH, magnesium, phosphate, potassium, and calcium should be closely monitored and replaced to the higher end of normal values. During the rewarming phase, the core temperature should increase at a rate of 0.25°C to 0.5°C per hour, with continued monitoring and replacement of electrolytes. Rapid rewarming can lead to increased catabolism and worse outcomes. The potential complications associated with TH include increased infections form leukocyte dysfunction, increased bleeding from platelets and clotting factors dysfunction, and arrhythmias (predominantly atrial fibrillation).

Post-resuscitation myocardial dysfunction is a transient reduction in left and right ventricular function that presents for 24 to 48 hours after cardiac arrest. It is now believed that TH may also have some beneficial effects in reducing the occurrence and severity of post-resuscitation myocardial dysfunction. Because the majority of out-of-hospital cardiac arrests occur as the result of acute coronary syndrome, these patients benefit from early coronary angiography and PCI.

Oxygenation

Observations from experimental models suggest that ventilation during and after resuscitation with minimal oxygen fractions to maintain oxygen saturation of 94% to 96% or PaO_2 of ~100 mm Hg would lead to a reduction in reperfusion injuries. In addition, in a multicenter cohort study, it was observed that adult patients with non–trauma-related cardiac arrest had a mortality odds ratio of 1.8 when hyperoxia (PaO_2 >300 mm Hg) was recorded as the initial blood gas value following arrest. Based on these principles and clinical evidence, the target oxygenation for the post-arrest patient should be 94% to 96% saturation, and not higher.

Fluids and Vasopressors

The resuscitation of patients with hemodynamic instability from hemorrhagic shock and sepsis is discussed in detail elsewhere in this book (Case 19, Sepsis). The Surviving Sepsis Campaign has provided guidelines for the use of fluids and vaso-pressors for septic patients. Similarly, military conflicts in the Middle East have led to development of resuscitation strategies for patients with hemorrhagic shock. What remains relatively undefined are the management strategies to minimize the harm associated with initial resuscitation of patients with various forms of shock. The administration of large amount of fluids and blood products for patients with clinical shock can produce generalized edema with excess extravasation of fluid into the extracellular tissue spaces. These fluid shifts produce edema and organ dysfunction, especially in the lungs and gastrointestinal tract. Resuscitation efforts directed at optimizing tissue oxygenation are most beneficial during the initial few hours following septic or hemorrhagic insults, whereas extended periods of excess fluid administration is potentially harmful. As soon as the patients begin to stabilize, it is important to cut back on excess fluids. For those patients who have received excess fluid initially, early administration of diuretic therapy can be highly beneficial. A randomized study comparing CVP endpoints for septic shock patients demonstrated that patients who were resuscitated with a target CVP of 4 mm Hg had better outcome than those patients resuscitation with CVP targets of 8 mm Hg. Another important benefit observed in patients who received limited fluid administration during resuscitation is improved early GI tract function and improved tolerance to enteral nutritional support.

Glucose Levels

Hyperglycemia is a common encounter in post-cardiac arrest patients. Recent observations suggest that strict glycemic control in ICU patients is associated with an increase in neurologic complications, and a randomized controlled trial has shown that there was no difference in mortality among out-of-hospital arrest patients managed with glucose levels of 72 to 108 mg/dL, versus those maintained with glucoses of 108 to 144 mg/dL. Taken together, these observations suggest that there is greater risk of harm to try to maintain glucose values in the "normal" range in the ICU patient population. The 2010 American Heart Association Guidelines for Cardiopulmonary Resuscitation and Emergency Cardiovascular Care recommends moderate glycemic control targeting glucose values between 144 and 180 mg/dL to avoid hypoglycemic episodes in these patients.

CLINICAL CASE CORRELATION

- See Case 3 (Scoring Systems and Patient Prognosis), Case 4 (Hemodynamic Monitoring), Case 19 (Sepsis), and Case 40 (Postoperative Care in the ICU).

COMPREHENSIVE QUESTIONS

39.1 Which of the following strategies has been shown to improve recovery from post-cardiac arrest syndrome?

A. Early echocardiography

B. Cooling of core body temperature to 28°C to 30°C

C. Maintaining oxygen saturations of 100%

D. Cooling of core temperature to 32°C to 34°C

E. Swan-Ganz catheter-directed goal resuscitation

39.2 Which of the following is the most accurate statement regarding glucose management in the post-cardiac arrest patient?

A. Hypoglycemia is a common cause of in-hospital cardiac arrest.

B. Glycemic control does not have any impact in the management of these patients.

C. Glycemic control targeting serum glucose values of 84 to 110 mg/dL is optimal.

D. Glycemic control targeting serum glucose values of 144 to 180 mg/dL is optimal.

E. Avoidance of glucose-containing intravenous fluid is preferred.

39.3 A 64-year-old man who was being treated in the hospital for acute cholecystitis is found to be unresponsive. He was noted to be in VF and underwent chest compressions for several minutes in addition to cardioversion. The patient has return of spontaneous rhythm and vital signs. Which of the following is an important treatment for this patient?

A. Target oxygen saturation of 91%

B. Target serum glucose level at 110 mg/dL

C. Percutaneous coronary angiography

D. Target core body temperature of 35°C to 36°C

E. Continue fluid resuscitation for 12 hours

39.4 Which of the following has been found to be a complication associated with therapeutic hypothermia treatment for patients following VF arrest?

A. TH is useful, but implementation requires the use of cardiopulmonary bypass machines.

B. Rewarming with rates greater than 0.25°C to 0.5°C/h is associated with worse outcome.

C. Hypermagnesia, hyperkalemia, and hyperphosphatemia are common complications associated with TH.

D. Acute kidney injury requiring temporary dialysis is common among patients treated with TH.

ANSWERS

39.1 **D.** Therapeutic hypothermia to cool core temperatures to 32°C to 34°C for 24 to 48 hours has been shown to improve neurologic outcomes in patients following VF arrests. Cooling of patient to 28°C to 30°C is associated with the increase in arrhythmia without additional improvements in neurologic outcomes. Maintaining oxygen saturation of 100% could result in hyperoxic injuries with an increase in mortality. Even though maintaining euvolemia improves outcome in the post-resuscitation patients, the use of a Swan-Ganz catheter has not been shown to provide benefits in these patients.

39.2 **D.** Hyperglycemia and hypoglycemia are common following resuscitation from cardiac arrest, and if unaddressed they can contribute to worse neurological outcomes. The AHA guidelines recommend moderate glycemic control targeting glucose values of 144 to 180 mg/dL. A randomized trial comparing glycemic control targeting levels of 80 to 110 mg/dL to target values of 110 to 140 mg/dL for post-cardiac arrest patients did not demonstrate a survival difference between the groups. Hypoglycemia in the post-resuscitation patient produces worse neurological outcomes; therefore, glucose-containing fluids may be indicated for patients with hypoglycemia.

39.3 **C.** Acute coronary syndrome is a likely cause for the VF arrest. Early cardiac intervention has been shown to improve prognosis in post-VF arrest patients. TH to target core temperatures of 32°C to 34°C and maintenance of serum glucose in the 144 to 180 mg/dL range are practices that have been reported to improve outcome. Resuscitation to achieve early hemodynamic goals (first 6 hours) has been shown to improve survival in septic patients; however, prolongation of resuscitation has not been shown to improve outcome. Intolerance of feeding, decreased pulmonary compliance, decreased oxygenation, and the development of abdominal compartment syndrome are associated with excess initial fluid administration and failure to reduce fluid administration following initial resuscitation from septic shock.

39.4 **B.** Rapid rewarming of patients under TH at rates that exceed 0.25°C to 0.5°C/h is associated with increase in catabolic rate and worse clinical outcome. Other complications that have been described associated with TH include increased infections, increased bleeding, hypomagnesemia, hypokalemia, and hypophosphatemia.

CLINICAL PEARLS

▶ There is improved neurologic recovery after successful resuscitation from VF arrests versus other cardiac rhythms.

▶ Core temperature cooling to 32°C to 34°C has been demonstrated in animal models to improve cardiac recovery following resuscitation from cardiac arrest.

▶ Oxygen saturation during and following resuscitation should be maintained in the 94% to 96% range.

▶ Hyperglycemia is common after resuscitation; however, aggressive glycemic control in these patients is associated with worse neurologic outcomes. The serum glucose should target the 144 to 180 mg/dL range.

▶ Goal-directed resuscitation has been shown to benefit some patients for the initial 6 hours, but prolongation of resuscitation efforts for any patient population has not been found to be beneficial.

REFERENCES

Abella BS, Leary M. Therapeutic hypothermia. In: Hall JB, Schmidt GA, Kress JP, eds. *Principles of Critical Care*. 4th ed. New York, NY: McGraw Hill Education; 2015:174-179.

Barnard S. Hypothermia after cardiac arrest: expanding the therapeutic scope. *Crit Care Med*. 2009; 37 Supplement:S227-S233.

Nolan JP, Soar J. Postresuscitation care: entering a new era. *Curr Opin Crit Care*. 2010;16:216-222.

Zia A, Kern KB. Management of postcardiac arrest myocardial dysfunction. *Curr Opin Crit Care*. 2011;17:241-246.

An 81-year-old man with an extensive past medical history including hypertension, type II diabetes mellitus, chronic obstructive pulmonary disease (COPD), and gout was admitted to the hospital with microcytic anemia and signs and symptoms of large bowel obstruction. The patient has lost approximately 10 lb (4.5 kg) over the past month. A colonoscopy revealed an obstructive carcinoma in the descending colon. The patient subsequently underwent an exploratory laparotomy and left colectomy. He is admitted to the ICU postoperatively.

▶ How would you optimally manage this patient's fluid status?
▶ How would you address the patient's nutritional status at this time?
▶ What are the possible complications related to his surgical disease processes, and how would you monitor and identify them?

ANSWERS TO CASE 40:

Postoperative Care in ICU

Summary: An 81-year-old man has an obstructing carcinoma in the descending colon. The mass was removed by an open left colectomy. The patient has extensive multiple medical comorbidities and is admitted to the ICU for close postop monitoring and management.

- **Management of fluid status:** This patient needs cautious balancing of his fluid status given his age and medical problems. Careful monitoring of urine output via Foley catheter and intravascular status with central venous pressure measurements will help to guide management.

- **Nutritional status:** The patient should be allowed to resume oral intake as soon as possible, generally within 48 hours if tolerated. If the patient is unable to take in adequate calories orally, he may require supplemental enteral nutrition.

- **Possible complications and the approach to monitoring and identification:**

  - **Cardiac:** Myocardial infarction, atrial fibrillation, other cardiac arrhythmias—identified by clinical examination, cardiac monitoring/EKG

  - **Respiratory:** Pulmonary edema, atelectasis, COPD exacerbation, acute respiratory distress syndrome (ARDS)—identified by clinical examination, CXR/chest CT, oxygen saturation, arterial blood gas

  - **Fluids/Electrolytes/Nutrition:** Third-space fluid shifts, stress-induced hyperglycemia, and poor nutritional status—identified by clinical examination, laboratory work up

  - **Gastrointestinal:** Surgical anastomostic leak, ileus, mechanical bowel obstruction— identified by clinical examination, imaging studies, laboratory work up

  - **Genitourinary:** Pre-renal azotemia, acute kidney injuries, and post-renal obstructive processes—identified by clinical examination, laboratory work up, imaging studies

  - **Endocrine:** Insulin-resistance, adrenal insufficiency—identified by clinical examination, laboratory work up

  - **Hematologic/Infectious:** Anemia, wound infection, systemic inflammatory response syndrome (SIRS), sepsis—identified by clinical examination, laboratory work up

  - **Musculoskeletal:** Gout flare—identified by clinical examination

ANALYSIS

Objectives

1. Learn the common complications that may develop in the postoperative patients.

2. Learn the disturbances produced by operative stress.

3. Learn patient assessment, risk stratification, and risk-reduction strategies in the preoperative and peri-operative settings.

Considerations

This patient has a descending colon cancer with anemia and large bowel obstruction. Large bowel obstruction from a mechanical cause has a poorer prognosis and higher morbidity since an emergency operation is needed. Additionally, the patient is already nutritionally depleted from the obstructive mass in the intestine as well as weight loss from malignancy. The added stress of operation will increase his baseline energy expenditure and his nutritional requirements. Attention must be paid to the patient's fluid status, as postoperative shifts will place stress on the cardiovascular and pulmonary systems, which are likely already affected by the patient's history of hypertension, anemia, and COPD. The presence of type II diabetes may mean that some degree of renal insufficiency is present and that there may be an increased risk for infection. An acute gout flare is possible from the catabolic state after surgery or as a result of the fluid shifts caused by surgery. To minimize this patient's postoperative complications and facilitate his postoperative recovery, meticulous ICU care will be important to monitor several important organ system functions.

APPROACH TO:
Postoperative Patients in the ICU

DEFINITIONS

CENTRAL VENOUS PRESSURE (CVP): The pressure in the superior vena cava, measured with a central venous catheter inserted into the internal jugular or subclavian vein. This estimates the right atrial pressure, reflecting the amount of the blood in the venous system returning to the heart.

ATELECTASIS: Collapse of lung alveoli or fluid consolidation that prevents effective gas exchange where the alveoli are deflated. This can affect varying proportions of the lungs and is commonly seen after injury or surgery, especially if breathing is restricted by pain or fatigue.

PULMONARY EDEMA: Fluid accumulation in the lung parenchyma either due to the inability of the heart to adequately remove fluid from the lung circulation (cardiogenic) or due to lung parenchyma injury (non-cardiogenic). It can be caused iatrogenically by over-infusion of intravenous fluid.

ACUTE RESPIRATORY DISTRESS SYNDROME (ARDS): Inflamed lung parenchyma associated with a systemic inflammatory response causing severe hypoxemia, often requiring mechanical intubation. It may be present by itself or as part of multiple organ dysfunction syndrome (MODS). It is defined as an acute process with a ratio of arterial partial oxygen tension (Pao_2) to fraction of inspired oxygen (Fio_2) below 200 mm Hg, with bilateral infiltrates on chest x-ray, in the absence of elevated cardiac filling pressures.

THIRD-SPACE FLUID LOSS: During inflammation, sepsis or shock, fluid can be sequestered in extravascular spaces as proteins and fluid move to interstitial compartments, depleting intravascular volume. Examples include pulmonary edema, bowel wall edema and fluid forced into the bowel lumen in cases of obstruction and retroperitoneal fluid sequestration with pancreatitis.

The intensive care providers in the ICU need to be familiar with the complications related to procedures, surgical diseases, and those caused by operative stresses. Understanding these issues is critical for the anticipation and treatment of complications, addressing the needs of the postoperative patients, and optimizing communications between the intensive care providers and the surgical specialists. Postoperative complications can range from being relatively minor to life-threatening. It is important for the clinician to be aware of the complications that can occur and to be vigilant about looking out for those that can cause serious morbidity and even mortality. The most important aspect to remember about postoperative complications is that complications in postoperative patients are nearly always related to operative procedures (known complications of the procedures and/or underlying disease conditions that necessitated the operations, and/or complications related to the exacerbation of one or more of the patient's comorbid conditions). Listed below are the various systems that can be affected by surgical stresses.

Complications Categorized by Systems

Cardiac complications include acute coronary syndrome, myocardial infarctions, cardiac arrhythmias and congestive heart failure. The increased stress on the heart increases the risk for myocardial infarction. Arrhythmias such as atrial fibrillation often occur due to fluid shifts throughout the body after an operation, placing more stretch on the atria of the heart. These fluid shifts can also cause or worsen congestive heart failure.

Pulmonary complications can be closely linked to cardiac dysfunction, in which the ability to adequately distribute intravascular fluid may be lost, causing a back up of fluid in the lungs, as in the case of pulmonary edema. Other common pulmonary complications include atelectasis, pneumonia, ARDS, and exacerbation of any underlying lung disease, such as COPD or emphysema.

Renal Complications mainly present as oliguria, or low urine output. Acute kidney injuries can be classified into pre-renal, renal and post-renal categories. Pre-renal causes are due to hypoperfusion of the kidney as seen in dehydration, fluid losses from vomiting/diarrhea or as a result of an operation, poor intake or inadequate repletion, and cardiogenic shock or significant blood loss. Insensible fluid losses are increased during an operation, especially if the abdomen is left open postoperatively. Bowel obstruction causes third spacing, further reducing intravascular volume. Renal causes of oliguria are from damage to the kidney itself, such as acute tubular necrosis from ischemia or medication toxicity. Post-renal causes are due to obstruction of urine flow, such as Foley catheter blockage, prostatic hypertrophy or compression from tumor, hematoma or fluid collection. If the FeNa (fractional excretion of sodium) is <1% along with other signs that the body is trying to retain water (high serum osmolality, low urine sodium), this indicates a pre-renal state. In contrast, proteinuria and cells or casts on urinalysis may point toward direct renal damage or acute tubular necrosis (ATN). Causes of post-renal (obstructive) oliguria can usually be found via physical examination or imaging.

Fever can be a sign of complications and can be divided into three categories based on timing. Immediately postoperative fever (<24 hours) may be a response to surgery or atelectasis, although in some cases a necrotizing wound infection (*Clostridium* or Group A *Streptococcus*) can be the cause. Fevers occurring from 24 to 72 hours may be residual atelectasis but should prompt a search for other sources of infection such as pneumonia, urinary tract infections (especially if a Foley catheter is in place) or IV line infection/phlebitis. After 72 hours, fever is likely due to the infectious sources mentioned above or wound infections, deep internal abscesses, anastomotic leaks, prosthetic infections or deep vein thrombosis. Rarely, entities such as acalculous cholecystitis, most often seen in critically ill patients, can also be a cause of fever. The work-up includes physical examination of the patient, the incision site and any IV lines or catheters as well as blood, sputum, urine and wound cultures. Imaging may be helpful, for example: checking a chest x-ray for signs of a pulmonary consolidation in pneumonia or an effusion, a Doppler ultrasound of the legs or chest CT to rule out deep vein thrombosis (DVT) or pulmonary embolus, or an abdominal CT scan to evaluate for deep abscesses. Appropriate treatment depends on the cause, varying from incentive spirometry and mobilization for atelectasis to removal of catheters and IVs, antibiotics and operative drainage of deep abscesses if necessary.

Wound complications may occur in any patient, although appropriate preoperative antibiotics, meticulous operative technique, and hemostasis are the most effective prevention. **There is no additional benefit in the extension of prophylactic antibiotics beyond the immediate postoperative period.** High-risk patients for wound complications are individuals with contaminated surgical fields, impaired blood flow to healing tissues from hypotension, diabetes, obesity or smoking and those who are immunocompromised. Wound complications include hematomas and seromas, infection in either superficial or deep spaces, and fascial dehiscence or incisional hernias. Wounds or hematomas/seromas that appear infected (tenderness, erythema, purulence) should be opened, drained, and packed loosely. Extensive wound dehiscence at the fascial level may require repair in the operating room. Close communication between the intensive care provider and the surgeons are critical for the management of wound-related complications.

Neurologic complications after operation are often related to the treatment of postoperative pain. While hypoxemia and stroke can cause neurological changes, electrolyte abnormalities and medications are also common causes. Medications for treatment of pain, including opiates, and sedatives in critically ill patients may cause delirium, agitation, and somnolence. Elderly patients tend to have greater susceptibility to these effects. Patients in the ICU may also experience delirium, ICU psychosis or "sundowning," which is contributed to by fragmented sleep patterns, disturbances in the day-night cycles, and loss of familiarity with one's surroundings.

Disturbances Produced by Operative Stress on the Various Systems

Cardiovascular: Due to increased postoperative metabolic demands, cardiac output increases, leading to higher oxygen requirements of cardiac myocytes. Operative stress coupled with hypovolemia, infection or traumatic injury, as well as any anesthetic or vasoactive medications, may prevent the patient's cardiovascular system from fully compensating for the increased demand, leading to myocardial ischemia, infarction, fluid overload, cardiac failure, and arrhythmias. Recent data suggest that postoperative acute coronary syndrome is just as likely to be produced by coronary artery plaque instability as by rupture. This is believed to be due to increased catecholamine and inflammatory mediators' responses in the postoperative period.

Pulmonary: Oxygen consumption demands are increased postoperatively due to increased metabolic demands. Ventilation and oxygenation problems in the postoperative period may arise from the combination of increased O_2 demand and compromised vital capacities. For example, upper abdominal and thoracic incisions have significant compromises on the patients' vital capacities secondary to pain associated with the respiratory effort; this can then result in subsequent atelectasis and increased susceptibility to pneumonia. Decreased mentation following general anesthesia and/or sedation medications may increase patients' susceptibilities to pulmonary aspirations. Lung parenchymal injuries may develop following systemic inflammatory response leading to Acute Lung Injury (ALI) and ARDS. Surgical stresses and immobility render the patients susceptible to venous thromboembolic complications. Conditions such as asthma or COPD can be exacerbated postoperatively and require treatment with steroids and/or broncho-dilators.

Metabolic: Patients' metabolic responses to surgery are variable and are related to the type and magnitude of the surgical stresses. Conditions such as trauma, sepsis, and burns further contribute to the increase in metabolic demands. Critically ill patients have accelerated breakdown of muscle protein for the reprioritization of acute-phase protein synthesis. Hyperglycemia in the postoperative patient is common and is caused by both increased glucose production by the liver and decreased uptake of glucose by insulin-dependent tissues. **Untreated hyperglycemia contributes to glycosuria, excess fluid loss, and impairment of leukocyte function leading to infections.** Glucose monitoring and treatment with insulin are essential in postoperative patients. Insufficient adrenal functions can be exacerbated by surgical stresses and/or sepsis. This may be manifested by hypotension that is unresponsive to standard fluid administration. In some instances, adrenal dysfunction can manifest as unexplained fever, hypoglycemia, confusion, lethargy and abdominal pain. By far the most common reason for adrenal insufficiency is iatrogenic. A patient with a history of long-term steroid medication use is susceptible to the development of adrenal insufficiency in the face of surgical stress, sepsis, or trauma.

Gastrointestinal: Patients who are not intubated can be expected to resume oral intake shortly after an operation. While the traditional practice is to maintain a nil per os (NPO) policy until there is return of bowel function documented by passage of flatus or bowel movement, a growing body of literature suggests that there are potential benefits to reinstating some form of oral intake within 48 hours of operations in patients who can tolerate it. In patients who are intubated and/or those who are not expected to take in adequate oral calories for prolonged periods, the need for supplemental nutrition via enteral tube should be anticipated and implemented. Operative manipulation of the bowel and medications for pain can contribute to ileus and delayed GI functions. **Narcotics can contribute to constipation and fecal impaction.** It is possible for adhesions to form and bowel obstructions to occur within days after surgery, although most obstructive complications secondary to adhesions occur later. Critically ill patients are also at risk for stress ulcers, as hypoperfusion, loss of host gastric barrier functions, and gastric acidity can produce mucosal injuries. ICU patients in shock, sepsis, respiratory, hepatic, renal or hematologic failure benefit from stress ulcer prophylaxis with H_2-antagonists or sucralfate.

Patient Assessment, Risk Stratification, and Risk-Reduction in the Preoperative and Peri-operative Settings

Patient Assessment: Many healthy patients are able to undergo operative procedures uneventfully. However, those who are medically compromised require more careful pre- and perioperative evaluations to assess for fitness for surgery and ensure favorable outcomes.

Several methods are commonly used to assess patients' medical status prior to an operation. The **American Society of Anesthesiologists' (ASA) classification** is based on the patient's condition. Class I patients are healthy, Class II have mild systemic disease, Class III have severe systemic disease which limits activity but is not incapacitating, Class IV have incapacitating systemic disease which is a constant threat to life, Class V are moribund patients not expected to survive 24 hours with or without operation and Class VI are organ transplant donors. The designation of "E" is added to any class if the case is an emergency.

Goldman calculated a **cardiac risk index** where a varying number of points are awarded for clinical factors present; the two biggest contributors to cardiac risk are 11 points for an S3 gallop/JVD and 10 points for a myocardial infarction within 6 months. The highest risk (Class IV) patients had a 22% incidence of major cardiac complications and a 56% mortality rate. More recently, Lee developed the Revised Cardiac Risk Index where six independent predictors of perioperative cardiac complications were established—ischemic heart disease, congestive heart failure, cerebrovascular disease, diabetes requiring preoperative insulin treatment, serum creatinine >2.0 mg/dL and whether the patient was undergoing a high-risk operation. A high-risk operation includes intraperitoneal, intrathoracic, or suprainguinal vascular (such as aortic) operations.

Risk Stratification: Preoperative evaluation provides the anesthesia and surgical teams' information regarding the patient's current medical status, risk profile, and recommendations for management during the perioperative period. Tests should only be ordered if the results could change the treatment and management plan. Examples include electrocardiogram (ECG) or a cardiac stress ECG to examine the patient's cardiac response to increasing oxygen demand with exercise, or dipyridamole-thallium scanning for those patients unable to exercise. Echocardiography gives an analysis of ventricular wall motion, ejection fraction, and ventricular hypertrophy. Pulmonary function tests are useful in patients who may need to undergo lung resection. On admission to the ICU, the APACHE (Acute Physiology and Chronic Health Evaluation) score may be used to risk-stratify patients and is calculated from 12 different physiological measurements. It is used for risk stratification and to compare the morbidity of patients, but due to its complexity it is cumbersome to use.

Risk Reduction: The ultimate goal of pre- and perioperative assessment is to optimize patient outcome. **Patients may certainly benefit from having their medical comorbidities optimized preoperatively,** such as having hypertension, cardiac arrhythmias, and diabetes well controlled. Improving the patient's preoperative nutritional status is also important. Percutaneous coronary intervention (PCI) and coronary artery bypass grafting (CABG) have not been shown to be effective in reducing perioperative cardiac morbidity except perhaps in patients with left main coronary artery disease. Use of β-blockers in at-risk patients has been shown to reduce the risk of perioperative cardiac ischemia and death, but the timing of stopping the β-blocker postoperatively remains controversial. If the patient does not have a condition that is an emergency, preoperative work-up may elucidate a need to modify the original anesthetic or operative plan and defer or change the operative approach. Intraoperative risk reduction strategies include keeping the patient warm, maintaining euglycemia, administration of perioperative antibiotics within an hour of skin incision and sequential compression devices for prevention of DVT. Postoperatively, patients should have continued DVT prophylaxis with sequential compression devices (SCDs), heparin, or low molecular weight heparin until they are able to mobilize. Other postoperative care includes oral hygiene, aspiration precautions, incentive spirometry to prevent atelectasis and pneumonia, frequent turning to prevent pressure sores and ulcer prophylaxis if indicated.

CASE CORRELATION

- See also Case 4 (Scoring Systems and Patient Prognosis).

COMPREHENSION QUESTIONS

40.1 Which of the following findings is most consistent with inadequate resuscitation of a 92-year-old, 45-kg patient?

A. Urine/serum creatinine ratio of 45

B. CVP of 13 mm Hg

C. Urine output of 25 mL in the last hour

D. Bilateral pulmonary crackles on auscultation

E. Fractional excretion of sodium of 1.3%

40.2 A 78-year-old patient develops a temperature of 101.4°F two days after undergoing an elective right hemicolectomy for a small, non-obstructing cancer that was found on colonoscopy. Which of the following is the LEAST likely cause of her fever?

A. Pneumonia

B. Urinary tract infection

C. Atelectasis

D. Wound infection

E. Intra-abdominal abscess

40.3 A 34-year-old obese man underwent an emergency midline laparotomy after sustaining a gunshot wound to the abdomen. A short segment of small bowel was resected due to damage from the bullet. Several days later the patient has made a good recovery. However, when he stands to walk to the bathroom, he experiences a large gush of serosanguinous fluid from his abdominal wound. Examination of the wound shows a 4-cm fascial dehiscence. The most appropriate management is:

A. Reapproximation of the wound with sterile tape

B. Abdominal binder and placing the patient on bedrest

C. Further opening of the wound to allow adequate drainage and packing with gauze

D. Return to operation room for repair

E. Culture of the wound fluid and antibiotic treatment

40.4 A 55-year-old patient has hypertension that is controlled with hydrochlorothiazide and metoprolol. What is his ASA classification?

A. I

B. II

C. III

D. IV

E. V

40.5 An elderly patient is an insulin-dependent diabetic with a history of stable angina and diverticuli seen on colonoscopy, and she takes chronic steroids for rheumatoid arthritis. She undergoes an emergency diverting colostomy for perforated diverticulitis with fecal spillage and is intubated in the ICU on broad-spectrum antibiotics. Two days postoperatively, she becomes acutely febrile to 102.6°F with confusion and lethargy. Her heart rate is 110 beats/min with a blood pressure of 79/58 mm Hg. She remains hypotensive despite fluid resuscitation, and vasopressors are started. Her laboratory tests show a glucose of 46 mg/dL. What is the most likely cause of her clinical picture?

A. Myocardial infarction

B. Diabetic ketoacidosis

C. Hypovolemia

D. Adrenal insufficiency

E. Sepsis

ANSWERS

40.1 **A.** In a hypovolemic patient, the CVP would be low (<5 mm Hg), she would not have bilateral crackles suggestive of pulmonary edema and the fractional excretion of sodium would be less than 1. The kidney would be trying to retain volume so the urine sodium would be low (<20 meq/L), the serum osmolality would be high (>500 mOsm/kg) and the urine/serum creatinine ratio would be >40. Although a urine output of 25 mL may seem low, for a patient weighing only 45 kg, 0.5 mL/kg/h equals an expected urine output of 22.5 mL/h.

40.2 **E.** The patient has developed a fever within 72 hours of undergoing surgery. This may still be due to atelectasis if the patient is not expanding her lungs well due to being in bed or to pain. However, infectious sources may be the culprit by this time frame. Pneumonia, urinary tract infection, wound infection and IV line infections may all be possibilities. Intra-abdominal abscesses generally take a few more days to form and are less likely at this relatively early time point.

40.3 **D.** This patient has experienced a fascial disruption with the serosanguinous fluid coming from the peritoneum. Because the dehiscence is larger than just 1 or 2 cm, the patient is at high risk for infection and evisceration as well as a ventral hernia. Prompt operative repair will minimize these risks and allow the patient to recover and resume normal activity sooner.

40.4 **C.** Hypertension is classified as a systemic disease. The patient requires medication to treat his disease, which makes his condition more serious than a class II. However, since his hypertension is controlled on his medications, he is ASA class III rather than class IV.

40.5   **D.** Acute adrenal insufficiency often presents as unexplained fever, persistent hypotension, mental status changes and hypoglycemia. This presentation can be similar to sepsis, but sepsis tends to present with hyperglycemia in its early stages. While the etiology of adrenal insufficiency can be primary in nature, abrupt cessation of steroids is the most common cause. Treatment consists of IV fluids and hydrocortisone 100 mg IV for adrenal crisis, with steroid taper as tolerated as the crisis resolves.

CLINICAL PEARLS

▶ Prophylactic antibiotics are not indicated past the immediate perioperative period.

▶ Most postoperative complications are related to the surgical procedure or the underlying diseases that led to the operation.

▶ Risk assessment in the preoperative setting helps identify patients who are at risk for specific complications and provide opportunities for the implementation of risk-reduction strategies.

▶ Older age and pre-existing conditions contribute to reduced functional reserve and increased susceptibility to injury-induced organ dysfunctions.

REFERENCES

Alali AS, Baker AJ, Ali J. Special considerations in the surgical patient. In: Hall JB, Schmidt GA, Kress JP, eds. *Principles of Critical Care*. 4th ed. New York, NY: McGraw Hill Education; 2015: 1046-1053.

Fleisher LA. Cardiac risk stratification for noncardiac surgery: Update from the American College of Cardiology/American Heart Assocation 2007 guidelines. *Cleve Clin J Med*. 2009;76 Suppl 4: S9-S15.

Marquardt DL, Tatum RP, Lynge DC. Postoperative management of the hospitalized patient. In: Souba WW, et al., eds. *ACS Surgery: Principles and Practice*. 7th ed. Philadelphia, PA: Decker Publishing. 2014.

Simmons J, Adam LA. Principles of postoperative critical care. In: Hall JB, Schmidt GA, Kress JP, eds. *Principles of Critical Care*. 4th ed. New York, NY: McGraw Hill Education; 2015:1060-1077.

Walsh F, Ali J. Chapter 88. Preoperative Assessment of the High-Risk Surgical Patient. In: Hall JB, Schmidt GA, Wood LDH, eds. *Principles of Critical Care*, 3rd ed. New York, NY: McGrawHill Education; 2005.

A 20-year-old man is brought to the ICU from the operating room following a damage-control operation for multiple gunshot wounds. The patient was reportedly unstable throughout the operation, where transection of the left superficial femoral artery (SFA) and multiple small bowel perforations were identified. During the operation, the patient had three small bowel segments resected and had placement of a temporary intraluminal shunt in the SFA to control the bleeding and re-establish blood flow to his leg. At the time of ICU arrival, his temperature is 34.6°C, pulse rate is 128 beats/min, and blood pressure is 90/70 mm Hg. He is intubated and mechanically ventilated. The patient is bleeding from his wounds and multiple intravenous catheter sites.

▶ What is the most likely diagnosis?
▶ What are the priorities in this patient's management?

ANSWERS TO CASE 41:

Hemorrhage and Coagulopathy

Summary: A 20-year-old man has a gunshot wound through his abdomen and extremity. The bowel injuries have been controlled with resection, and the vascular injury has been controlled with a temporary shunt. His presentation to the ICU is consistent with shock and coagulopathy.

- **Most likely diagnosis:** Coagulopathy of trauma/hemorrhage
- **Priorities in management:** Warm the patient, resuscitate with packed red blood cells, fresh frozen plasma, and platelets to correct coagulopathy and acidosis

ANALYSIS

Objectives

1. Learn the principles of massive transfusion.
2. Learn the conditions that contribute to coagulopathy following massive transfusions.
3. Understand the limitations of laboratory studies for the evaluation of patients with this condition.

Considerations

This patient suffered significant penetrating trauma that required a damage-control operation and temporary shunting of the SFA. On admission to the ICU, he is hypotensive, tachycardic, and is bleeding from his wounds and catheter sites. His surgical bleeding site has been controlled (shunting of the SFA), but he is continuing to bleed from his wounds, indicating that he has a significant coagulopathy. During the operation, he has lost not only red blood cells, but also the coagulation factors that are present in his plasma. Additionally, he is **hypothermic**, which is common among trauma victims.

The hypothermia usually starts in the emergency department during the initial resuscitation and continues while in the operating room. Trauma patients have all of their clothes removed and are infused with normal saline and packed red blood cells that may not be warm. In the operating room, their chest and/or abdomen may be open, increasing their heat loss. They also may be paralyzed for intubation, which prevents shivering. All of these mechanisms can lead to profound hypothermia. The hypothermia actively slows down the coagulation process, leading to an increase in coagulopathy and continued nonsurgical bleeding (ie, bleeding that cannot be controlled by suture ligation). It is likely that this patient is also acidotic from incomplete resuscitation, which can increase the coagulopathic state. **The combination of acidosis, hypothermia, and coagulopathy is often referred to as the "Triad of Death."**

APPROACH TO:
Hemorrhage and Coagulopathy

DEFINITIONS

HEMOSTATIC RESUSCITATION: Hemostatic resuscitation is a relatively new concept that evolved largely based on clinical observations from injuries managed during the conflicts in Iraq and Afghanistan. This begins with limitation of fluids in the field, application of tourniquets, and administration of hemostatic agents for direct bleeding control. Once victims arrive to the medical care facility, the resuscitation is directed to preserve coagulation functions rather than restoring normal vital signs.

MASSIVE TRANSFUSION: The often-used definition is the transfusion of >10 units of pRBC (packed red blood cells) in 24 hours. Patients who require massive transfusion have suffered a large amount of blood volume loss and therefore require the replacement of packed red blood cells, fresh frozen plasma, and platelets in a short time period. These components are often given in a ratios that mimic whole blood concentrations.

FACTOR VII: Coagulation factor that can be made in recombinant fashion and administered to patients who are coagulopathic.

THROMBOELASTOGRAPHY: Method for real time measurement of coagulation status. The results report the time to clot formation and the clot strength. The results can be used for goal directed administration of blood products.

CLINICAL APPROACH

Massive Transfusion Principles

Hemorrhage remains one of the leading causes of preventable death in trauma patients. The cause of death goes beyond just exsanguination. Up to one-third of all trauma patients who present to the hospital already have a coagulopathy. This coagulopathy is due to tissue injury, hypoperfusion, and loss of clotting factors and platelets via hemorrhage. Accentuation of this initial coagulopathy may also be mediated by an increase in fibrinolysis via a protein C pathway. Surgical control of the hemorrhage is the primary therapy of ongoing bleeding. Until surgical control of hemorrhage is obtained, the patient should be resuscitated with volume. Historically, the correction of the hypovolemia caused by hemorrhage was infusion of large volumes of crystalloids. Normal saline was the crystalloid of choice, but infusion of large volumes of normal saline has untoward complications. Dilutional coagulopathy, thrombocytopenia and hyperchloremic acidosis from large crystalloid infusions increases coagulopathy. Ongoing hemorrhage affects all three components of the "Triad of Death" and increases the coagulopathy.

The complications of resuscitating a patient with large volumes of crystalloid has lead to a "hemostatic resuscitation" approach, that is, resuscitating the patient with blood and blood products that will help mitigate the coagulopathy of trauma until definitive control of the bleeding is achieved.

The goal of a hemostatic resuscitation is to give the patient fluid that approximates the blood that they have lost. This hemostatic resuscitation is often referred to as a "massive transfusion," as it includes large volumes of packed red blood cells, fresh frozen plasma, and platelets. There is no one single definition of what constitutes a massive transfusion, but several definitions have been proposed. These include:

1. Replacement of one entire blood volume within 24 hours

2. Transfusion of greater or equal to 10 units of pRBCs in 24 hours

3. Transfusion of greater or equal to 20 units of pRBCs in 24 hours

Also, there are definitions of "dynamic massive transfusion," including

1. Transfusion of >4 units of pRBCs in 1 hour when ongoing need is foreseeable or

2. Replacement of 50% of total blood volume within 3 hours

When a patient receives a blood transfusion, they are actually receiving a transfusion of packed red blood cells (pRBCs). This is the end product of whole blood (taken from a donor) that has been centrifuged so that the heavier components (the red blood cells) can be separated from the lighter components (the plasma and platelets). The coagulation factors remain in the plasma component. When a patient is transfused, they receive red blood cells to increase oxygen carrying capacity but do not receive any coagulation factors. Multiple transfusions of packed red blood cells without addition of coagulation factors will lead to a dilutional coagulopathy. Thus, during massive transfusions, when patients are going to be given large volumes of pRBCs, they are also given fresh frozen plasma (FFP) to provide hemostatic factors. The exact ratio of PRBCs to FFP to provide the perfect hemostatic scenario is not known. However, **most experts would agree that a 1:1:1 ratio of pRBCs:FFP:platelets is the best formula for a hemostatic resuscitation.** One unit of platelet pheresis is approximately 6 to 10 random platelet packs, so 1 unit of platelets is transfused for 6 units of pRBCs and FFP.

Coagulopathy Following Massive Transfusions

Up to one-third of trauma patients with significant injury will present to the trauma bay with a coagulopathy already in progress. This is in part due to loss of coagulation factors from bleeding, as well as tissue injury and hypoperfusion.

To understand the conditions that affect coagulopathy after massive transfusions, it is first important to understand the normal process of coagulation. The major physiologic events that occur during coagulation are vasoconstriction, platelet plug formation, fibrin formation, and fibrinolysis. During platelet plug formation, the coagulation factors interact with the surface of the platelets to form a fibrin lattice that provides support to the platelet plug.

During and after massive transfusion, many of the factors associated with normal coagulation are altered. Thrombocytopenia limits the amount of platelet plug that can be formed at the site of injury. Initially, this is caused by absolute loss of platelets from hemorrhage and dilution from crystalloid administration. The infusion of large volumes of crystalloid contributes to coagulopathy during massive transfusions. Therefore, crystalloid infusion should be limited during massive transfusions. Then, during the massive transfusion, packed red blood cells and FFP are administered, which contain minimal amounts of platelets. This can lead to a further drop in the platelet count. Often times, the number of platelet transfusions available at the hospital is limited due to the short shelf life of platelets. This can lead to a delay in the administration of platelets, even during massive transfusions given by protocol.

The storage solution for blood products contains citrate as a preservative to keep the products from clotting during storage. Citrate is a strong binder of calcium and when large volumes of pRBCs are given, intravascular stores of calcium can be depleted. Coagulation defects can be seen when ionized calcium levels drop below 0.7 mmol/L.

Despite administration of all blood components (RBC, FFP, platelets), coagulopathy can still be seen in some patients during massive transfusion. It is thought that administration of specific coagulation factors can help the coagulation process. Factor VII can be made in a recombinant fashion and administered intravenously. The administration of rFVII is still controversial. In a randomized controlled trial, rFVII was shown to decrease the pRBC use by 20% in trauma patients who required massive transfusions. The administration of rFVII contributes to a prothrombotic state, which could increase the risk of venous thromboembolic events. In recent studies, there does not appear to be an increased risk for thromboembolic events in trauma patients.

Other life-threatening problems that increase coagulopathy are hypothermia and acidosis. These three problems combined are often referred to as the "Triad of Death," and each problem exacerbates the other. Hypothermia often begins in the trauma bay and continues to progress through the operating room and even into the ICU. Hypothermia directly affects the coagulation cascade by inhibiting the initiation of clot formation and increasing the time it takes for thrombin levels to reach normal. It is extremely important to keep all trauma patients warm by warming the fluids administered (including blood products) and keeping the patient covered with warm blankets or other warming devices. Acidosis is often started by hypoperfusion of tissue after blood loss, but it can be exacerbated by administration of large volumes of normal saline. The chloride content of normal saline (154 mEq/L) can lead to a hyperchloremic acidosis. The acidosis impairs the ability of thrombin to participate in hemostasis. The acidosis severely inhibits the activity of enzyme complexes on lipid surfaces.

Laboratory Studies

The clinical evaluation of the patient in the scenario at the beginning of the chapter clearly indicates that he is coagulopathic. The continued oozing from his wounds after surgery, as well as oozing from nonsurgical sites (such as his IV sites), indicates that he is coagulopathic. The actual determination of the severity of his coagulopathy by laboratory studies is more difficult.

Current management of patients undergoing massive transfusions include frequent laboratory monitoring of arterial lactate to assess adequacy of resuscitation, ionized calcium, and electrolytes. The laboratory values that are used to determine the coagulation status of the patient are prothrombin time (PT), partial thromboplastin time (PTT), and international normalized ratio (INR). These tests are problematic in trauma patients because the trauma patient's actual coagulopathic state is in constant flux, as they are continuously receiving large volumes of blood, plasma, and platelets. The standard coagulation laboratory examinations take time to analyze, so the result reported does not necessarily reflect the patient's current coagulation state when the results are returned. Also, in order to run the PT/PTT tests, the patient's blood sample is warmed to 37°C and mixed with platelet-poor plasma. Trauma patients are often hypothermic, so this analysis again does not reflect the patient's actual coagulation status; nor does it reflect the cellular interactions of clotting.

Evidence is starting to show that rotational thromboelastometry (ROTEM) or thromboelastograms (TEG) are superior to standard coagulation measurements in trauma patients. These laboratory tests can be performed in a near real-time analysis and return rapid results. This allows for immediate analysis and goal-directed therapy of the coagulation disorder. The thromboelastograms (Figure 41–1) is measured on a small aliquot of whole blood and measures the clotting time (R value), clot formation (a angle), clot strength (MA: maximum amplitude), and clot lysis (LY 30). The clotting time measures the time to onset of clot formation. An increase in the clotting time represents a deficiency of coagulation factors. The kinetics of the clot formation are represented by the alpha angle. This represents the rate of fibrin build up and cross linking. The maximum amplitude is a measurement of the overall clot strength. The clot strength is a representation of platelet and fibrin interactivity. The use of TEG has shown to decrease the mortality rate and improve transfusion practices in patients receiving massive transfusions.

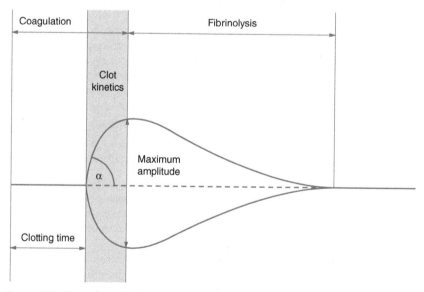

Figure 41–1. Figure of viscoelastic test for clotting.

> CASE CORRELATION
>
> ● See also Case 21 (Acute GI bleeding), Case 28 (Blunt Trauma), and Case 33 (Multi-organ dysfunction).

COMPREHENSION QUESTIONS

41.1 A 20-year-old man is shot in the right upper quadrant of his abdomen. On admission to the trauma bay, the paramedics inform you that he has two large bore IVs in each arm and has been given 2 L of normal saline en route to the hospital. His airway is patent, he is breathing spontaneously with saturations of 99% on 2 L O_2 per nasal cannula. His blood pressure is 80/40 mm Hg and his heart rate is 120 beats/min. He has a missile wound to the right upper quadrant of the abdomen. His abdomen is very tender, and he is cold and diaphoretic. The best next step in treatment for this patient is:

A. Administer 500 mL of 5% albumin

B. Administer 2 L of lactated Ringer's solution

C. Give 2 units of type-specific blood

D. Give 2 units of non–type-specific blood (O negative)

E. Warm the patient and send coagulation laboratories

41.2 A 37-year-old woman is brought in by paramedics after sustaining a severe crush injury of her right lower extremity. She is taken to the operating room (OR) where her lower extremity is explored, washed out, has an external fixation device placed, and a wound vacuum device placed over the open wound. The surgery takes several hours, and she is admitted to the ICU after the surgery. Her wound vacuum output is 1.5 L of frank blood over the next 4 hours. She received 2 units of pRBCs during the surgery and has received 3 more units since arriving in the ICU, and one more unit is being transfused now. Her heart rate is 120 beats/min and blood pressure is 90/60 mm Hg. Her current hemoglobin concentration is 7 g/dL and platelet count is 475,000/mm³. Her INR is 1.9. Her temperature is 35°C. The best next step in management of this patient is:

A. Transfuse platelets

B. Transfuse FFP and recheck INR in 2 hours

C. Take patient to OR for continued bleed from wound

D. Decrease the wound vacuum suction

E. Transfuse two more units of blood and recheck hemoglobin

41.3 A patient is undergoing a massive transfusion during an operation for a Grade IV liver laceration. He has received 9 units of pRBCs and 8 units of FFP. The best next step in treating this patient is:

    A. Four more units of pRBCs

    B. 2 L of crystalloid

    C. 1 unit of platelet pheresis

    D. 6 units of platelet pheresis

    E. 1 unit of cryoprecipitate

41.4 A 63-year-old woman is undergoing a colectomy for severe diverticulitis. During the operation, there is a significant amount of bleeding from an unidentified mesenteric vessel. The surgeons have stated that they are having difficulty getting control of the vessel and have called for a vascular surgeon. While the surgeons have been working to get surgical control of the bleeding, she has been transfused 6 units of pRBCs in the last hour. She is still bleeding and intermittently hypotensive. The next step in management is:

    A. Continue to transfuse red blood cells based on whether she is still hypotensive

    B. Continue to work on surgical control of bleeding and begin a massive transfusion protocol

    C. Check her INR and transfuse FFP only if INR >2.0

    D. Administer rFVII and normal saline intravenously

ANSWERS

41.1 **D.** This patient has a gunshot wound to the right upper quadrant and is hypotensive and tachycardic. His appearance is consistent with a high grade of shock. He is breathing and has normal saturations, so it is unlikely that he has an injury to his chest. His abdomen is tender, and he most likely has blood in his abdomen. In this patient who has already received 2 L of normal saline before reaching the hospital and is still hypotensive, it is appropriate to start giving the patient blood. In the initial trauma setting, it is inappropriate to wait for type-specific blood. The first blood transfusions should be non-type and crossed blood (Type O). A sample of the patient's blood should be sent for analysis so that future transfusions can be cross-matched. While it is important to start warming the patient as soon as possible, immediate resuscitation with blood and blood products predicates the warming and evaluation of coagulation status.

41.2 **C.** This patient suffered a significant injury to her lower extremity that required an operation, fixation device, and wound vacuum placed over her open wound. After being admitted to the ICU, she continues to have several problems. Her bleeding has not stopped, she has low blood concentrations and elevation in her coagulation, and she is cold. The most concerning aspect of this patient is her continued bleeding, as noted by the high output of blood in her wound vacuum. When faced with a patient who does not respond appropriately to resuscitation, it is important to consider that the cause is inadequate "source control." In this case the acute surgical bleeding must be stopped so that she can be adequately resuscitated. It is likely that she will need more blood, FFP, and possibly platelets while the bleeding is being controlled, but the first step is to control surgical bleeding.

41.3 **C.** During a massive transfusion, the goal is to achieve a hemostatic resuscitation. This is best achieved in a 1:1:1 ratio of blood products, and one pack of platelet pheresis equal 6 to 10 packs of pooled platelet packs. Thus, after 6 to 8 units of pRBCs and platelets are given, 1 unit of platelets should be administered.

41.4 **B.** This patient has required 6 units of pRBCs in the last hour, and there is anticipation that the patient will have ongoing transfusion requirements. This meets the definition of a dynamic massive transfusion need. While the surgeons are gaining surgical control of the bleeding, a massive transfusion should begin so that hemostatic resuscitation can be started to decrease the probability that the patient will become coagulopathic.

CLINICAL PEARLS

► Up to one-third of all trauma patients who arrive to the emergency department are already coagulopathic.

► The "Triad of Death" is the presence of coagulopathy, acidosis, and hypothermia. Each of these detrimental conditions exacerbates the other and should be preempted by active warming of the patient and the use of hemostatic resuscitation.

► The current recommendation for massive transfusions is that it should be done in a 1:1:1 ratio of pRBCs:FFP:platelets.

► 1 unit of platelet pheresis is equal to 6 units of pooled platelet packs.

► Standard coagulation laboratory studies lag behind in severely injured trauma patients undergoing massive transfusions. TEG or ROTEM analysis is likely a better representation of the patient's actual coagulation status.

REFERENCES

Jasti N, Streiff MB. Coagulopathy in the critically ill patient. In: Cameron JL, Cameraon AM, eds. *Curr Surg Ther.* 11th ed. Philadelphia, PA: Elsevier; 2014:1290-1304.

Johansson PI, Ostrowski SR, Secher NH. Management of major blood loss: an update. *Act Anaesthesiol Scand.* 2010;54:1039-1049.

Sihler KC, Napolitano LM. Complications of massive transfusion. *Chest.* 2010;137:209-220.

A 46-year-old man is admitted to the ICU for management of severe acute pancreatitis. The patient develops acute respiratory insufficiency requiring intubation and mechanical ventilator support. His respiratory status remains unimproved on hospital day number four. At this point, his hemodynamic status has improved, and the patient is no longer requiring vasoactive agents for support of his blood pressure. Because of the pancreatitis, the patient cannot have any enteral feedings.

▶ How would you initiate nutritional support for this patient?
▶ What are the potential limitations in your ability to deliver nutritional support?
▶ What are factors that contribute to the increase in this patient's nutritional requirements?

ANSWERS TO CASE 42:

Nutritional Issues in ICU

Summary: A 46-year-old man with severe acute pancreatitis is now hemodynamically stable but still requiring ventilatory support on hospital day four.

- **Nutritional support:** Begin appropriate enteral nutritional support based on his nutritional status and projected needs. This nutrition plan will take into account his ongoing severe inflammatory response and his associated respiratory dysfunction.

- **Potential limitations in your ability to deliver nutritional support:** For this patient with severe acute pancreatitis requiring mechanical ventilator support and large volume fluid resuscitation, traditional nutritional intake by mouth may not be possible. In addition, the intestinal edema associated with his resuscitation may contribute to impaired intestinal motility and absorption.

- **Factors that contribute to the increase in this patient's nutritional requirements:** Hypermetabolism and increase catabolism from his pancreatitis will contribute to marked increased in amino acid requirement and decreased ability to utilize glucose.

ANALYSIS

Objectives

1. Learn the approaches to nutritional assessments and strategies of monitoring responses to nutritional support.

2. Learn the nutritional management of patients with pancreatitis and renal insufficiency (with and without concurrent hemodialysis).

3. Learn the principles of nutritional support specifically designed for the modulation of host inflammatory and immune responses.

Considerations

The severe inflammatory response in pancreatitis can generate large fluid shifts between the intravascular and extravascular space, leading to hemodynamic instability as well as edema and respiratory failure. Patients with severe pancreatitis require aggressive fluid resuscitation to maintain adequate intravascular volume to maintain end-organ perfusion. This patient's hypotension did not respond initially to fluid resuscitation alone and required pressor support but has now improved. Patients like this usually have a large net positive fluid balance that the lungs are most sensitive to, especially in the setting of acute respiratory distress syndrome (ARDS). This type of lung injury requires prolonged mechanical respiratory support beyond the initial resuscitation phase. In addition, his initial hypotension may have decreased his end-organ perfusion, which can lead to acute kidney injury.

This patient's source of acute pancreatitis is unknown, but based on statistics, alcoholic pancreatitis is highly probable. If his pancreatitis is due to alcohol, he may also have a poor baseline nutritional status due to chronic excess alcohol consumption. He may also have deficiencies that would benefit from specific vitamin and mineral supplementation in addition to caloric and protein provision. Enteral nutritional support will target the delivery of 25 to 30 kcal/kg of non-protein calories and 1.5 to 2.0 g/kg of proteins per day. Close monitoring to avoid hyperglycemia (glucose >140-160 mg/dL) should be implemented. Similarly, if nasogastric feeding is initiated, the patient should be closely monitored for signs of intolerance, such as abdominal distention and/or high gastric residual volumes (>500 mL).

APPROACH TO:
Nutrition Issues in ICU

DEFINITIONS

ENTERAL NUTRITION: Nutrition provided through the gastrointestinal tract via a tube, catheter, or stoma that delivers nutrients distal to the oral cavity

PARENTERAL NUTRITION: The intravenous administration of nutrition, either via central or peripheral access

PROTEIN-CALORIE MALNUTRITION: Recent weight loss of greater than 10% to 15% or actual body weight <90% of ideal body weight

TROPHIC FEEDING: Low volume enteral feeding (usually 10-30 mL/h) meant to prevent mucosal atrophy but insufficient to provide adequate calorie and protein requirements

CLINICAL APPROACH

Critical illness is associated with a catabolic response due to changes in the hormonal milieu related to cytokine responses that occur following major physiological insults. The increased metabolic response continues into a later anabolic phase of tissue healing. Both of these increase the patient's need for nutritional supplementation. The goals of nutrition therapy are to modify (most cases downregulate) the metabolic response to stress, to prevent oxidative cellular injury, and to up-regulate the host immune responses. Initiation of early nutritional support, primarily enteral nutrition, is a proactive strategy directed at reducing some of the deleterious effects produced by the host's hypermetabolic responses, which in turn should reduce complications, ICU length of stay, and mortality.

When choosing a route for nutritional therapy, it is important to consider that in the majority of critically ill patients, it is practical, safe, as well as less expensive to utilize enteral nutrition over parenteral nutrition. Results from various clinical trials comparing enteral versus parenteral nutrition in critically ill patients have shown that enteral nutrition is associated with a reduction in infectious complications, specifically central line infections and pneumonia. Enteral nutrition is also associated with cost savings from reduced adverse events and reduced hospital length of stay. **It appears that critically ill ICU patients with hemodynamic compromise and requiring high doses of vasoactive agents and a large volume of blood products may have an increased risk of intolerance to enteral nutritional support and increased risk of gut-related complications. Therefore, it is generally advisable to withhold enteral feeding until these patients are fully resuscitated.**

Enteral nutrition utilizes the gut barrier to control water and electrolyte absorption. It also supports the functional integrity of the gut by maintaining tight junctions between the intraepithelial cells, stimulating blood flow and inducing the release of trophic endogenous agents (ie, cholecystokinin, gastrin, bombesin, and bile salts). Furthermore, the structural integrity of the gut, including the villous height and mass of secretory IgA-producing immunocytes, is better maintained with enteral nutrition. Loss of functional integrity can adversely affect gut permeability, producing increased bacterial challenge, perpetuation of systemic inflammatory response syndrome (SIRS), increased risk for systemic infection, and increased likelihood of multi-organ dysfunction syndrome (MODS) development.

In a previously healthy patient with no evidence of malnutrition, the use of parenteral nutrition may be withheld until after 7 to 10 days of hospitalization without nutrition. This is mostly due to concerns with infectious complications associated with parenteral nutrition. If, however, there is pre-existing protein-calorie malnutrition and enteral nutrition support is not feasible, it is appropriate to initiate parenteral nutrition much earlier after adequate resuscitation has taken place. Parenteral nutrition is indicated primarily for patients in whom enteral nutrition is not feasible or not tolerated and for severely malnourished patients who are about to undergo major upper GI surgery.

Initiating nutritional therapy first requires an assessment of the patient's nutritional status by determining weight loss and previous nutrient intake prior to admission, level of disease severity, comorbid conditions and function of the gastrointestinal (GI) tract. Estimates of calorie requirement for the patient's basic metabolic rate is done with the Harris-Benedict equation; this formula uses the patient's weight and activity level. This can also be measured via indirect calorimetry with the aid of a respiratory therapist. Protein requirements are estimated from the patient's degree of illness and monitored with 24-hour nitrogen-balance measurements. **Traditional markers (albumin, prealbumin, trasnferrin, retinol-binding protein) are a reflection of the acute phase response and do not accurately represent nutrition status in the ICU patient.** These markers by themselves have too low specificity but may, together with body weight changes, provide an estimate of general nutrition status. Enteral nutrition should be started within 24 to 48 hours following admission or as soon as fluid resuscitation is completed and the patient is hemodynamically stable. Feeding started within this time frame is associated with less gut permeability and diminished activation and release of inflammatory cytokines. It has also been shown to reduce infectious morbidity and hospital length of stay. Either gastric or small bowel feeding is acceptable in the ICU patient, but small bowel is preferable in patients with a high risk of aspiration and patients with severe brain injury, as intracranial hypertension is associated with decreased gastric emptying.

The use of "trickle" or trophic feeds may prevent mucosal atrophy but has not been shown to actually improve outcomes from the standpoint of immune-modulating. Feedings should be advanced toward at least 50% to 65% of the caloric goal over the first 48 to 72 hours following initiation for maximal benefits. Gastric residuals <500 mL in the absence of other signs of intolerance are acceptable and do not increase the risk of aspiration or pneumonia. **In critically ill patients, protein is the most important macronutrient for supporting immune function and wound healing.** Assessment of the adequacy of protein nutrition is estimated from nitrogen balance (needs to be 1.2-2.0 g/kg/d) or non-protein calorie:nitrogen ratio (70:1-100:1). Phosphate levels should be monitored closely and replaced when needed in respiratory failure patients for optimal pulmonary function.

Many enteral formulations are available to meet the needs of different patients. In patients with ARDS or lung injury, enteral formulations characterized by an anti-inflammatory lipid profile and antioxidants should be used (ie, omega-3 fish oils, borage oil) because they have been shown to reduce ICU length of stay, duration of mechanical ventilation, organ failure and mortality. Patients with respiratory failure can receive calorically dense formulations if fluid restriction is needed. Antioxidant vitamins (including vitamin E and ascorbic acid) and trace minerals (including selenium, zinc, and copper) may also improve ICU patient outcomes. Thiamine and folate supplementation for individuals with a history of chronic alcohol abuse is important. Formulations with low glucose concentrations are available for diabetics as well to improve glycemic control.

Special considerations regarding enteral nutrition should be made for patients with renal failure. Acute kidney injury (AKI) usually develops in the setting of multiple organ failure in the critically ill. These patients also require the standard enteral formulations described previously with continued adherence to the protein and calorie provisions as before. If significant electrolyte abnormalities develop, formulations with appropriate electrolyte profiles may be considered. **In AKI patients receiving renal replacement therapy (RRT), increased protein provision should be considered. RRT results in amino acid loss of approximately 10 to 20 g/d depending on the method, length of time, and type of filters used. These patients require formulations with 1.5 to 2.0 g/kg/d of protein, with some studies suggesting as high as 2.5 g/kg/d of protein to preserve a positive nitrogen balance.**

In acute pancreatitis, patients with severe acute pancreatitis should have a nasogastric (NG) tube placed on admission and enteral nutrition started as soon as fluid volume resuscitation is complete. Three meta-analyses showed that use of enteral nutrition compared to parenteral nutrition reduces infectious morbidity, hospital length of stay, need for surgical interventions, multiple organ failure, and mortality. Outcome benefits are seen in patients with acute pancreatitis when enteral nutrition is initiated within 24 to 48 hours. There has been no significant difference seen in outcomes of feeding by the gastric versus jejunal route; however, jejunal feeding may be better tolerated in these patients, as severe pancreatitis can be associated with poor gastric emptying. To improve tolerance to enteral nutrition higher in the GI tract, low fat elemental formulations in continuous infusion rather than bolus feeding should be used.

COMPREHENSION QUESTIONS

42.1 For which of the following would parenteral nutrition be inappropriate?

A. A 72-year-old woman on her eighth ICU day with sepsis from a ventilator-associated pneumonia requiring two vasoactive agents for support of her blood pressure.

B. A 62-year-old malnourished man with an obstructing esophageal cancer about to undergo an Ivor-Lewis esophagectomy.

C. A 75-year-old healthy man who 7 days ago underwent an uncomplicated right hemicolectomy for a malignancy. He is ambulating but still has abdominal distention and has not had flatus yet.

D. A 26-year-old man with multiple gunshot wounds to the abdomen and extensive small bowel injury who has just undergone extensive small bowel resection and now has only 45 cm of small bowel left and no ileo-cecal valve.

E. A 60-year-old woman who underwent a subtotal gastrectomy for stage II adenocarcinoma of the stomach 8 days ago and has developed an anasta-motic leak.

42.2 Which of the following methods is the best for assessing nutritional status in a critically ill patient?

A. History and physical examination

B. Albumen, prealbumin and retinol-binding protein

C. Triceps skin fold

D. Harris-Benedict equation

E. Percent body fat estimation

42.3 Which of the following is most accurate regarding enteral and parenteral nutrition?

A. Both enteral and parenteral nutrition help preserve structural integrity of the gut.

B. The majority of the cost benefit for the healthcare system of using enteral nutrition versus parenteral nutrition is from the direct cost of the cheaper generic enteral solutions versus the more expensive individualized parenteral nutrition solutions, which are made to order and mixed in the hospital.

C. There is a clear mortality benefit of using enteral nutrition versus parenteral nutrition in the ICU patient.

D. In severe acute pancreatitis, enteral rather than parenteral nutrition is the preferred method of nutrition.

E. Peripheral TPN administration is associated with lower complications than enteral nutritional support.

42.4 A 57-year-old woman who weighs 132 lb (60 kg) is admitted to the ICU for acute pancreatitis complicated by acute kidney injury. She is requiring hemodialysis every other day. Which of the following is the best nutrition regimen for this patient?

A. Place a nasojejunal (NJ) tube and feed continuous enteral 2000 kcal/d solution containing 120 g of protein daily.

B. Place NG tube and feed continuous enteral 2000 kcal/d solution containing 80 g of protein daily.

C. Place surgical jejunostomy tube and feed enteral 2000 kcal/d solution containing 115 g of protein daily in bolus fashion.

D. Place a peripherally inserted central line and give parenteral 2000 kcal/d solution containing 120 g of protein daily.

E. Place an NG tube and begin feeding to deliver 1800 kcal/d and 60 g of protein daily.

42.5 A 56-year-old man is admitted in the ICU for respiratory failure due to acute lung injury after a motor vehicle accident. The patient is placed on the ventilator. Which of the following is the more accurate principle in the management of this patient?

A. Calorie-dense, low volume enteral solutions should be used.

B. Anti-inflammatory lipid profile and antioxidants like omega-3 fish oils and borage oil are typically avoided.

C. Uric acid supplementation as needed to help with ventilation.

D. High caloric intake and hyperglycemia are usually not issues in this type of patient.

E. Close aspiration monitoring and cessation of enteric feeding if gastric residuals are >100 mL are necessary.

ANSWERS

42.1 **C.** In a previously healthy patient with no evidence of malnutrition, the use of parenteral nutrition should not be given until after 7 to 10 days of hospitalization without nutrition if the duration of parenteral nutrition is expected to be greater than 5 to 7 days. This can be started earlier if there is evidence of malnutrition. Enteral nutrition should be given unless patients do not have a functioning GI tract or if they have hemodynamic compromise, specifically those requiring high dose catecholamine agents or large volume of fluids or blood products. Parenteral nutrition is also recommended in patients in whom enteral nutrition is not feasible and who are about to undergo major upper GI surgery under the following conditions: (1) If the patient is malnourished, give parenteral nutrition 5 to 7 days preoperatively and continue postoperatively. (2) If normal nutrition, begin parenteral nutrition 5 to 7 days postoperatively should enteral nutrition continue not to be feasible and duration of parenteral nutrition is expected to be greater than 5 to 7 days. Special circumstances like short bowel syndrome and high output proximal GI enterocutaneous fistulas would also be indications for parenteral nutrition.

42.2 **A.** Assessment of nutritional status is done best by evaluating patient's weight loss and previous nutrient intake prior to admission, level of disease severity, comorbid conditions, and function of the gastrointestinal tract. Albumin, prealbumin, trasnferrin, and retinol-binding protein are a reflection of the acute phase response and do not accurately represent nutrition status in the ICU. Triceps skin fold and other anthropometry may be affected by edema. The Harris-Benedict equation is an estimation of basal metabolic caloric requirements based on weight, not an assessment tool for nutritional status.

42.3 **D.** Even in severe acute pancreatitis, initiation of enteral nutrition after acute resuscitation is the preferred method of nutrition delivery. Only enteral nutrition helps preserve villous height and structural integrity of the gut. The majority of cost savings from enteral nutrition is from its decreased infection rate and hospital stay. There is a clear infectious benefit with enteral nutrition, but no clear mortality benefit has been found.

42.4 **A.** The ideal regimen for a renal failure patient undergoing renal replacement therapy in the ICU is one with 1.5 to 2.0 g/kg/d of protein. In severe acute pancreatitis, enteral nutrition is preferred, and there is no outcome difference between using gastric versus jejunal feeding; however, placing surgical jejunostomy tubes carries its own inherent risks. Furthermore, patients tolerate continuous feeds easier than they tolerate bolus feeding in this situation.

42.5 **A.** The feedings should be calorie-dense, low-volume enteral solutions. Enteral solutions characterized by an anti-inflammatory lipid profile and antioxidants like omega-3 fish oils and borage oil are desirable. Phosphate supplementations (not uric acid) are utilized to help with ventilation. Excess caloric intake and hyperglycemia should be avoided to decrease infectious complications. Gastric residuals <500 mL in the absence of other signs of intolerance are acceptable and do not increase the risk of aspiration or pneumonia.

CLINICAL PEARLS

▶ Enteral nutrition is practical, safe, less expensive, and leads to fewer infections than parenteral nutrition.

▶ Enteral nutrition should be started within 24 to 48 hours following admission or as soon as fluid resuscitation is completed and the patient is hemodynamically stable.

▶ In patients receiving renal replacement therapy (RRT), increased protein should be considered.

▶ Markers such as albumin, prealbumin, trasnferrin, and retinol-binding protein are a reflection of the acute phase response and do not accurately represent nutrition status in the ICU patient; however, the serial measurements can help determine progress with nutritional therapy.

REFERENCES

Latifi R. Nutritional therapy in critically ill and injured patients. *Surg Clin N Am.* 2011;91:579-593.

McClave SA, Martindale RG, Vanek VW, et al. Guidelines for the provision and assessment of nutrition support therapy in the adult critically ill patient: Society of Critical Care Medicine and American Society for Parenteral and Enteral Nutrition. *Crit Care Med.* 2009;37:1-30.

Neal MD, Sperry JL. Nutritional support in the critically ill. In: Cameron JL. Cameron AM, eds. *Current Surgical Therapy.* 11th ed. Philadelphia PA: Elsevier Saunders; 2014:1284-1289.

Ramprasad R, Kapoor MC. Critical care nutrition. *J Anesthes Clinical Pharmacol.* 2012.doi 10.410310970-9185.92401.

Review Questions

The following are strategically designed review questions to assess whether the student is able to integrate the information presented in the cases. The explanations to the answer choices describe the rationale, including which cases are relevant.

REVIEW QUESTIONS

R-1. A 68-year-old man is admitted to the ICU for an exacerbation of congestive heart failure (CHF). He has hypertension, diabetes, and hyperlipidemia. Which of the following uses the patient's age for prognostic scoring on mortality for this patient in the ICU?

   A. Apache I

   B. Apache II

   C. Apache III

   D. Glasgow coma scale

   E. Model for end-stage liver disease (MELD) score

R-2. A 46-year-old woman is admitted to the ICU with fever, hypotension, and a diagnosis of streptococcal cellulitis of the thigh. She is treated with IV antibiotics with cefazolin, cefipime, and vancomycin. The BP persists in the 60/40 mm Hg range with HR in the 140 beats/min range despite infusion of 3 L IV of normal saline. Which of the following is the best next step in the treatment of this patient?

   A. Add metronidazole to the antibiotic regimen

   B. Surgical excision of the cellulitis

   C. Initiate norepinephrine infusion

   D. Initiate isoproterol infusion

R-3. A 57-year-old woman is admitted to the ICU for respiratory failure from an overwhelming pneumococcal pneumonia. She is intubated and placed on a ventilator and on propofol for IV sedation. After 12 hours, she is noted to have red-brown colored urine. Her creatine phosphokinase (CPK) level is 2,000 IU/L. Which of the following is the most likely diagnosis?

   A. Hemolysis

   B. Myocardial infarction

   C. Nephrolithiasis

   D. Rhabdomyolysis

R-4. A 65-year-old man is being evaluated in the emergency department for acute onset of chest pain of 1 hour duration. He was discharged from the hospital 7 days ago with an inferior wall ST-segment MI. Which of the following is the best method of diagnosing reinfarction?

A. Chest radiography

B. Echocardiography

C. Serum Troponin I levels

D. Serum CPK-MB levels

R-5. A 68-year-old man is taking digoxin for his congestive heart failure. His other medications include lisinopril, furosemide, and atenolol. He calls his physician because he begins to feel nauseated, fatigued, and his vision has a "yellow haze." When he arrives to his physician's office, he is found to have ventricular tachycardia. Which of the following is most likely to predispose to this arrhythmia in this patient?

A. Hypokalemia

B. Hypocalcemia

C. Hyponatremia

D. Hypophosphatemia

R-6. In the patient in R5, in addition to correction of any electrolyte problems, which of the following is the best initial treatment?

A. Alpha interferon

B. Amiodarone

C. Immunoglobulin fragments

D. Quinidine

E. Verapamil

R-7. A 45-year-old woman is admitted to the ICU from the emergency department for acute upper GI bleeding. She has ascites and jaundice. The intensivist is suspecting variceal bleeding. In addition to esophagoduodenoscopy, which of the following is the most appropriate therapy for this patient?

A. Albuterol

B. Corticosteroids

C. Octreotide

D. Vasopressin

R-8. A 32-year-old man is admitted to the neuro ICU after a motor vehicle accident with multiple blunt traumas, including concussion. The Glasgow coma score is 7. Which of the following is the most important intervention in this patient?

A. IV fluid hydration with lactated Ringer solution

B. Maintain BP of 140/90 mm Hg

C. Intubation and ventilation

D. IV mannitol

R-9. A 39-year-old man was admitted to the hospital for acute appendicitis and appendectomy. On hospital day two, he is found to be disoriented and hallucinating. His oxygen saturation is 95%, and fingerstick glucose is 90 mg/dL. On examination, he is found to have a temperature of 100.0°F, BP of 150/90 mm Hg, HR 120 beats/min, and tremulousness. His only medication per his wife is a sleep medication. He is currently on IV ampicillin/sulbactam. Which of the following is the most likely diagnosis?

  A. Benzodiazepine withdrawal

  B. Hypoxic encephalopathy

  C. ICU psychosis

  D. Penicillin-induced altered mental status

R-10. A 28-year-old woman who is pregnant at 30 weeks' gestation is seen in the emergency department for a seizure of 2 minutes' duration. It was described as a tonic-clonic seizure. The patient had no seizure history. Currently, the patient is postictal and has no neurological deficits. Which of the following is the best therapy for this patient?

  A. IV phenytoin

  B. IV magnesium sulfate

  C. IV diazepam

  D. IV carbamazepine

ANSWERS

R-1. **C.** The APACHE score is a general prognostication for ICU mortality. The Apache score uses physiological parameters such as temperature, HR, BP, and the APACHE III expanded the parameters using age, race, and end-organ function. The Glasgow coma scale is a measure of neurological function; the MELD score is used in liver insufficiency.

See also Case 2 (Transfer of the critically Ill patient), and Case 3 (scoring systems and patient prognosis).

R-2. **C.** This patient has sepsis due to infection-related hypotension. The priorities are the ABCs, meaning oxygenation and circulation must be addressed. The BP of 60/40 mm Hg is incompatible with life and must be elevated. IV norepinephrine is the pressor agent of choice in sepsis-related hypotension. Metronidazole is not indicated in this instance due to a streptococcal infection. Surgical excision is not indicated in cellulitis but would be necessary in necrotizing fasciitis. Isoproterenol is not indicated, especially with the HR already at 140 beats/min.

See also Case 4 (Hemodynamic monitoring), and Case 5 (Vasoactive drugs).

R-3. **D.** One of the side effects of propofol is rhabdomyolysis, breakdown of muscle. This causes the red-brown colored urine and markedly elevated CPK levels. Acute MI does lead to elevated CPK levels but not in the range of 1000s IU/L. Nephrolithiasis would not be associated with high CPK levels. Hemolysis can cause a red-brown urine but with elevated bilirubin levels, not CPK levels.

See also Case 9 (Ventilator management) and Case 10 (respiratory weaning).

R-4. **D.** CPK-MB should be drawn. Troponin I levels are very sensitive for myocardial ischemia/infarction but persist to be elevated for 10 to 14 days. Thus, these markers are not the best to diagnose reinfarction. Instead, CPK-MB is preferred since these levels are usually elevated for about 3 days. Chest x-ray may show cardiomegaly or pulmonary edema but are not useful to rule out MI. Echo may show heart failure or dyskinesis of the heart but again do not diagnose MI.

See also Case 14 (Acute coronary syndromes).

R-5. **A.** This patient has the clinical picture of digoxin toxicity with GI side effects, lethargy or confusion, and visual abnormality (classically a yellow or green tint). Digoxin has a very small therapeutic index and high toxicity related to inhibition of the Na/K ATPase pump; the toxicity is accentuated by hypokalemia. Since digoxin binds to the ATPase pump on the same side as potassium, if K levels are low, then digoxin can more easily bind to the ATPase pump and exert inhibitory effects and leading to higher toxicity.

See Case 15 (Cardiac arrhythmias) and Case 16 (Acute cardiac failure).

R-6. **C.** Digoxin-specific immunoglobulin fragments (DigiFab) is effective in binding and clearing digoxin quickly and has improved survival from digoxin toxicity dramatically. When given as an IV infusion, improvements in the cardiac rhythm can be seen within 20 to 30 minutes. Quinidine exacerbates digoxin toxicity and should not be given. In fact, quinidine nearly doubles the digoxin concentration due to decreased renal clearance. Answers B (amiodarone) and E (verapamil) also increase digoxin concentrations. Answer A (interferon) has no effect on digoxin.

See Case 15 (Cardiac arrhythmias), and Case 16 (Acute cardiac failure).

R-7. **C.** Vasopressin can dramatically decrease the splanchnic blood flow and reduce upper GI bleeding. However, vasopressin and vasopressin analogues are now in disfavor due to the systemic vasoconstrictive effects, and for that reason octreotide is a preferred adjunctive therapy in conjunction with EGD for variceal upper gastrointestinal hemorrhage patients. Prior to endoscopy, octreotide (loading dose 50 μg, followed by 25-50 μg/h × 5 days) should be administered and may reduce the risk of bleeding. Octreotide can also be used as adjunctive therapy if endoscopy is unsuccessful, contraindicated, or unavailable. β-blocking agents can help to reduce portal hypertension, but albuterol has no place in this therapy. Corticosteroids have no efficacy in variceal bleeding.

See Case 21 (Acute GI bleeding) and Case 22 (Acute liver failure).

R-8. **C.** Patients with severe brain injury (GCS ≤ 8) require early intubation for protection of their airway. This also allows for the provision of increased oxygen administration to reduce hypoxia. Additionally, the minute ventilation can be controlled and the patient can be hyperventilated to decrease the $Paco_2$ and thus cause vasoconstriction. This will decrease both the cerebral blood flow and cerebral blood volume. The decrease in blood volume can aid in the acute decrease of elevated ICP. Potential benefits of controlled hyperventilation are probably most prominent in the first 24 to 48 hours after injury, so hyperventilation to decrease ICP should be used with extreme caution and only for short periods of time. IV hydration should be employed using normal saline rather than LR or hypotonic solution to avoid cerebral edema. The BP should be maintained above 90 mm Hg systolic. IV mannitol is useful in conditions of increased ICP, but intubation and protection of the airway is more important.

See also Case 27 (Traumatic brain injury) and Case 8 (Airway management).

R-9. **A.** This patient likely has benzodiazepine withdrawal, which presents similarly to alcohol withdrawal. Clinically, the patient will have tremulousness, tachycardia, elevated BP, and possibly hallucinations and seizures. The treatment is a low-dose short-acting benzodiazepine, such as lorazepam, and supportive care. Meanwhile, a diligent search for other causes of delirium and altered mental status should be undertaken. With a normal oxygen saturation, hypoxic encephalopathy is unlikely. ICU psychosis is possible but typically presents in older patients. Penicillin usually is not associated with AMS.

See also Case 30 (Altered mental status) and Case 37 (Poisoning).

R-10. **B.** This is a pregnant woman without a seizure history who has a tonic-clonic seizure. Without any other history, this is eclampsia until otherwise proven, with the best therapy being magnesium sulfate, usually with a 4 to 6 g IV load and then infusion of 2 g/h. If the patient had a prior seizure history, then other agents such as phenytoin could be considered. Diazepam is usually not given due to the long half-life and respiratory depression. A CT of the head may be considered in this case to rule out an intracerebral process. If eclampsia is diagnosed, the treatment is delivery and continued magnesium sulfate.

See also Case 35 (Hypertensive emergencies in obstetrics) and Case 31 (status epilepticus).

Page numbers followed by *f* or *t* indicate figures or tables, respectively.

9 781637 510247